Enhancing Children's Wellness

Issues in Children's and Families' Lives

AN ANNUAL BOOK SERIES

Drawing upon the resources of Child and Family Agency of Southeastern Connecticut, one of this nation's leading family service agencies, **Issues in Children's and Families' Lives** is designed to focus attention on the pressing social problems facing children and their families today. Each volume in this series will analyze, integrate, and critique the clinical and research literature on children and their families as it relates to a particular theme. Believing that integrated multidisciplinary approaches offer greater opportunities for program success, volume contributors will reflect the research and clinical knowledge base of the many different disciplines that are committed to enhancing the physical, social, and emotional health of children and their families. Intended for graduate and professional audiences, chapters will be written by scholars and practitioners who will encourage readers to apply their practice skills and intellect to reducing the suffering of children and their families in the society in which those families live and work.

Volume 1: Family Violence: Prevention and Treatment
LEAD EDITOR: Robert L. Hampton
CONSULTANTS: Vincent Senatore, *Child and Family Agency, Connecticut*; Ann Quinn, *Connecticut Department of Children, Youth, and Family Services, Connecticut*

Volume 2: The Family-School Connection
EDITORS: Bruce A. Ryan and Gerald R. Adams

Volume 3: Adolescent Dysfunctional Behavior
EDITORS: Gary M. Blau and Thomas P. Gullotta

Volume 4: Preventing Violence in America
EDITORS: Robert L. Hampton, Pamela Jenkins, and Thomas P. Gullotta

Volume 5: Primary Prevention Practices
AUTHOR: Martin Bloom

Volume 6: Primary Prevention Works
EDITORS: George W. Albee and Thomas P. Gullotta

Volume 7: Children and Youth: Interdisciplinary Perspectives
EDITORS: Herbert J. Walberg, Olga Reyes, and Roger P. Weissberg

Volume 8: Healthy Children 2010: Enhancing Children's Wellness
EDITORS: Roger P. Weissberg, Thomas P. Gullotta, Robert L. Hampton, Bruce A. Ryan, and Gerald R. Adams

Volume 9: Healthy Children 2010: Establishing Preventive Services
EDITORS: Roger P. Weissberg, Thomas P. Gullotta, Robert L. Hampton, Bruce A. Ryan, and Gerald R. Adams

Healthy Children 2010

Enhancing Children's Wellness

Editors

Roger P. Weissberg
Thomas P. Gullotta
Robert L. Hampton
Bruce A. Ryan
Gerald R. Adams

Vol. 8 *Issues in Children's and Families' Lives*

SAGE Publications
International Educational and Professional Publisher
Thousand Oaks London New Delhi

For information:

SAGE Publications, Inc.
2455 Teller Road
Thousand Oaks, California 91320
E-mail: order@sagepub.com

SAGE Publications Ltd.
6 Bonhill Street
London EC2A 4PU
United Kingdom

SAGE Publications India Pvt. Ltd.
M-32 Market
Greater Kailash I
New Delhi 110 048 India

Printed in the United States of America
Library of Congress Cataloging-in-Publication Data
Main entry under title:

Healthy children 2010: ENHANCING CHILDREN'S WELLNESS / editors, Roger P. Weissberg . . . [et al.].
p. cm.—(Issues in children's and families' lives; vol. 8)
Includes bibliographical references and index.
ISBN 0-7619-1091-3 (cloth: acid-free paper).—
ISBN 0-7619-1092-1 (pbk.: acid-free paper).
1. Health promotion—United States. 2. Health behavior in children—United States. 3. Health behavior in adolescence—United States. 4. Health education (Elementary)—United States. 5. Health education (Secondary)—United States. I. Weissberg, Roger P., 1951- . II. Series: Issues in children's and families' lives; v. 8.
RJ102.E54 1997 97-4750
362.1'083'0973—dc21

97 98 99 00 01 02 03 10 9 8 7 6 5 4 3 2 1

Acquiring Editor: C. Deborah Laughton
Editorial Assistant: Eileen Carr
Production Editor: Astrid Virding
Production Assistant: Karen Wiley
Typesetter/Designer: Marion S. Warren
Cover Designer: Lesa Valdez
Print Buyer: Anna Chin

The sponsoring organization for this book series, Child and Family Agency of Southeastern Connecticut, traces its history to that period of time in the early 1800s when benevolent charitable societies developed. We are fortunate in that the unselfish philanthropic spirit which led to the volunteerism of that time continues to the present. This book is deservingly dedicated to a group of individuals who over the years have helped to make Child and Family Agency the very special place it is for children and their families.

Mrs. Miriam Angell
Ms. Johnatha Bennett
Mrs. Joyce Brennan
Mrs. Lee Buckley
Mrs. Martha Burd
Mrs. Peggy Callahan
Mrs. Suzie Canning
Mrs. Margaret Cosgrove
Mrs. Sue Curtiss
Mr. Lowell Daniels
Mrs. Lillian Erb
Mrs. Jane Fagan
Ms. Alva Greenberg-Gahagan
Mrs. Judi Honiss
Mrs. Parthenia Johnson
Mr. Ward Johnson
Mr. Ken Kenerson
Mrs. Ellie Krusewski
Mrs. Jeanne Lena
Mrs. Diane MacFadyen
Mr. Stephen McGuire
Mrs. Kate Peal
Mrs. Virginia Perry
Mrs. Cynthia Rowley
Mrs. Patricia Rogerson
Mrs. Valerie Shickel
Ms. Wendy Traub

Contents

Foreword

In 1996, the American Medical Association published a report—organized and written by Missy Fleming—called *Healthy Youth 2000: A Mid-Decade Review.* This refreshingly candid report makes no effort to gloss over the snail's pace at which we are crawling toward the goal of improving the health of our youth. The present volume focuses on recent advances in research-based approaches to promote the *wellness* of children. What can we do for all children that not only will help them cope better with the many transitions and exigencies of contemporary living but also will maximize their chances to manifest and exploit their abilities and interests? Distinctive about this volume is its treasure trove of studies, projects, and programs demonstrating the positive consequences of the wellness orientation. A fair number of the chapters describe systematic efforts through years and even decades, efforts informed by methodological rigor and the rules of evidence.

We are given here not only ideas but ideas that have demonstrable practical, positive effects. I am happy and proud to be able to say this because this book contains evidence that more than a few thinkers and researchers have freed themselves from orientations riveting on the pathological. These words should not be construed as in any way derogating efforts to prevent this or that pathological or antisocial condition. It is my way of saying that we have far too long given only lip service to the promotion of wellness. Wellness is not for this or that group; it is a goal we seek for everyone.

For some people, the concept of wellness may sound vague, too global, or gooey. A Supreme Court justice once said that he could not define pornography precisely but he sure as hell knew it when he saw it. As individuals, we know when we lack the feeling of wellness. That is true for everyone, young or old. We have learned a great deal about the commonalities among feelings that are the opposite of wellness. This volume gives us a beginning, firm basis for the promotion of wellness that instills in our youth attitudes, styles of thinking, and non-self-defeating social skills. I say *beginning* because that is where we are. Wellness is an individual phenomenon, but it is always embedded in an interpersonal, social-familial, or institutional context. How can contexts promote wellness? What features of context are obstacles to the sense of wellness?

Are schools context for the promotion of wellness? The rhetoric says yes. The evidence makes a mockery of that rhetoric. Inevitably, the concept of wellness directs our attention to contexts, a point well illustrated in many chapters of this book. In the course of reading this book, I found myself asking this question: What if I sat in an elementary school classroom every day for a week, interested only in noting instances of any type that I consider opportunities for the teacher to do or say something consistent with a wellness orientation? For decades, I have sat in hundreds of classrooms but usually with a focus on individual children who were considered to be problems, for example, too aggressive, too retiring, unmotivated, or fearful of failure. The question I ask now includes, but goes beyond, those instances. I used the word *opportunities* because it includes instances that are not "clinical" or problematic in nature. They are part of the "normal" social-behavioral flow of the modal classroom. They go unremarked. I venture the opinion that during any one day, the teacher has many opportunities to do or say something reflective of a wellness orientation. I also predict that it would not occur to the modal teacher to exploit these opportunities. Why not? The answer is that nothing in the preparation of teachers, and little or nothing in the culture of the school, makes wellness orientations salient. Teachers are problem oriented; they operate in the repair mode. My point is that wellness cannot be defined or promoted independent of context.

This is an important book that deserves a wide audience. I also hope that it will be put into the hands of policymakers, too many of whom cannot distinguish between prevention of pathological conditions and prevention based on a wellness orientation. I want to express my personal thanks and appreciation to Dr. Weissberg and his colleagues for the exemplary manner in which they organized and brought this book to completion.

—Seymour B. Sarason
Professor of Psychology, Emeritus,
Yale University

Reference

Fleming, M. (1996). *Healthy youth 2000: A mid-decade review.* Chicago: American Medical Association, Department of Adolescent Health.

Acknowledgments

Many people contributed to this volume. On behalf of my coeditors, I thank the outstanding authors of the foreword and the 10 chapters. At the outset, the editors invited top scholars and leaders in the fields of health promotion and preventive mental health. We are particularly grateful for their efforts to produce thoughtful, high-quality work. In addition, we appreciate that these busy people turned in their manuscripts on schedule and responded with grace and effectiveness to editorial feedback. I am also indebted to Tom Gullotta, senior editor of the series on Issues in Children's and Families' Lives and a coeditor of this volume. He is a great, energetic collaborator and a delight to work with because of his creative, optimistic, problem-solving approach to life and productive scholarship. I also express my appreciation to Carol Bartels Kuster, who assisted in bringing closure to this book with scholarship, organizational skill, and sound judgment.

Several organizations and individuals have generously provided financial and intellectual support for our efforts to disseminate information about ways to promote children's social, emotional, and physical health. We acknowledge the contributions of the Surdna Foundation, the Fetzer Institute, the University of Illinois at Chicago, Daniel Goleman, Eileen Growald, Robert Sherman, Timothy Shriver, David Sluyter, Serita Winthrop, and colleagues from the Collaborative for the Advancement of Social and Emotional Learning (CASEL). Recently, I became executive director of CASEL, and I am delighted and optimistic by the constructive, leading role that the organization will play in supporting the widespread establishment of effective programs that enhance the wellness of children. I also thank the National Institute of Mental Health's Prevention Research Branch and Office on AIDS for their support and funding of the University of Illinois at Chicago Prevention Research Training Program in Urban Children's Mental Health and AIDS Prevention (1-T32-MH19933), the Irving B. Harris Grandchildren Charity Trust, the Ounce of Prevention Fund, the University of Illinois at Chicago Great Cities Program, and the Office of Educational Research and Improvement of the U.S. Department of Education through a grant to the Mid-Atlantic Laboratory for Student Success at the Temple University Center for Research in Human Development and Education. These funding sources allow my colleagues, students, and me to develop and evaluate innovative school and community health enhancement and prevention programs.

One goal of this volume is to influence our nation's policies and practices regarding children's health in the future by raising awareness about effective and theoretically based prevention programs and strategies. The contributors identified empirically based preventive interventions that schools and communities may implement to enhance children's social, emotional, and physical wellness. It becomes more feasible to foster childrn's successful development when concerned individuals collaborate to share their collective wisdom, energy, and commitment. We thank the fine people at Sage for helping us bring this volume to fruition and share our information and perspectives with others.

—Roger P. Weissberg
University of Illinois at Chicago

• *CHAPTER 1* •

Introduction and Overview: Let's Make "Healthy Children 2010" a National Priority!

ROGER P. WEISSBERG

CAROL BARTELS KUSTER

Healthy People, the first *Surgeon General's Report on Health Promotion and Disease Prevention,* was a landmark document (U.S. Department of Health, Education, and Welfare, Public Health Service, 1979). It summarized the nation's dramatic health accomplishments since 1900 and contended that further improvements would require the widespread implementation of effective health promotion and disease prevention strategies. A decade later, the Office of Disease Prevention and Health Promotion (ODPHP) coordinated a broad-based national effort to develop a second report, *Healthy People 2000: National Health Promotion and Disease Prevention Objectives* (U.S. Department of Health and Human Services, Public Health Service [DHHS], 1991). *Healthy People 2000* identified more than 300 health objectives, organized into 22 priority areas, to be accomplished by the year 2000. These objectives have guided health promotion and disease prevention policies and programs at the federal, state, and local levels during the 1990s.

The seeds for editing the current volume, *Healthy Children 2010: Enhancing Children's Wellness,* were planted almost a decade ago. Work on *Healthy People 2000* began in 1987 with the convening of a consortium of almost 300 national membership organizations and all 50 state health departments (DHHS, 1991). As planning for *Healthy People 2000* was under way, the National Mental Health Association (NMHA) invited the senior editor (R. P. Weissberg) to comment at an ODPHP-sponsored meeting on objectives for children in the priority area of "Mental Health and Mental Disorders." The NMHA has a distinguished history of advocacy for children's preventive mental health programs (Report of the National Mental Health Association Commission on the Prevention of Mental-Emotional Disabilities, 1986). It expressed concern that *Healthy People 2000* placed inadequate emphasis on children's mental health outcomes and on establishing objectives for the dissemination of family- and community-based primary prevention programs.

Our assessment of *Healthy People 2000* (DHHS, 1991) concurs with the NMHA's concerns about insufficient coverage for children's mental health needs and scientifically based preventive mental health interventions. Overall, *Healthy People 2000* proposed 14 mental health objectives; only 2 identified health status goals for children ("Reduce by 15 percent the incidence of injurious suicide attempts among adolescents aged 14 to 17"—Objective 6.2, p. 211; "Reduce to less than 10 percent the prevalence of mental disorders among children and adolescents"—Objective 6.3, p. 211). Only one mentioned a secondary prevention service goal ("Increase to at least 75 percent the proportion of providers of primary care for children who include assessment of cognitive, emotional, and parent-child functioning, with appropriate counseling, referral, and followup, in their clinical practices"—Objective 6.14, p. 219). In this book and in a companion volume, *Healthy Children 2010: Establishing Preventive Services* (Weissberg, Gullotta, Hampton, Ryan, & Adams, 1997), we strongly recommend that *Healthy People 2010* increase the number of child-focused objectives and the specificity and accuracy of these objectives and include program, service, and policy objectives related to children's mental health as well as to their physical health and social functioning.

Kolbe, Collins, and Cortese (in press) pointed out that our country's most severe and costly health and social problems are caused, in large part, by behavioral patterns that develop during childhood and adolescence. These problems include tobacco use, drug and alcohol abuse, sexual risk behaviors, violence, poor nutrition, and behaviors and environmental circumstances that result in injuries. Yet examination of the 692-page *Healthy People 2000* report reveals that these priority areas, similar to mental health and mental disorders, received sparse coverage in this agenda-setting document.

On the positive side, *Healthy People 2000* places considerable emphasis on establishing quality school health education programs that target multiple health outcomes (DeFriese, Crossland, Pearson, & Sullivan, 1990; Kolbe et al., in press; McGinnis & DeGraw, 1991; Weissberg & Elias, 1993). A core recommendation calls for an "increase to at least 75 percent the proportion of the Nation's elementary and secondary schools that provide planned and sequential kindergarten through 12th grade quality school health education" (Objective 8.4, p. 255). Related objectives encourage increases in the proportion of schools nationwide—"preferably as part of quality school health education"—that provide education regarding: (a) tobacco use (Objective 3.10, p. 147) and alcohol and other drugs (Objective 4.13, p. 173); (b) sexuality (Objective 5.8, p. 198), HIV (Objective 18.10, p. 488), and sexually transmitted disease transmission (Objective 19.12, p. 505); (c) nonviolent conflict resolution (Objective 7.16, p. 239); (d) nutrition (Objective 2.19, p. 127); and (e) injury prevention and control (Objective 9.18, p. 285).

The chapters in this volume and its companion, *Healthy Children 2010: Establishing Preventive Services* (Weissberg et al., 1997), make clear that many additional, critically important recommendations for child health outcomes and preventive services could be offered. We hope that the publication of these volumes in 1997 will promote early discussion regarding objectives about children's social, emotional, and physical wellness in *Healthy People 2010.* We believe that the interests of the nation's young people would be best served if the government next published two reports: *Healthy Children 2010* and *Healthy Adults 2010.* The value of separately emphasizing the health needs of children and youth in *Healthy People 2000*—thus making them more salient—has been highlighted constructively in publications of the American Medical Association (1990; Fleming, 1996).

Available data on the social circumstances and health status of our nation's children offer compelling support of the view that enhancing children's wellness must be given greater priority (National Commission on Children, 1991). Findings regarding children's substance use, high-risk sexual behavior, delinquency, suicide, and school performance indicate that unacceptably large numbers of young people experience problems and engage in multiple risk behaviors that may limit their potential to develop into constructive, contributing members of society (Dryfoos, 1990). In addition, indicators about divorce, children who grow up in single-parent homes, two-career couples, and poverty suggest that too many children are growing up without adequate family support and guidance, increasing their vulnerability to involvement in health-damaging behaviors (DHHS, 1996).

Currently, approximately 69 million young people under the age of 18 live in the United States. That number is projected to increase to 74 million by the year 2010, the largest absolute number of youth in the nation's history (U.S. Bureau of the Census, 1993). America's population is also becoming more racially and ethnically diverse, largely because of immigration and differential birthrates. When *Healthy People* was published, approximately 74% of people under 18 were White, 15% were Black, 9% were Hispanic, 2% were Asian American, and 1% were from other racial or ethnic groups. By 2010, the proportion of White young people will decline to 58%, whereas there will be a slight increase to 17% for Blacks and larger increases to 18% for Hispanics and 7% for Asian Americans (DHHS, 1996). Language barriers, poverty, and cultural isolation affect the social and health needs of many minority children. When combined with population growth, sociodemographic shifts, and diminishing support by adults for children, these problems will lead to increased numbers of children who engage in problem behaviors and consequently experience negative behavioral outcomes (Snyder & Sickmund, 1995; Zill & Nord, 1994).

During the past decade, several reviews have described the progress made in the prevention of children's social and health problems (e.g., Botvin, Schinke, & Orlandi, 1995; Carnegie Council on Adolescent Development, 1995; Consortium on the School-Based Promotion of Social Competence, 1994; Dryfoos, 1990; Durlak, 1995; Institute of Medicine, 1994; Millstein, Petersen, & Nightingale, 1993; Moore, Sugland, Blumenthal, Glei, & Snyder, 1995; Price, Cowen, Lorion, & Ramos-McKay, 1989; Simeonsson, 1994; Tolan & Guerra, 1994; Weissberg & Greenberg, 1997). Given this progress, it is timely to review empirically based prevention programs for young people and to identify priorities for new child health objectives for the year 2010. The chapters in this volume share the latest research and theories about family, school, and community prevention and health promotion programs to improve the health status of children during the next decade. These provide a foundation for increasing the quantity and quality of children's health objectives in 2010.

Summary of Chapters

Chapter 2: The Prevalence of Problem Behaviors: Implications for Programs (Joy G. Dryfoos)

Joy Dryfoos summarizes current prevalence data for problem behaviors among adolescents across five areas: substance use, sexual behavior, delinquency and violence, depression and suicidal ideation, and school failure. A sampling from her findings powerfully indicates why the dissemination of effective prevention and health promotion programs for children and youth must receive greater emphasis nationally: (a) about 30% of 14- to 17-year-olds have smoked cigarettes, 30% have engaged in binge drinking, and 18% have smoked marijuana within the past 30 days; (b) approximately 53% of high school students report that they have had intercourse, and almost 20% report having four or more sex partners; (c) at least 18% of males and 5% of females admitted that they had carried a gun, knife, or club on school grounds during the past 30 days; (d) about 24% of high school students self-reported that they thought seriously about attempting suicide, 19% made a suicide plan, and 9% actually attempted suicide during the past year; and (e) about 25% of 10th graders have already been retained in grade, and almost 12% of all young people drop out of school. Assessing the likelihood of reaching objectives established in *Healthy People 2000* and the *1995 Midcourse Review* (DHHS, 1991, 1995), Dryfoos pessimistically notes that during the 1990s, rates of the following have increased: cigarette, alcohol, and marijuana use; the proportion of females aged 15 to 17 who are sexually active; suicide and suicide attempts; and interpersonal violence.

Dryfoos reviews studies indicating that these problem behaviors often co-occur in young people and that common risk and protective factors influence the development of social and health problems. She estimates that 30% of 14- to 17-year-olds engage in multiple problem behaviors placing them at high risk of extremely negative consequences; about 35% are experimenting with various risky activities that jeopardize their futures; and the final 35% are at low risk from their current behaviors. On the basis of her analysis of findings from prevalence studies, risk and protective factor research, and preventive-intervention research, she concludes,

> Evidence is clear from the experiments of the past that more powerful comprehensive approaches are required, that we cannot continue to treat troubled young people in categorical efforts that do not deal with the social and psychological environment that gives rise to these problems. (p. 44, this volume)

She recommends focusing preventive interventions on the settings and structures that so powerfully affect outcomes among youth, including families, schools, and neighborhoods; health, welfare, and justice systems; and employment and training.

Chapter 3: School-Based Drug Abuse Prevention Strategies: From Research to Policy and Practice (Linda Dusenbury and Mathea Falco)

The adolescent problem behavior that has received perhaps the greatest amount of attention is drug use. Numerous "wars" against drugs, involving media campaigns, policy formation and reformation, and intervention-prevention program development, have been waged in the past 20 years. We now know a great deal about the causes, effects, and consequences of drug abuse, as well as the key ingredients in effective drug prevention-intervention programs. Despite these advances in awareness and responsiveness, however, and despite the seeming proliferation of school-based programs, reports of drug use among youth have been increasing in recent years. Indeed, little progress has been made toward reaching many of the drug use reduction goals of *Healthy People 2000*. For example, rates of tobacco, marijuana, alcohol, and illicit drug use are rising, whereas levels of disapproval and perceived harmfulness of drugs are decreasing among youth.

Why are we losing ground in our efforts to stem drug use among children? One answer is that we are not using effectively what we know. Linda Dusenbury and Mathea Falco offer reasons why some of our most promising programs are not widely used while some relatively ineffective programs are widely disseminated. On the basis of their extensive review of available drug prevention programs, evaluation evidence, and interviews with leading experts in the field, they describe key ingredients for drug prevention programs, identify state-of-the-art programs and practices, and elaborate guidelines for choosing effective programs. Among their key findings, they conclude that school-based drug prevention programs are most effective when they (a) reflect proven prevention theory and research; (b) provide developmentally appropriate information about tobacco, alcohol, and drugs; (c) employ interactive teaching techniques; (d) provide adequate coverage and sufficient follow-up training for students; (e) are culturally sensitive; (f) offer teacher training and support for high-quality implementation; (g) include supplemental components designed for the family, community, and media; and (h) demonstrate their effects on drug use behavior in rigorous evaluation. In their view, drug use does not occur in isolation of other problems, and our best course is to include drug prevention as part of comprehensive health education and broader personal and social skills training.

Chapter 4: Preventing High-Risk Sexual Behavior, Sexually Transmitted Diseases, and Pregnancy among Adolescents (Lynda M. Sagrestano and Roberta L. Paikoff)

In earlier decades, prior to the AIDS epidemic, interventions aimed at adolescent sexual behavior focused on pregnancy and sexually transmitted disease (STD) prevention. Although these problems presented clear health risks, they were not necessarily debilitating or fatal. With the rise in rates of STDs and particularly HIV/AIDS among adolescents, however, the need for effective prevention programs has become critical. In their chapter, Lynda Sagrestano and Roberta Paikoff review the limited progress made toward the three *Healthy People 2000* goals related to adolescent sexual behavior. These goals are (a) reduce early sexual behavior by encouraging abstinence and delaying onset of first sexual intercourse, (b) reduce early pregnancies, and (c) increase contraceptive use among adolescents. Unfortunately, national data indicate that since 1990, proportionally more adolescents are sexually active, sexual initiation is occurring at younger ages, and rates of adolescent pregnancy have increased, particularly among minority youth. There is evidence of one promising trend, however—an increase in the proportion of sexually active adolescents who later choose abstinence and/or use contraceptives.

Sagrestano and Paikoff identify methodological, developmental, and contextual considerations for interventions with both sexually active and nonsexually active adolescents. They identify characteristics of several successful primary and secondary prevention programs and outline recommendations for improving methodological rigor in prevention programs targeted toward adolescent sexuality. On the basis of their developmental-ecological theoretical perspective, they argue compellingly that primary prevention programs must start with preadolescents and continue through the years to address the changing nature of family, school, peer, and community risk factors as youth progress developmentally through adolescence. Specifically, they emphasize three recommendations: (a) intervene early—prevention of sexually risky behavior must focus on primary prevention (before the onset of sexual behavior) because preventive interventions have been much less successful with nonvirgins; (b) follow up with developmentally appropriate booster sessions throughout adolescence; and (c) include secondary prevention efforts that focus on safe sex or abstinence for those youth who are sexually active.

Chapter 5: Violence Prevention for the 21st Century (Mary E. Murray, Nancy G. Guerra, and Kirk R. Williams)

Many problems affecting children and youth are regarded as the particular province of youth and those adults, such as their parents and teachers, directly concerned with their healthy development. One problem, by its very nature, however, is a threat to the well-being not only of youth but of the general population—the problem of youth violence. As Mary Murray, Nancy Guerra, and Kirk Williams make clear, this is truly a threat to the public health that is becoming increasingly serious each year. Although the current generation of youth may not be violent more often than previous generations, the results of their violent behaviors are more often lethal.

Murray, Guerra, and Williams review empirical data on violence-related prevention programs and identify implications for violence prevention efforts that recognize the importance of developmental stages, type of violence, and setting or location. They organize their review developmentally, describing exemplary programs involving pre- and postnatal services to families, preschool enrichment programs, interventions during the elementary school years, and programs for adolescents. They suggest that violence may be best understood through an ecological model of life course development in which violent/aggressive behavior is seen as the result of unmet developmental needs. Ensuring that these needs are met in appropriate ways thus becomes the foundation of violence prevention efforts. The chapter concludes with a critique of *Healthy People 2000* goals and highlights several instructive empirically and theory-based directions to guide the establishment of improved objectives for 2010. They recommend, for example, that future objectives should (a) discriminate among types of violence, (b) focus on serious and lethal violence, (c) address the problem of juvenile gangs, (d) link violence reduction goals to specific strategies that address the multiple causes of violence, and (e) build a comprehensive response that addresses the range of risk factors common to many problems, including violence.

Chapter 6:
Prevention of Depression (Bruce E. Compas, Jennifer Connor, and Martha Wadsworth)

Those youth susceptible to drug abuse, unhealthy sexual behavior, violence/aggression, suicide, and other problems are often the same youth who are experiencing depression. The tendency for depression to co-occur with other debilitating conditions is explored in a scholarly review by Bruce Compas, Jennifer Connor, and Martha Wadsworth. They describe the current state of definition and diagnosis of depression in children and adolescents, provide startling prevalence data, and discuss the deleterious effects of depression in childhood. Given the widespread, lasting, and often devastating effects of depression, surprisingly few prevention efforts specifically target depression or evaluate their impact on depressive symptoms. Recently, however, pioneering efforts to prevent depression in children have produced promising results. Some notable programs have reduced levels of depressive symptoms, for example, by focusing on improving academic achievement, cognitive skills, and/or social problem-solving techniques.

Compas, Connor, and Wadsworth recommend that interventions at the universal, indicated, and selected levels can work in complementary fashion to deliver appropriate "doses" of prevention. Further, they suggest that interventions should include both person-centered and context-centered foci. Such broadly based efforts likely will be needed to adequately encompass the large number of risk factors associated with depression.

Compas and colleagues note that depression during childhood and adolescence was given relatively little attention in *Healthy People 2000*. They contend that the growing evidence regarding the prevalence, severity, course, and correlates of depression make clear that depression should be a high priority for preventive services that are a part of *Healthy People 2010* objectives. They also point out that the *Healthy People 2000* goal of reducing suicide among youth will be assisted by addressing depression's role as an important risk factor for suicide.

Chapter 7: Prevention of Youth Suicide (John Kalafat)

As the goals of *Healthy People 2000* make clear, one of the primary threats to adolescent health is self-inflicted injury. Suicide is currently ranked within the top three leading causes of death for adolescents between 15 and 19 years of age. In his chapter, John Kalafat provides an overview of what schools may do to address this problem. Given the large array of risk factors associated with suicide and suicide attempts among youth, Kalafat argues that interventions should target general protective factors rather than individual risk factors. For example, identifying barriers to help seeking among troubled adolescents can lead to the development of efforts to reduce these barriers, thereby encouraging youth to seek out and use adult help for a variety of problems, including suicidal ideation. Naturally, such programs will also need to ensure the availability of responsive and able adults.

As a first step toward maximizing general protective factors, Kalafat identifies barriers to help seeking in one of the natural environments of children—the schools. He also describes ways in which these obstacles may be overcome, such as reorganizing schools to provide students with longer and enhanced interactions with teachers, increasing peer involvement and support, and reducing the isolation and alienation common to many large schools. He highlights the importance of increasing the general availability of adult support in schools and incorporating instruction in social problem-solving skills to interrupt the trajectory toward suicide, drug abuse, and other related negative outcomes.

Chapter 8: Promoting Healthy Dietary Behaviors (Cheryl L. Perry, Mary Story, and Leslie A. Lytle)

With the increasing prominence of salient health threats such as violence, physical abuse, and drug use among youth, one important cause of morbidity and mortality is often overlooked—poor nutrition. Cheryl Perry, Mary Story, and Leslie Lytle emphasize the importance of establishing healthy eating patterns early in life. These early patterns are highly predictive of adult eating behavior, which is directly linked to adult morbidity and mortality. Their review of school-based programs indicates that simply educating children about nutrition is not enough to alter their eating behavior. The authors discuss the role of social norms about desirable foods, the influence of media directed at children, and changes in family structure in determining eating patterns.

Perry, Story, and Lytle note that most of the eight *Healthy People 2000* nutrition objectives for children and adolescents will not be met despite the introduction of the food guide pyramid, new food labels, and revised dietary guidelines. They recommend that *Healthy People 2010* place greater emphasis on policies and environments that encourage healthier decisions among young people. Specifically, they call for wider dissemination of nutrition education programs that have been effective in research trials. They also note that healthier eating behaviors among children are likely to be sustained when classroom-based behavioral education is complemented by school food service changes, parental involvement, and community-wide change. In other words, future efforts to promote good nutrition and healthy eating behavior will need to expand their focus to those elements of the social environment that promote or discourage good nutritional habits.

Chapter 9: Prevention and Control of Injuries (Barbara S. Tuchfarber, Joseph E. Zins, and Leonard A. Jason)

One goal of *Healthy People 2000* was the reduction of accidental injury. Although such injury among children and youth is still a primary threat to well-being, some reduction in injury rates has been achieved. Barbara Tuchfarber, Joseph Zins, and Leonard Jason point out that most "accidents" among children and youth are not unpredictable twists of fate but results of predictable behaviors among identifiable high-risk groups. These authors describe ways in which child, parent-family, and environmental factors interact to determine to whom an "accident will happen." For example, children's high level of social competence combined with appropriate parental modeling of safe behaviors and the enforcement of safety-related legislation are associated with lower levels of child injury.

Tuchfarber, Zins, and Jason review the leading causes of injury across age groups and describe prevention strategies that can help continue the trend toward reducing unintentional injury among children. Specifically, they recommend (a) federal, state, and local policies that require bicycle safety helmets and changes in handgun design; (b) mandated social competence training in schools that focus on interpersonal violence and unintentional injury; and (c) organized efforts of pediatricians, child care providers, psychologists, and public health experts to increase the scope of injury prevention endeavors.

Chapter 10: Academic Performance and School Success: Sources and Consequences (J. David Hawkins)

Healthy People 2000 (DHHS, 1991) offers risk reduction objective 8.2, which proposes to "increase the high school graduation rate to at least 90 percent, thereby reducing risks for multiple problem behaviors and poor mental and physical health" (p. 253).

Conceptually, this objective is important because it highlights a continuing theme in this volume that many problem behaviors in youth co-occur and have common risk and protective factors. Improving social and environmental forces that influence positive youth development and health outcomes represents a critical, cost-effective set of strategies for enhancing children's wellness and preventing multiple problems. One socializing institution with obvious importance to children's lives is school. Ideally, schools are places of safety, learning, and nurturance in which students maximize their potential. As most agree, many schools fall short of this ideal. Although it may not be possible to realize this ideal in all instances, it is possible to develop schools that approximate this goal.

In his chapter, David Hawkins discusses the relationship between a child's success in school and success in later life. He argues persuasively that success in school can be a powerful buffer against many of the risk factors described earlier by Dryfoos. His concept of school success is not limited to a child's mere academic performance. Rather, he sees school success as the formation of a positive bond between a child and school personnel. Such "bonding to the school" involves the development of a child's commitment to succeed in school on the basis of a school culture favorable to learning and feelings of attachment to teachers. Hawkins describes characteristics of schools that promote the formation of a bond to school and thereby learning and academic achievement. He illustrates several effective interventions that demonstrate that schools *can* be reorganized to maximize bonding. Hawkins notes that when schools fail to create the conditions that bond students to school, they fail to foster a powerful protective factor against health risk behaviors. He concludes with an optimistic and apt objective for his chapter and our book on enhancing children's wellness: "We can and should ensure that all American public schools are effective in promoting the academic competence, emotional competence, and healthy behaviors of all students" (p. 301, this volume).

Conclusion

In summary, as comprehensive as *Healthy People 2000* is, it does not go far enough in addressing the health problems and needs of children and youth. The present volume makes clear that the widespread dissemination of effective health promotion practices and policies to foster social and environmental supports for children's social, emotional, and physical wellness are our best bet toward improving their current functioning as well as their health as adults. Given that most of the risky behaviors in which children engage are preventable, family-, school-, and community-based prevention efforts are an appropriate and necessary focus for our commitment. This volume and its companion, *Healthy Children 2010: Establishing Preventive Services,* are intended to make salient the importance of addressing risk and protective factors for children and youth and to describe promising directions for such efforts. Those who read these chapters will benefit from the latest integrative reviews of theoretically based and empirically supported programs to enhance children's health and social development. By disseminating this information, we hope to improve current services and policies for children and also to inform discussion about objectives for *Healthy People 2010.* We hope that this contribution will have tangible effects on planning and practice so that the nation pursues and reaches ambitious but attainable health objectives for children by 2010.

References

American Medical Association, Department of Adolescent Health. (1990). *Healthy youth 2000: National health promotion and disease prevention objectives for adolescents.* Chicago: Author.

Botvin, G. J., Schinke, S., & Orlandi, M. A. (1995). School-based health promotion: Substance abuse and sexual behavior. *Applied & Preventive Psychology, 4,* 167-184.

Carnegie Council on Adolescent Development. (1995). *Great transitions: Preparing adolescents for a new century: Concluding report of the Carnegie Council on Adolescent Development.* New York: Carnegie Corporation.

Consortium on the School-Based Promotion of Social Competence. (1994). The school-based promotion of social competence: Theory, research, practice, and policy. In R. J. Haggerty, L. R. Sherrod, N. Garmezy, & M. Rutter (Eds.), *Stress, risk, and resilience in children and adolescents: Processes, mechanisms, and interventions* (pp. 268-316). New York: Cambridge University Press.

DeFriese, G. H., Crossland, C. L., Pearson, C. E., & Sullivan, C. J. (Eds.). (1990). Comprehensive school health programs: Current status and future prospects. *Journal of School Health, 60,* 127-190.

Dryfoos, J. G. (1990). *Adolescents at risk: Prevalence and prevention.* New York: Oxford University Press.

Durlak, J. A. (1995). *School-based prevention programs for children and adolescents.* Thousand Oaks, CA: Sage.

Fleming, M. (1996). *Healthy youth 2000: A mid-decade review.* Chicago: American Medical Association, Department of Adolescent Health.

Institute of Medicine. (1994). *Reducing risks for mental disorders: Frontiers for preventive intervention research.* Washington, DC: National Academy Press.

Kolbe, L. J., Collins, J., & Cortese, P. (in press). Building the capacity of schools to improve the health of the nation: A call for assistance from psychologists. *American Psychologist.*

McGinnis, J. M., & DeGraw, C. (1991). Healthy schools 2000: Creating partnerships for the decade. *Journal of School Health, 61,* 292-297.

Millstein, S. G., Petersen, A. C., & Nightingale, E. O. (Eds.). (1993). *Promoting the health of adolescents: New directions for the twenty-first century.* New York: Oxford University Press.

Moore, K. A., Sugland, B. W., Blumenthal, C., Glei, D., & Snyder, N. (1995). *Adolescent pregnancy prevention programs: Interventions and evaluations.* Washington, DC: Child Trends.

National Commission on Children. (1991). *Beyond rhetoric: A new American agenda for children and families.* Washington, DC: U.S. Government Printing Office.

Price, R. H., Cowen, E. L., Lorion, R. P., & Ramos-McKay, J. (1989). The search for effective prevention programs: What we have learned along the way. *American Journal of Orthopsychiatry, 59,* 49-58.

Report of the National Mental Health Association Commission on the Prevention of Mental-Emotional Disabilities. (1986). *The prevention of mental-emotional disabilities.* Alexandria, VA: National Mental Health Association.

Simeonsson, R. J. (Ed.). (1994). *Risk, resilience, and prevention: Promoting the well-being of all children.* Baltimore: Paul H. Brookes.

Snyder, H. N., & Sickmund, M. (1995). *Juvenile offenders and victims: A national report.* Washington, DC: Office of Juvenile Justice and Delinquency Prevention.

Tolan, P. H., & Guerra, N. G. (1994). Prevention of delinquency: Current status and issues. *Applied & Preventive Psychology, 3,* 251-273.

U.S. Bureau of the Census. (1993). *Population projections of the United States by age, sex, race, and Hispanic origin: 1993 to 2050* (Current Population Reports, Series P-25-1104). Washington, DC: Author.

U.S. Department of Health and Human Services. (1996). *Trends in the well-being of America's children and youth: 1996.* Washington, DC: Author.

U.S. Department of Health and Human Services, Public Health Service. (1991). *Healthy people 2000: National health promotion and disease prevention objectives* (DHHS Publication No. PHS 91-50212). Washington, DC: U.S. Government Printing Office.

U.S. Department of Health and Human Services, Public Health Service (1995). *Healthy people 2000: Midcourse review and 1995 revisions.* Washington, DC: U.S. Government Printing Office.

U.S. Department of Health, Education, and Welfare, Public Health Service. (1979). *Healthy people: The surgeon general's report on health promotion and disease prevention* (DHEW Publication No. PHS 79-55071). Washington, DC: U.S. Government Printing Office.

Weissberg, R. P., & Elias, M. J. (1993). Enhancing young people's social competence and health behavior: An important challenge for educators, scientists, policy makers, and funders. *Applied & Preventive Psychology, 3,* 179-190.

Weissberg, R. P., & Greenberg, M. T. (1997). School and community competence-enhancement and prevention programs. In I. E. Sigel & K. A. Renninger (Eds.), *Child psychology in practice* (Handbook of Child Psychology, Vol. 4, 5th ed.). New York: John Wiley.

Weissberg, R. P., Gullotta, T. P., Hampton, R. L., Ryan, B. A., & Adams, G. R. (Eds.). (1997). *Healthy children 2010: Establishing preventive services* (Issues in Children's and Families' Lives, Vol. 9). Thousand Oaks, CA: Sage.

Zill, N., & Nord, C. W. (1994). *Running in place: How American families are faring in a changing economy and an individualistic society.* Washington, DC: Child Trends.

• *CHAPTER 2* •

The Prevalence of Problem Behaviors: Implications for Programs

JOY G. DRYFOOS

My interest in problem behaviors started off in one specific categorical domain, the prevention of teenage pregnancy. By the 1980s, it was becoming clear that early unprotected sexual intercourse was not an isolated behavior but had to be viewed in relationship to what else was going on in the young person's life and in the settings in which a young person lived. One simple cross-tabulation changed my perspective. On the basis of data from the 1980 National Longitudinal Survey of Youth, it was shown that among 16- to 19-year-old females, about 21% to 23% of those who were both below average in basic skills and poor became teen mothers, compared with 3% to 5% of those who had average or better basic skills and were not poor (Pittman, 1986). The proportions were almost the same for White, African American, and Hispanic young women.

If school failure and poverty were so strongly related to early childbearing, were other problem behaviors also related to those factors? With this question in mind, I began to explore the interrelationships among behaviors relating to substance use, delinquency, sexual activity, and school performance. I wanted to ascertain the risk status of American adolescents to have a better fix on the design of prevention programs. My goal was to quantify the number of young people who "did it all," "did some of it," and those who were not apparently in danger of any negative outcomes from their social activities or their school performances. This work was published in *Adolescents at Risk: Prevalence and Prevention* (Dryfoos, 1990).

I found, like many other researchers, that risk behaviors did indeed cluster and that a number of common factors could be identified across behavioral domains that either put young people at risk or protected them from the consequences. At that time, I estimated that 10% of all 10-to 17-year-olds were at extremely high risk—already in the juvenile justice system—and another 15% were involved in the whole array of high-risk behaviors such as using drugs and alcohol, having unprotected sexual intercourse, and failing in school. Another 25% were on the brink, experimenting and vulnerable. Half of all young people appeared to be relatively safe from negative consequences of their behaviors—as long as their families, schools, and neighborhoods remained stable.

This estimate was somewhat speculative because no one source of data included all the categories of interest. From the few studies that went beyond a single variable, I had pieced together a "simulated" estimate, extrapolating from various sources to create a construct of the distribution of high-risk behaviors among the adolescent population. Since 1990, a virtual explosion of data has become available relating to high-risk adolescents. Not only has interest been piqued in young people with various problems, but a new field of research has emerged that looks at resiliency and healthy youth development, the flip side of high-risk behavior. The problem behavior territory has been expanded to include risk for HIV infection, adding measurements such as number of sexual partners, sex with drug-using partners, and condom use. My own comprehension of "high riskness" now encompasses mental health variables such as depression and stress.

The terms *high risk* and *low risk* are used in the broadest sense in this work. In the literature, researchers have individual sets of definitions, usually differentiating one group from another by selected (and different) criteria. Some studies use family characteristics (e.g., single-headed household, low socioeconomic status) to define high-risk status; others use school performance (achievement scores) or problem behaviors (substance abuse). Some researchers look at early acting out such as aggressiveness in preschool, or even shyness, as predictors of future problems. My definition of high risk is this: having the attributes of a young person with low probabilities of gaining an education, getting a job, effectively parenting, or being able to participate in the political process.

This chapter moves toward fleshing out that definition, because it is those characteristics of high-risk youth that should shape prevention methodology. But first, five "snapshots" are presented of the latest information on the prevalence of the five categorical behaviors of interest. Then recent attempts to examine the interrelationships between and co-occurrences among these behaviors are summarized. Using the latest data, the estimates of high-risk status are revisited, focusing this time on 15 million youth aged 14 to 17. The age range has been narrowed from 10 to 17 to fine-tune the estimate and target high school age youth. Adolescence is also the time when risky behaviors appear to peak. Risk factors or predictors are examined to determine the attributes of high-risk youth across behavioral domains.

Observations about the shaping of prevention programs are offered in the context of *Healthy People 2000* (U.S. Department of Health and Human Services, Public Health Service [DHHS], 1995), a volume that sets out behavioral objectives that young people were expected to meet. This review of the trends in prevalences of risky behaviors during the past decade is not encouraging, suggesting the need for much more intensive and large-scale replication of effective prevention programs, using proved components that cut across categorical domains.

Categorical High-Risk Behaviors

The term *categorical* is well understood by program developers because most funding for youth programs derives from categorical sources—funding streams that are dedicated to one type or category of problem behavior such as drug abuse, alcoholism, teen pregnancy, HIV/AIDS, suicide, and conflict. The current mode of program planning leans much more in the direction of *comprehensiveness,* putting together various components of categorical efforts to address co-occurring behaviors.

Sources of Data

A unique tool for tracking the prevalence of categorical behaviors became available to researchers in the early 1990s when the Centers for Disease Control and Prevention's (CDC) Division of Adolescent and School Health (DASH) launched the Youth Risk Behavior Surveillance System (YRBS; Kolbe, Kann, & Collins, 1993). A government panel was brought together to review the leading causes of mortality and morbidity among youth and to devise a questionnaire. This survey instrument was approved by a wide range of other scientists and potential gatekeepers, particularly school personnel. The system that emerged from this collaborative process entails three complementary components: a national probability sample of 9th to 12th graders; state and local school-based surveys; and a national household-based survey attached to the health interview survey that gathers information on school dropouts as well as current students.

The YRBS is unique in many ways. First of all, it focuses primarily on behaviors, rather than on knowledge and attitudes. It provides an annual portrait of youth at the national, state, and local levels that can guide practitioners and researchers in shaping interventions. This survey has been designed to capture information on 26 of the national health objectives and several of the national educational goals. The data discussed below derive from the 1993 report based on high school students from the national survey, 24 states, and nine localities (CDC, 1995). Additional data are presented from other surveys in the various categorical domains.

Substance Use

About one third of all in-school adolescents currently (within 30 days of the survey) smoke, half use alcohol, and almost one fifth use marijuana. Approximately 1% to 2% use cocaine, with little difference between use by males and by females.

Smoking. In regard to smoking, about 70% of all students have tried at least a puff or two, and 14% are frequent users. Use goes up with higher grade levels, but not dramatically. White students are most likely to report smoking (34%), African American students the least likely (15%), with Hispanic students falling in between (29%). Prevalence of other forms of tobacco use is significant only among White, non-Hispanic males—26% reported using chewing tobacco or snuff during the 30 days preceding the survey.

Drinking. About 81% of all high school students have ever had a drink. Differences in current alcohol use (past 30 days) by grade are not large. About 41% of 9th graders are current drinkers, compared with 56% of 12th graders. Differences by race/ethnicity are not marked. Hispanic males have the highest rates (55%), and African American females the lowest rates (37%). Episodic heavy drinking is measured by the reported consumption of five or more drinks on at least one occasion during the past 30 days. Fully 30% of all high school students report this extremely high level of alcohol use, sometimes referred to as binge drinking. This rate increases with grade from 22% of 9th graders to 39% of 12th graders and is particularly high among Hispanic (39%) and White (36%) males.

Drugs. One third of all students have ever tried marijuana. Current use rises with grade, from 13% of 9th graders to 22% of 12th graders, and is most prevalent among African American and Hispanic males (24%). Hard drug use has low reported prevalence in the YRBS, but still 5% of all students have ever tried cocaine, and among Hispanic youth, 10% of females and 12% of males have done so. This difference is reflected among current cocaine users (past 30 days) with 6% of Hispanic youth reporting use. The same pattern is seen in youth who have ever used crack, with Hispanic youth showing higher rates (6%). Less than 2% of students reported ever having injected drugs, with higher rates among males than among females.

The YRBS asked questions about use of substances on school property within the past 30 days. Some 15% of students acknowledged smoking, 5% using alcohol, and 6% using marijuana at school. Almost one fourth reported that they had been offered, sold, or given an illegal drug on school property.

Substance use among adolescents has been tracked for several decades by the University of Michigan and through the National Household Survey on Drug Use. Although these surveys use different methodologies and definitions from the YRBS, they are useful for tracking trends. Although substance use declined significantly in the 1980s, an increase in marijuana and cocaine use has been reported in recent years, as well as an upturn in the amount of binge drinking. Students report less concern about the consequences of substance use than in the past and greater access to the sources of supply in school and out in the community. Peer disapproval of marijuana has also declined, from a high of 70% among high school seniors in 1992 to 58% in 1994 ("Health Update," 1995).

Sexual Behavior

More than half of high school students report that they have ever had sexual intercourse, and 37% say that they have had intercourse during the 3 months preceding the survey. Differences between females and males are significant in 9th grade (32% of females ever had sex compared with 44% of males), but by 12th grade, the rate nears equity (66% of females and 70% of males). African American students are much more likely to report sexual intercourse (70% of females and 89% of males) than are White students (47% of females and 49% of males). Gender differences were shown among Hispanic students, with 48% of females and 66% of males so reporting.

One measure of high-risk behavior in the YRBS is having four or more sex partners during one's sexual "career." Almost one in five students reports this behavior, but the differences between groups are striking. Among African American students, 57% of males and 27% of females report four or more partners, more than twice the rate of Hispanics or Whites. The rate goes up with age, as would be expected.

More than half of the currently sexually active students report that they used a condom during their most recent act of sexual intercourse, and 12% reported the use of birth control pills. Males were more likely to report condom use: 59% of males did so, with highest rates among African Americans (64%). Still, 46% of females reported condom use, with the highest rates also among African Americans. Some 22% of sexually active females used birth control pills at last intercourse, with highest rates among White females (24%) and lowest rates among Hispanic females (15%).

The rates of sexual activity among adolescents have increased dramatically during the past several decades, particularly among White youth, who have almost "caught up" with African American youth and girls with boys. In recent years, the prevalence has leveled off and condom use has increased, perhaps in response to concerns about contracting HIV. The adolescent birthrate dropped in the early 1980s, rose in the early 1990s, and now appears to be diminishing slightly.

Delinquency: Violence

The YRBS provides measures of weapon carrying and fighting, reflecting behaviors that are clearly related to violence and conduct disorders. Almost one in four students carried some type of weapon within 30 days of the survey, and 8% acknowledged carrying a gun. In this domain, gender differences are significant. Some 34% of male respondents carried a weapon, 14% a gun, whereas 9% of females carried a weapon, 2% a gun. Gun carrying was reported more frequently by African American males (21%) than Hispanic (17%) or White males (12%). Students in the 9th grade were more likely to report carrying a gun than 12th graders (9% versus 7%), indicating that the potential for violence is already in place as students leave middle school and go to high school.

Students were asked whether they had carried a weapon such as a gun, knife, or club on school property within the past 30 days. At least 18% of males and 5% of females admitted that they had done so. Some 9% of males and 5% of females reported that they had been threatened or injured with a weapon on school property. It is not surprising that students feel too unsafe to go to school. About 10% of Hispanic, 7% of African American, and 3% of White high school students reported high levels of fear about their safety. More than a third of all students have had property stolen or damaged at school.

Male students were also more often in fights: More than half of the males reported this behavior within the past year, compared with 32% of females. Here, there were differences by race/ethnicity for females but not for males. About 42% of African American, 34% of Hispanic, and 30% of White female students were in physical fights.

Some of these young people turn up in juvenile court. According to the Department of Justice, almost 1.5 million delinquency cases were handled in 1992, a dramatic increase from 1988, when there were fewer than 1.2 million cases (U.S. Department of Justice, 1994). About 5% of all 10- to 17-year-olds were arrested, with the rate reaching 11% at age 16. More than 9% of 14- to 17-year-olds were involved with the courts. Males were almost five times more likely to be arrested than females (9% versus 2%), and the rate for African American youngsters (11%) was more than twice the rate for White youth (5%). One in five of those arrested was detained in secure facilities.

Depression: Suicidal Ideation

The YRBS provides insights into students' mental health through a series of questions on suicidal ideation. One in four high school students disclosed to the YRBS serious thoughts about attempting suicide within the past year, 19% made a suicide plan, and 9% actually attempted suicide. This behavior, highly indicative of depression and stress, is much more likely to be reported by females than by males (30% of females thought about suicide, compared with 19% of males). The prevalence among Hispanic and White students is similar (26% and 24%, respectively), higher than among African American students (20%). Hispanic female students, however, report a strikingly high rate of suicidal ideation (34%) and a 20% prevalence rate for attempts. Attempts appear to decrease with age, ranging from 10% of 9th graders to 7% of 12th graders.

A smaller study of middle school students provides more detail on mental health indicators (Millstein et al., 1992). More than a third of 6th- to 8th-grade students reported being bothered by feelings of anger, 26% said they were depressed, and 23% acknowledged that they were having problems getting along with others.

According to a recent review of the health of adolescents, the prevalence of developmental, behavioral, or emotional problems among youth under age 18 ranges from 17% to 22% (Ozer, Brindis, Irwin, & Millstein, n.d.). It is estimated that approximately 5 million adolescents aged 12 to 17 have emotional or behavioral problems.

School Failure

Measures of dropout, achievement, and school attendance rates are not typically included in surveys of high-risk behaviors. For example, the YRBS does not include any measures of school performance, although a special survey was conducted of school dropouts relating school problems to other categorical problems. For prevalence rates on school variables, one can look at the National Education Longitudinal Study (NELS), the U.S. Department of Education's enlightening longitudinal study tracking eighth graders since 1988 (National Center for Education Statistics, 1995).

When the NELS respondents were in 8th grade, almost one in five was not proficient at the basic level in mathematics, and 14% could not read at the most basic level (Hafner, Ingels, Schneider, & Stevenson, 1990). Significant racial/ethnic differences occur in school performance, with Asian and White students achieving higher scores, whereas African American, Hispanic, and American Indian students score much lower. Reading scores are the lowest for students who do not speak English at home. Children from low socioeconomic status homes are the least successful. Grades are mirrored in these scores, with minority students, especially males, having lower scores and grades. Among all 8th graders, 18% have already been held back a year.

By 10th grade, many of these low-performing students drop out. Rumberger (in press) conducted a unique analysis of the NELS data showing that during the 2-year period from 8th (middle school) to 10th (high school), 9% of Hispanic, 10% of African American, and 5% of White students dropped out. Students who had been held back were 11 times more likely to drop out than those who were not. By 10th grade, 26% of Hispanics, 33% of African Americans, and 19% of White high school students had been retained at least once. Those who were still in school by 10th grade were still in great jeopardy of not graduating. One can calculate rates of retention from census data by examining the proportion of each age cohort that is older than the norm. About 5% of all high school-age students are 2 or more years older than their peers, and 25% are 1 year older (U.S. Bureau of the Census, 1993, Table A-3).

The U.S. Census reports dropout statistics for the general population. In 1994, one in eight 16- to 24-year-olds no longer in school was without high school credentials (National Education Goals

Panel, 1995). The dropout rate for Hispanics was 30%, substantially higher than the rate for African Americans (13%) and for Whites (8%). This measure has changed little during recent years, lowering slightly among African Americans and Whites but rising for Hispanics, probably attributable to the continuing immigration.

The Monitoring the Future survey asked students whether they had skipped school or classes within the past 4 weeks (National Education Goals Panel, 1995). Some 11% of 8th graders had skipped school and 14% skipped class, whereas 31% of 12th graders skipped school and 37% skipped class. All the reported rates were highest among Hispanic students and lowest among Whites, following the pattern of dropout rates.

Summary of High-Risk Behaviors

Almost every adolescent appears to have tried some form of risky behavior. Nearly all high school students have tried smoking and drinking, and many regularly use cigarettes, alcohol, and marijuana. Gender differences are insignificant. These behaviors appear to be well established by 9th grade, with relatively small differences between those students and 12th graders. Race/ethnicity differences do appear, notably in the higher prevalence of marijuana and cocaine use among Hispanic males.

More than half of all high school students have experienced sexual intercourse. Higher-grade and African American students have the highest prevalence and are most likely to have had sex with multiple partners. Condom use among sexually active students is quite frequent, but the rates decline with grade as birth control pill use increases.

High school students report serious vulnerability to the consequences of violent behavior, not surprising because a third of all males and almost 1 in 10 females carry some type of weapon. That almost 14% of male students report carrying guns is mind-boggling. Physical fights are prevalent, and many students are afraid to go to school because of the threat of injury, property destruction, or worse. More than 9% of 14- to 17-year-olds were arrested and entered the juvenile justice system in a year.

One in four high school students reports having contemplated suicide within the past year, and almost 9% actually attempted it. Rates were significantly higher among females, particularly Hispanics. One in five Hispanic females reported a suicide attempt within the year. But even so, one in five male high school students reported thinking about suicide, and 5% actually tried it.

Finally, one in five 8th graders cannot do math, and one in seven can barely read. About one fourth of 10th graders have been retained in a class, a powerful determinant of dropping out. Some 12% of all young people did not finish high school. All the measures relating to school issues point toward the greater vulnerability of poor, minority youth, particularly when they are situated in segregated schools.

Table 2.1 summarizes these findings among the current population of 14- to 17-year-olds (N = 14,600,000). Large numbers of young people are involved with problems that may have hazardous consequences.

Co-Occurrence of High-Risk Behaviors

Many young people report that they are involved with risky behaviors. These behaviors do not occur randomly. They come in packages. An expansive literature has emerged that describes these interrelationships reflecting the availability of multivariable data sources such as the YRBS and the advances in computer technology.

Summary of Co-Occurring Behaviors

Many published analyses that interrelate the various behaviors of interest have been reviewed here. Because most of these data bases are cross-sectional, rather than longitudinal, researchers are careful not to draw causal inferences from the correlations. It is clear, however, that these high-risk behaviors do come in packages, some youth do "do it all," and some do little.

Substance abuse is closely related to delinquency. Almost all adjudicated youngsters report some involvement with drugs. Heavy alcohol, smoking, and marijuana use appears to co-occur with early unprotected intercourse and multiple partners. Nonusers are less likely to initiate risky sexual relationships. Heavy smokers are much more likely to contemplate suicide.

Table 2.1 Percentage of 14- to 17-Year-Olds With Categorical Risk Behaviors, Circa 1993

Indicator	*Percentage*
Total	100.0
Substance use	
Current drinking	48.0
Binge drinking	30.0
Current smoking	30.5
Current marijuana	17.7
Hard drugs	1.9
Sexual activity	
Sexually active	53.0
No condom use, sexually active	25.0
Teen mother (females)	2.7
Delinquency	
Adjudicated	9.4
Carry guns	7.9
Truant	20.0
Depression/suicidal	
Suicide attempt	8.6
Suicidal thoughts	24.1
School	
Dropout	4.9
Two years behind in school	5.0
One year behind in school	25.0
No reported high-risk behaviors	15.0

Young people who initiate sex at early ages, have multiple partners, and do not use protection are often under the influence of alcohol and/or drugs when they participate in sexual activity. Nonvirgins report much higher rates than do virgins of delinquent behavior such as fighting or weapon carrying and trouble in school. Early sexual initiation is a strong indicator of multiple partners, not using condoms, having been pregnant or causing a pregnancy, and, among females, feeling depressed and having a sexually transmitted disease.

Violent behavior is highly related to other negative outcomes such as substance use and unprotected sex. Cocaine use is one of the most significant predictors of carrying a gun to school. The most delinquent youth are much more likely to be involved in any form of drug use, to have dropped out or be failing, to have poor mental health, and among girls, to have early pregnancies. The link between delinquency and being held back in school appears as early as first grade.

Dropouts appear to be involved with sex, drugs, and violence to a much greater degree than enrolled high school students. School dropouts are much more likely to have had sexual intercourse with multiple partners, to smoke daily and use marijuana, and to carry weapons and fight. Falling behind in school and frequent truancy are strong predictors of dropping out and are associated with all the high-risk behaviors. Dropouts report frequent suspensions, arrests, and significant time spent in juvenile homes or shelters.

Depression and stress, as measured by suicidal ideation, are strongly related to early intercourse. Sexual abuse is implicated in this pathway because it is related to unprotected sex, drug use, and depression. Reported incest and extrafamilial sex abuse are strikingly high among chemically dependent adolescents. Young people who contemplate suicide are more likely to use alcohol and other drugs. The most significant association is between the most serious suicide attempts and the most illicit drugs such as cocaine.

Numbers of Risk Behaviors

A number of studies have addressed what I call the "packaging" issue, the cumulative effects of multiple risk behaviors. Others have looked at numbers of nonpersonal factors that increase risk—demographic and family variables that appear to put young people in jeopardy of negative consequences such as dropout.

Co-occurrence of problem behaviors was measured by Ellickson, Saner, and McGuigan (in press) for both the most violent youth and those who reported only occasional activities. Among the half of the youth who were delinquent in the less stringent definition, more than half reported at least one other problem behavior (also broadly defined), 9% had only one other problem, 23% had two others, 16% had three others, and 5% had four other problem behaviors.

In 1990, Search Institute, a nonprofit research organization, conducted a survey of more than 46,000 youth in grades 6 to 12. Although the sample was heavily Midwestern and 90% White, on key indicators such as those found in the YRBS, the findings were quite similar. Benson (1993) used these data to produce a unique analysis of at-risk behaviors, defined as "choices that potentially limit psychological, physical, or economic well-being during adolescence or adulthood" (p. 39). Benson selected 20 at-risk indicators in the domains of substance use, sex, depression/suicide, antisocial behavior, school, vehicle safety, and bulimia. Almost a third of the students reported four or more at-risk indicators, rising from 6% of 6th graders to 50% of 12th graders. Boys had higher rates of multiple risk involvement than did girls. Of 6th graders, however, 40% were not at risk in any of the domains, decreasing to 11% of 12th graders.

Table 2.2 presents the patterns derived from the Search Institute study of co-occurrences among selected high-risk behaviors for students in grades 9 to 12. The indicators measure the riskiest of behaviors: For alcohol, it is binge drinking; for tobacco, daily or frequent use; for illicit drugs, six or more times a year; for sexual intercourse, more than twice; frequent depression or attempted suicide; for antisocial behavior, two or more incidents of vandalism, theft, fighting, trouble with the police, or weapon use. School problems are measured by two or more absences in a month and/or the desire to dropout.

Table 2.2 clearly demonstrates the significant overlap between these behaviors. For example, almost all the students who report that they use illicit drugs also report that they are sexually active (84%). The youth who are having trouble in school are likely to binge on alcohol (62%), be sexually active (72%), and have some delinquency problems (53%). Everyone who does one thing, however, does not always do another. Thus, among self-reported illicit drug users, apparently 16% are not yet sexually active. Among youth with school troubles, 38% do not binge on alcohol, 28% are not sexually active, and 47% are not delinquent.

Hahn (1995) used a database created by *Phi Delta Kappa* to examine the clustering of 24 risk indicators (measuring personal pain, academic factors, and family factors). He found that 85% of the respondents had at least 1 of the risk indicators. By 10th grade, almost 31% had 3 or more risks, 14% had 5 or more risks, and 1.2% reported 10 or more risk factors. The prevalence of certain risk factors increased dramatically with age, as expected, giving further evidence of the importance of what Hahn calls the "nipping in the bud" approach to early intervention.

Table 2.2 Co-Occurrences of Problem Behaviors

If at Risk in This Area	*Percentage of 9-12 Graders at Risk in This Domain*	*Alcohol*	*Tobacco*	*Illicit Drug Use*	*Sexuality*	*Depression/ Suicide*	*Antisocial Behavior*	*School*
Alcohol	31	—	42	27	70	33	49	23
Tobacco	20	66	—	35	77	39	53	26
Illicit drugs	11	72	60	—	84	46	61	32
Sexuality	44	49	34	22	—	34	41	19
Depression/Suicide	25	41	30	21	59	—	38	18
Antisocial behavior	28	54	37	24	64	34	—	22
School problems	12	62	43	31	72	40	53	—

SOURCE: Adapted from *The Troubled Journey: A Portrait of 6th-12th Grade Youth* (Figures 5.6 and 5.9), by P. Benson, 1993, Minneapolis, MN: Search Institute. Adapted with permission by P. Benson, President, Search Institute.
NOTE: This table should be read as follows: 31% of students are at risk of alcohol abuse. If a student is at risk in the area of alcohol use, then the probability that the student uses tobacco is 42%, uses illicit drugs is 27%, is sexually active is 70%, and so on.

Vanderschmidt, Lang, Knight-Williams, and Vanderschmidt (1993) investigated five risk behaviors (violence, sexual activity, and alcohol, cigarette, and drug use) among a sample of inner-city middle school students. Prevalence rates were high (11% had carried a gun, and 46% were sexually active). Almost 80% of the students reported past or present risk in one or more of the categories. Among those with two or more past or present risks, 80% included violence and 71% included sexual activity. When only current risk was considered, the prevalence reached 94% for violence and 85% for sexual activity. In this sample, 20% reported no risk behaviors ever, and one third said they were not currently involved.

A number of studies have looked at runaway youth in shelters or homeless youth who are by definition high risk. A survey of street youth in Los Angeles, New York, and San Francisco exhibited high prevalences: 52% to 71% were sexually active but not using protection, 41% to 68% were hustling, drug dealing, and/or stealing, and 77% to 96% were involved with drugs (Kennedy, Greenberg, Clatts, Kipke, & Mills, 1994). One in four in San Francisco, almost a third of the Los Angeles respondents, and almost half of the New York group did it all. Only 2% to 13% of street youth were not involved in any of those risky behaviors.

Sequencing of High-Risk Behaviors

I have abstained from entering the extensive debate over the sequencing of problem behaviors and which of these behaviors comes first. My own view is that early initiation of any of the behaviors predicts trouble ahead across domains. Young children with conduct disorders are identifiable in preschool classes. If they are not treated, they have high probabilities of getting involved at early ages with sex, drugs, and/or violence. Whether children have sex at 10 (many boys report that they do!), smoke at 8, or get drunk for the first time at 11 does not make much difference. Any of those acts is quite likely to lead to the others. Early sexual acting out among young girls frequently leads to school failure (long before the unintended pregnancy that often follows). Being left back in school predicts trouble, and being left back twice guarantees failure.

Estimates of Risk Status Groups

On the basis of the findings presented here, it is possible to estimate the numbers of young people aged 14 to 17 who fall into groupings of problem behaviors, from the highest risk to no risk at all. Although much more information is available than in the past, this is also a simulated estimate, taking existing data from several sources and forcing the numbers and ratios into cells according to the patterns that have emerged. The percentages of young people involved in each one of the categories were shown in Table 2.1. Table 2.2 and the summary of co-occurrence studies in the text provide insights into how these behaviors overlap and can be aggregated.

Table 2.3 shows the estimates of the distribution of 14- to 17-year-olds according to risk status. About 15% of high school age youth are at very high risk of extremely negative consequences. Another 15% are involved in similar behaviors that will place them in great jeopardy of never "making it." About 35% of contemporary youth are experimenting with various high-risk activities, and they can go either way, to success or failure. The rest of the young people (35%) are at very low risk or not at risk because of their behaviors. Thus, for the purposes of targeting programs and understanding the current ecology of youth behavior, the teen population can be divided roughly into thirds.

Table 2.4 shows the distribution of the categorical behaviors according to risk groups. A review of the prevalence of problem behaviors for the total population shows that 25% of all 14- to 17-year-olds are behind grade, and 5% have already dropped out.

Table 2.3 Estimates of Numbers and Percentages in Each Risk Status Group

Status	*Percentage*	*Number (000s)*
Total in population	100%	14,600
Very high risk	15	2,200
High risk	15	2,200
Medium risk	35	5,000
Low risk	20	2,900
No risk	15	2,200

Table 2.4 Distributions of Categorical Behaviors According to Risk Status Group

	Total With Problem: Percentage of 14- to 17-Year-Olds	*Percentage of Very High Risk*	*Percentage of High Risk*	*Percentage of Medium Risk*	*Percentage of Low Risk*	*Percentage of No Risk*
Current drinking	48	80	70	60	24	—
Current smoking	31	60	50	35	10	—
Current marijuana	18	40	40	16	—	—
Sexually active	53	90	80	60	34	—
Sexually active/No condom use	25	68	52	20	—	—
Adjudicated	9	62	—	—	—	—
Carry guns	8	52	—	—	—	—
Truant	20	45	45	18	—	—
Suicide attempt	9	18	18	8	—	—
Suicidal thoughts	24	40	40	35	—	—
Dropout	5	33	—	—	—	—
Two years behind	5	33	—	—	—	—
One year behind	25	20	75	31	—	—

NOTE: This table should be read as follows: 48% of all 14- to 17-year-olds currently drink. Among *Very High Risk* youth, 80% drink, among *High Risk* youth, 70% drink, and so on.

Some 18% to 48% are involved in some form of substance use, and 53% are sexually active. More than 9% have been adjudicated as delinquents, 22% carry weapons, and 21% report truancy. Almost a fourth have suicidal thoughts, and 9% report having made an attempt. But these prevalences are different in the various risk groups.

High-Risk Youth

According to this distribution (Tables 2.3 and 2.4), *Very High Risk* youngsters are those who have been within the juvenile justice system within the past year, carry guns, and/or use illegal drugs such as cocaine. About 15% of all 14- to 17-year-olds fall into this category. It is estimated that among these 2.2 million young people, more than 60% would have been arrested at least once during a year. More than half would have access to guns. At least 80% would drink, 40% would be users of illegal drugs, and 90% would be sexually active, mostly unprotected. About 40% would be depressed, and many would have attempted suicide. About one third would have already dropped out of school and another third would be 2 or more years behind. The remainder would be 1 year behind.

Another 15% of all adolescents are at *High Risk* much like the first category, but they have not yet been adjudicated. Some of them might be identified as *High Delinquency Risk*. They are heavily involved with drinking, smoking, and marijuana; are behind modal grade in school and often truant; and frequently have unprotected intercourse. Others might be identified as *High Mental Health Risk* adolescents with some of the same behaviors as the group above, but they also are extremely depressed, as indicated by suicide attempts. These 4.4 million high-risk youngsters, almost one third of the youth population, are in great jeopardy unless they receive immediate, intensive interventions.

Medium-Risk Youth

Medium Risk young people make up the largest category. About 35% of all 14- to 17-year-olds—some 5 million youngsters—are involved in one or two high-risk behaviors, but less intensely. They may be behind in school (31%) and occasionally truant (18%), or drink once in a while (60%), or experiment with marijuana (16%), or have sex (60%) without contraception sometimes, or have suicidal thoughts from time to time (35%). These young people are clearly vulnerable because of their behaviors and need considerable support to not deepen their involvement to the degree that their futures are in jeopardy.

Low- and No-Risk Youth

About 10% are at *Low Risk*. They might take a drink once in a while (24%) or cut a class, but they are not in any jeopardy because of their behaviors. About a third are sexually active, and they always use contraception. At least 15% of all 14- to 17-year-olds are at *No Risk*. They report no high-risk behaviors, no depression, and no school problems.

These 5 million young people, more than a third of the youth population, are currently protected from the most deleterious consequences of the new morbidities. But they are surrounded by many of the negative factors that may promote antisocial behavior. They are also in jeopardy of being victimized by other youth. Their resilience may be dependent on the stability of their families, the quality of their schools, and the safety of their neighborhoods, all factors subject to change.

New Estimates Yield Higher Risk Rates

This estimate differs from the previous one in several ways. First of all, it encompasses only 14- to 17-year-olds, the time when most of the risk indicators peak. The previous estimate included 10- to 13-year-olds as well, which lowered the aggregate prevalences significantly. Also, in several domains, the prevalences have risen among 14- to 17-year-olds since the mid-1980s. Juvenile crime rates have increased slightly, reflecting more violent acts and more weapons offenses. Binge drinking and current smoking rates have gone up, but current drinking has come down, and the rest of substance-using behavior has stayed about the same. Sexual activity is near the same level, although condom use has improved. School dropout rates and school failure rates for this age group have changed little.

Approximately one third of all adolescents fall into the high-risk group in this iteration, compared with one fourth in the earlier version. One third are at medium risk, compared with one fourth previously. One third are at low or no risk, compared with one half. The point here is not scientific accuracy but rather the creation of rough calculations for the purposes of understanding the need for targeted interventions for high-risk youth.

Attributes of High-Risk Youth

A strong case can be made for targeting for immediate and powerful interventions those youngsters who "do it all" or, at least, do most of it. Almost one in three adolescents falls into this grouping. How can those children be recognized? Many studies verify the power of certain common variables as predictors or precursors of the different outcomes.

The NELS longitudinal study of eighth graders identified a group of factors that predicted school failure, focusing on family structure and status (National Center for Education Statistics, 1995). Some 26% of eighth-grade students in 1988 had one of the factors, and 20% had two or more, including single-parent homes, family incomes of less than $15,000, older sibling who had dropped out, parents who did not finish high school, limited proficiency in English, or being at home for 3 hours a day or more without supervision.

Two years later, 15% of the students with two or more of these factors had dropped out, compared with 2% of those with no factors. By 1992, when they were seniors, 33% with two or more factors were no longer enrolled in school, compared with 8% of those with none. By graduation time, 24% of the group with multiple factors were classified as dropouts, compared with only 4% of those with no factors. Those who had multiple family factors in 1988 were much more likely to have a child by 1992 (19% versus 5%) and to have been suspended or arrested.

A review of the studies cited above (see also Howell & Bilchek, 1995; Roth, 1995) that delineate factors that predict categorical high-risk behaviors yields a list of variables that appear to be the most common precursors across domains.

Family:
- Lack of supervision
- Lack of attachment and bonding
- Parental substance use
- Abuse and neglect
- Absence of cultural resources
- Frequent moving

School:
- Low expectations for success
- Little commitment to education
- Being behind in school
- Low grades

Community:
- Poverty
- Gangs
- Access to guns

Individual:
- Susceptibility to peer influences
- Lack of social competency
- Tolerance of deviance/unconventionality

Protective Factors

Despite living in a risky society, all young people are not in jeopardy of failure to grow into responsible adults. As this chapter has noted, some are not involved in any behaviors with potentially negative consequences, and a good many more are experimenting in quite responsible ways, for example, having protected sex in what they perceive as serious, long-term relationships. Most young people who use marijuana do not go on to become active drug abusers. Some researchers have suggested that experimentation is a healthy aspect of youth development. Shedler and Block (1990) suggest that "experimental use of drugs may be considered a normative behavior among U.S. teenagers in terms of prevalence, and from a developmental task perspective" (p. 613).

Protective factors are the flip side of risk factors. Young people who have "made it" despite all odds have been studied by several prominent researchers (Garmezy, 1985; Werner & Smith, 1982).

Four factors have been frequently mentioned that foster resiliency or invulnerability to the consequences of high-risk behaviors.

Attachment to a Caring Adult. The best documented fact in the extensive literature on youth is the importance of social bonding between a young person and an adult. The responsible adult may be either or both parents (single mothers can perform this function very well), a grandparent, teacher, or any other mentor. Consistency, caring, encouragement, and maintenance of contact through childhood and adolescence are all important factors. According to Resnick, Harris, and Blum (1993), the single most powerful explainer of emotional well-being in adolescents is a variable they call *family connectedness.* Adolescents who perceive a meaningful, caring relationship in their lives, either from their families or from another caring adult, are quite resistant to the negative consequences of drugs, sex, and delinquency. They are not immune, however, to the consequences of violence, for example, drive-by shootings or in-school episodes.

Independence and Competency. Many children who make it despite all odds appear to have a strong streak of independence. They can make decisions and solve problems on their own, seeming to have a built-in competence that helps them overcome barriers as they arise in poor social environments. Others describe them as having "sunny personalities." During periods of stress, resilient youth appear to be able to distance themselves from their troubled families.

High Aspirations. Autobiographical accounts contribute to the understanding of how the dreamer becomes the doer, for example, the disadvantaged youngster who wants to become a scientist and finds out how to get on the achievement track at the earliest age. Usually, an adult is involved in helping turn the aspirations into reality.

Effective Schools. A supportive and challenging school can act as a significant influence in the life of a disadvantaged youngster. As researchers express it, "the effect of all the other variables is through education," meaning that when other factors such as family structure, socioeconomic status, and race are taken into consideration, the bottom line is having access to a strong educational system.

Caring teachers with high expectations for students can act as buffers against the outside world and assist young people in achieving their goals.

Implications for Programs

The review of behavioral patterns, risk status, and risk and protective factors should serve as a framework for designing more effective prevention programs. All young persons are entitled to a supportive family, strong schools, and a safe environment, but some need more support than others. All young people are not at equal risk of failure. One third of adolescents need powerful targeted interventions that will change their life courses as soon as possible, or they will never be able to succeed. Intervention has to start early enough to head off these risky behavioral patterns. Given the knowledge of the patterning of problem behaviors, it is possible to identify youth at early ages with individual, family, school, and community attributes that place them at risk.

Do we know how to change the life courses of high-risk youth? My answer is a tentative "yes." Program evaluation is still in its early stages, producing many preliminary results from demonstration projects typically evaluated by the people who design them. Few of the successful models have been replicated and evaluated by outsiders. But the state of the art is far enough advanced to have a good idea about how to proceed.

Programs that address the underlying causes of the problems that youth encounter are more likely to help them change and succeed than those that focus only on single categorical behaviors. Proved interventions focus on approaches such as one-on-one support from a responsible adult (e.g., mentoring, tutoring, advocacy, and case management), family counseling, cognitive skills enhancement, training in social competency, community service, and youth involvement. Schools are fundamental building blocks in prevention of problem behaviors, first, as the purveyors of essential cognitive skills, and second, as the hub for one-stop centers. Comprehensive multicomponent school-community efforts have proved effects across domains. Outreach in the form of home visiting and street work is an important component when working with the highest-risk youth. Media can play an important role in shaping community attitudes regarding health promotion and prevention of high-risk behaviors. Programs that are directed toward policy issues (such as gun control and taxation on cigarettes and alcohol), as well as services, have shown excellent results.

Attention to Settings

Concern is shifting from trying to alter individual behaviors to changing the settings that either promote or discourage healthy youth development. This position was spelled out in *Losing Generations,* a report of the National Research Council Panel on High-Risk Youth (1993), which recommended moving the locus of attention away from the personal attributes of adolescents and their families and toward the settings that so profoundly influence outcomes—families, neighborhoods, schools, health and welfare systems, employment and training, and the justice system. Researchers and practitioners (but not politicians) have reached a consensus that poverty and racism are major determinants of the declining status of children and that these issues must be dealt with for young people to have equal access to success in this society.

Early Identification

One method of early identification of children in high-risk settings is to target those who are behind their modal grade. Research has substantiated the negative consequences of being older than one's classroom peers. The further behind students fall, the more likely they are to fail and to become involved in activities with potentially negative consequences. This approach to early identification does not require extensive research or expenditure for new needs assessments. The age and grade of the child are one fact that is universally available. Schools with high grade retention rates are prime targets for intervention.

Replication

Many program models of effective schools and youth organizations do exist, but they have not been widely replicated. A recent review of selected categorical prevention programs identified a number of common factors driving replication (Dryfoos, 1996).

Strong evaluation and clear documentation of changed behavioral outcomes establish a program's reputation for success. And, of course, publication of evaluation findings in a peer-reviewed journal is de rigueur. A number of large-scale replications, however, have taken place without strong research findings. Some rely on the charisma of the leader. Qualities such as eloquence, evidence of commitment, being personable, and conveying a sense of authority give programs an aura. Having political know-how, building board membership that involves prominent business leaders, and knowing the "right" people help raise funds. Having an "in" with government agencies leads to high visibility, for example, inclusion in conferences, public hearings, and media events. Several programs have been written into legislation, moving from the demonstration project phase to becoming models for states (e.g., Parents as Teachers in Missouri, Family Life Education in New Jersey, and Primary Mental Health Project in California) and for federal grant programs (e.g., DARE in Drug Free Schools and Cities-in-Schools in Department of Justice and Department of Labor). Others enjoy foundation favor with large multisite grants that stimulate rapid dissemination, at least of the program concepts.

The marketing of program manuals, training videos, and prevention curricula is a big business. The expectation that social skills programs and substantive curricula can be faithfully replicated by teachers and other workers merely by supplying them with manuals and videos has not been born out by experience. Experience has shown, however, that replication can take place in a much more orderly way if training is organized and presented directly by the program developers. On-site facilitators and coaches have been used effectively in building second-generation programs. National youth organizations such as Girls Inc. and Boys and Girls Clubs have been particularly successful at disseminating effective models through their capacities to provide training and technical assistance to their affiliates. National research organizations and think tanks such as RAND and Public/Private Ventures also have the ability to employ program developers, conduct research, disseminate their own publications, and offer technical assistance. Several of the major replications of prevention projects are administered by university centers, but the majority of the replicated programs are managed by nonprofit agencies, national or even local youth organizations, and research-program development groups.

Program models designed to address the needs of various populations such as African American males and Hispanic youth are in demand by community-based organizations. Certain programs are attractive to practitioners because they are new, cutting-edge, imaginative, dynamic, or otherwise exciting.

Some programs with high-quality evaluations do not get replicated. The successful Midwestern Prevention Project developed by Pentz (1993) and colleagues at the University of Southern California program included five components: school-based curricula, parent programs, community organization, social policy change, and mass media components. Despite documentation of positive effects and a heavy exposure through conferences and publications, this project is not being replicated. The program is believed to be too complicated to implement without considerable financial support as well as sustained technical assistance (M. Pentz, personal communication, 1995).

Some programs with negative evaluations showing that the program has limited effect do get replicated. In some cases, the evaluation is used to change the model to improve the potential. In other cases, the evaluation is ignored, and the program is marketed with no change (Ringwalt et al., 1994). The latter is most observable in the substance abuse field, with huge sales of manuals and training time despite the adverse information (to which the public does not have access). Some popular interventions that have shown no effect on changing high-risk behaviors include self-esteem workshops, peer counseling, parent workshops, ability grouping, unstructured mentoring, and employment and training programs that do not include an educational component.

Evaluating Progress Through *Healthy People 2000*

One instrument for measuring success in preventing high-risk behavior among adolescents is the monitoring of progress through the national *Healthy People 2000* objectives. A midcourse review was conducted that documented some improvement in health outcomes but not as much advancement as might be hoped for among young people (DHHS, 1995). A look at the five categorical domains addressed here is not encouraging. Following declines during a decade, cigarette, alcohol, and marijuana use among youth began to increase in the mid-1990s, making it less likely that the rates will be reduced to the year 2000 objectives. The proportion of females aged 15 to 17 who are sexually active, as well as pregnancy rates, has increased. Suicide attempts and suicide rates are elevating. Violence rates continue to increase. The dropout rate, although stabilized, has not fallen significantly.

Those who have worked in the field of prevention have a difficult time accepting that high-risk behavior continues to shape the lives of millions of adolescents. The rates seem unchangeable, no matter how hard practitioners labor to intervene. One problem is turnover: Every year, a new cohort of young people arrive in middle school, ready to experiment if they have not begun already. Efforts have to remain constant. Demonstration projects may work for 2 or 3 years, but they have no effect on succeeding generations except to provide guidance on effective programming. Evidence is clear from the experiments of the past that more powerful comprehensive approaches are required, that we cannot continue to treat troubled young people in categorical efforts that do not deal with the social and psychological environment that gives rise to these problems.

Just as the behaviors come in packages, so must the prevention and treatment. Young people who are failing in school, using drugs, carrying guns, and having unprotected sex are not likely to be influenced by sporadic classroom-based prevention curricula delivered by harassed teachers. These high-risk youngsters need a set of integrated components that have been identified through research and experience.

References

Benson, P. (1993). *The troubled journey: A portrait of 6th-12th grade youth.* Minneapolis, MN: Search Institute.

Centers for Disease Control and Prevention. (1995, March 24). CDC surveillance summaries. *Morbidity and Mortality Weekly Review, 44*(SS-1), 1-56.

Dryfoos, J. (1990). *Adolescents at risk: Prevalence and prevention.* New York: Oxford University Press.

Dryfoos, J. (1996). *"Adolescents at risk" revisited: Continuity, evaluation and replication of prevention programs.* Report to Carnegie Corporation, New York.

Ellickson, P., Saner, H., & McGuigan, K. (in press). Profiles of violent youth: Substance use and other concurrent problems. *American Journal of Public Health.*

Garmczy,, N. (1985). Stress-resistant children: The search for protective factors. In J. Stevenson (Ed.), *Recent research in developmental psychopathology* (pp. 213-233). Oxford, UK: Pergamon.

Hafner, A., Ingels, S., Schneider, B., & Stevenson, D. (1990). *A profile of the American eighth grader: NELS:88 student descriptive study.* Washington, DC: National Center for Education Statistics.

Hahn, A. B. (1995). *America's middle child: Making age count in the development of a national youth policy.* Waltham, MA: Brandeis University.

Health update. (1995, January 11). *Education Week,* p. 10.

Howell, J., & Bilchek, S. (1995). *Guide for implementing the comprehensive strategy for serious, violent, and chronic juvenile offenders.* Washington, DC: Office of Juvenile Justice and Delinquency Prevention.

Kennedy, M., Greenberg, J., Clatts, M., Kipke, M., & Mills, S. (1994, November). *Patterns and correlates of high-risk behavior among street youth.* Paper presented at the annual meeting of the American Public Health Association, Washington, DC.

Kolbe, L. J., Kann, L., & Collins, J. L. (1993). Overview of the Youth Risk Behavior Surveillance System. *Public Health Report, 108,* 2-9.

Millstein, S. G., Irwin, C. E., Adler, N. E., Cohn, L. D., Kegeles, S. M., & Dolcini, M. M. (1992). Health-risk behaviors and health concerns among young adolescents. *Pediatrics, 3,* 422-428.

National Center for Education Statistics. (1995). *Statistics in brief* (NCES 95-736). Washington, DC: U.S. Department of Education.

National Education Goals Panel. (1995). *Data volume for the National Education Goals Report: Volume One. National Data.* Washington, DC: U.S. Government Printing Office.

National Research Council Panel on High-Risk Youth. (1993). *Losing generations: Adolescents in high-risk settings.* Washington, DC: National Academy Press.

Ozer, E., Brindis, C., Irwin, C., & Millstein, S. (n.d.). *The health of adolescents in the U.S.: 1994.* San Francisco: University of California, Institute for Health Policy Studies, National Health Information Center.

Pentz, M. (1993). Benefits of integrating strategies in different settings. In A. Elster, S. Panzarine, & K. Holt (Eds.), *American Medical Association State-of-the-Art Conference on Adolescent Health Promotion: Proceedings* (NCEMCH Research Monograph, pp. 15-34). Arlington, VA: National Center for Education in Maternal and Child Health.

Pittman, K. (1986). *Preventing adolescent pregnancy: What schools can do.* Washington, DC: Children's Defense Fund.

Resnick, M., Harris, L., & Blum, R. (1993). The impact of caring and connectedness on adolescent health and well-being. *Journal of Paediatrics and Child Health, 29*(Suppl. 1), S3-S9.

Ringwalt, C., Greene, S., Ennett, S., Iachan, R., Clayton, R., & Leukefeld, C. (1994). *Past and future directions of the D.A.R.E. program: An evaluation review.* Research Triangle Park, NC: Research Triangle Institute.

Roth, S. (1995, March). *Teenage motherhood and high school dropouts: The role of school experiences.* Paper prepared for poster at the annual meeting of the American Educational Research Association, San Francisco.

Rumberger, R. W. (in press). Dropping out of middle school: A multilevel analysis of students and schools. *American Educational Research Journal.*

Shedler, J., & Block, B. (1990). Adolescent drug use and psychological health: A longitudinal inquiry. *American Psychologist, 45,* 612-630.

U.S. Bureau of the Census. (1993, October). *School enrollment: Social and economic characteristics of students* (Current Population Reports, Series P-20, No. 479). Washington, DC: U.S. Government Printing Office.

U.S. Department of Health and Human Services, Public Health Service. (1994). Current trends. *Morbidity and Mortality Weekly Report, 43*(9), 129-132.

U.S. Department of Health and Human Services, Public Health Service. (1995). *Healthy people 2000: Midcourse review and 1995 revisions.* Washington, DC: U.S. Government Printing Office.

U.S. Department of Justice. (1994). *OJJDP update on statistics: Offenders in juvenile court* (Juvenile Justice Bulletin). Washington, DC: Office of Juvenile Justice and Delinquency Programs.

Vanderschmidt, H. F., Lang, J. M., Knight-Williams, V., & Vanderschmidt, G. F. (1993). Risks among inner-city young teens: The prevalence of sexual activity, violence, drugs, and smoking. *Journal of Adolescent Health, 14,* 282-288.

Werner, E., & Smith, R. (1982). *Vulnerable but invincible: A longitudinal study of resilient children and youth.* New York: McGraw-Hill.

• *CHAPTER 3* •

School-Based Drug Abuse Prevention Strategies: From Research to Policy and Practice

LINDA DUSENBURY
MATHEA FALCO

This chapter reviews school-based drug abuse prevention and proposes new directions for prevention research that will move toward the goals of *Healthy People 2000* (U.S. Department of Health and Human Services, Public Health Service [DHHS], 1991, 1995). Drawing on the most current research, we identify key ingredients of successful prevention programs, analyze the 46 most widely available drug abuse prevention curricula for relative effectiveness, and suggest various ways to improve program design and implementation. We conclude with policy recommendations for *Healthy People 2010* designed to make effective prevention an integral part of adolescent education.

Healthy People 2000 Objectives for Youth

The *Healthy People 2000* (DHHS, 1991) objectives include prevention of tobacco, alcohol, and drug use as well as treatment, reduction of alcohol-related traffic accidents, and increased regulation of tobacco and alcohol advertising. Specific objectives targeting youth include the following:

3.5. Reduce the initiation of cigarette smoking by children and youth so that no more than 15% have become regular cigarette smokers by age 20.

3.9. Reduce smokeless tobacco use by males aged 12 through 24 to a prevalence of no more than 4%.

4.1b. Reduce deaths among people aged 15 to 24 caused by alcohol-related motor vehicle crashes to no more than 18 per 100,000.

4.5. Increase by at least 1 year the average age of first use of cigarettes, alcohol, and marijuana for ages 12 through 17 (Baseline: Age 11.6 for cigarettes, age 13.1 for alcohol, and age 13.4 for marijuana in 1988).

4.6. Reduce the proportion of young people who have used alcohol, marijuana, and cocaine in the past month as follows:

Substance/Age	*Baseline 1988*	*Target 2000*
Alcohol/ages 12-17	25.2%	12.6%
Alcohol/ages 18-20	57.9%	29.0%
Marijuana/ages 12-17	6.4%	3.2%
Marijuana/ages 18-25	15.5%	7.8%
Cocaine/ages 12-17	1.1%	0.6%
Cocaine/ages 18-25	4.5%	2.3%

4.7. Reduce the proportion of high school seniors and college students engaging in recent occasions of heavy drinking of alcoholic beverages to no more than 28% of high school seniors and 32% of college students.

4.8. Reduce alcohol consumption by people aged 14 and older to an annual average of no more than 2 gallons of ethanol per person.

4.9. Increase the proportion of high school seniors who perceive social disapproval associated with the heavy use of alcohol, occasional use of marijuana, and experimentation with cocaine, as follows:

Behavior	*Baseline 1989*	*Target 2000*
Heavy use of alcohol	56.4%	70%
Occasional use of marijuana	71.1%	85%
Trying cocaine once or twice	88.9%	95%

4.10. Increase the proportion of high school seniors who associated risk of physical or psychological harm with the heavy use of alcohol, regular use of marijuana, and experimentation with cocaine, as follows:

Behavior	*Baseline 1989*	*Target 2000*
Heavy use alcohol	44.0%	70%
Regular use of marijuana	77.5%	90%
Trying cocaine once or twice	54.9%	80%

4.11. Reduce to no more than 3% the proportion of male high school seniors who use anabolic steroids. (pp. 144-147, 164-175)

A primary service objective of *Healthy People 2000* relating to youth is to provide children with tobacco, alcohol, and drug prevention curricula as part of quality school comprehensive health education. Comprehensive health education is a broad spectrum approach that provides a variety of school-based programs and services to promote general competence as well as mental, physical, and social health (Weissberg & Elias, 1993).

There are sound empirical reasons for providing drug abuse prevention as part of a comprehensive approach to health education as opposed to discrete programs that focus on a single risk behavior (e.g., smoking *or* drug use *or* premature sexual behavior). Strong intercorrelations have been observed for different types of substance use (e.g., smoking, drinking, and drug use) as well as between different types of health-compromising behaviors (e.g., substance use and premature sexual behavior). In addition, these behaviors have been observed to correlate with psychosocial risk factors, which include environmental as well as personality variables, suggesting a common underlying cause (Jessor & Jessor, 1977). Finally, these behaviors appear to be moderated by common prevention strategies (resistance skills training).

There are also good policy reasons for providing drug abuse prevention as part of comprehensive health education. Increasing demands on class time make it difficult for teachers to add discrete programs to their class time. Discrete programs also are less likely than comprehensive programs to be maintained by a school (Johnson, MacKinnon, & Pentz, 1996).

Progress Toward Reaching *Healthy People 2000* Goals for Youth

A major accomplishment noted in the midcourse review was that declining death rates among 15- to 24-year-olds in alcohol-related traffic fatalities had already reached the *Healthy People 2000* objectives (Fleming, 1996). This objective therefore was revised to make it more challenging.

The National Household Survey on Drug Abuse (DHHS, 1993) suggests that there may have been some progress toward meeting the goals concerning average age of initiation for marijuana, although retrospective data from the Monitoring the Future Study (National Institute on Drug Abuse [NIDA], 1991-1996) are not consistent with this finding. According to the National Household Survey, the average age of initiation for marijuana has increased since 1988, with the most dramatic increase occurring between 1992 and 1993; at 13.9 years in 1993, it was halfway to the targeted 2000 objectives of 14.4 years. In contrast, according to the Monitoring the Future Survey, in 1995, 5.3% of 8th graders reported that they had used marijuana by the 6th grade, compared with 2.4% of 10th graders.

Unfortunately, little progress has been made toward increasing the average age of initiation for tobacco use or alcohol use, which remain well below their 2000 targets (Fleming, 1996). Initiation of tobacco use has remained fairly stable in the National Household Survey at around 11.7 years since 1988 (it was 11.6 in 1988). The average age of initiation for alcohol use, 12.9 in 1993, was slightly lower than the 13.1 years it was in 1988.

Considerable progress has been made in recent years toward some of the other objectives (for example, expanding no-smoking rules within the workplace). The National Household surveys (DHHS, 1993) and Monitoring the Future surveys (Johnston, O'Malley, & Bachman, 1995), however, reveal disturbing trends in adolescent alcohol, tobacco, and drug use, which have been increasing rapidly since 1992. During the same period, beliefs about the risks and disapproval of drug use (which have been shown to be important inhibitors of use) have declined.

The most recent Monitoring the Future survey (NIDA, 1996) revealed that in 1996, cigarette smoking rose for the 5th year in a row for 8th and 10th graders, and for the 4th year in a row for high school seniors. Since 1991, the proportion of 8th and 10th graders who reported smoking in the past month increased by up to 50% (from 14% to 21% for 8th graders, and from 21% to 30% for 10th graders). Among high school seniors, the proportion of students reporting smoking in the past month increased more than one fifth (from 28% to 34%). Between 1993 and 1995, the proportion of 10th and 12th graders perceiving smoking as harmful has declined significantly (from 61% to 57% among 10th graders, and from 70% to 66% among 12th graders).

Since 1991, the rate of illicit drug use also has increased among 8th, 10th and 12th graders. From 1991 to 1996, the proportion of 8th graders who had used any illicit drug in the past month increased from 5.7% to 14.6%. During the same period, monthly illicit drug use by 10th graders increased from 11.6% to 23.2%, and by 12th graders from 16.4% to 24.6%. Between 1991 and 1996, monthly marijuana use has more than tripled among 8th graders (from 3.2% to 11.3%), more than doubled for 10th graders (from 8.7% to 20.4%) and increased by more than half for 12th graders (from 13.8% to 21.9%).

The rate of alcohol use has tended to be more stable in the past few years, although it remains unacceptably high. In 1996, 26% of 8th graders reported that they have had a drink in the past month, compared with 40% of 10th graders and 51% of seniors. In 1995, the rate of binge drinking (five or more drinks in a row within the past 2 weeks) was 15% for 8th graders, 24% for 10th graders, and 30% for 12th graders.

Data in 1995 show that although the majority of young people still disapprove of using illicit drugs, the intensity of disapproval has grown weaker. For example, disapproval of trying marijuana declined significantly for 8th and 10th graders between 1991 and 1995 (from 85% to 71% among 8th graders and from 75% to 60% among 10th graders).

The proportion of students seeing drug use (including use of marijuana and cocaine) as dangerous has also declined since 1991 for 8th, 10th, and 12th graders. Between 1991 and 1995, there were significant declines in perceived harmfulness of trying marijuana (from 40% to 29% among 8th graders, from 30% to 22% among 10th graders, and from 27% to 16% among 12th graders) and in perceived harmfulness of trying cocaine (from 56% to 45% among 8th graders and from 59% to 54% among 10th graders).

Observed increases in tobacco, alcohol, and drug use across age and ethnic groups are likely the result of influences that extend across U.S. society (NIDA, 1995, 1996). Why have things gotten worse recently? A major influence operating in recent years is waning public and political attention to the problem of drugs, which has resulted in less-balanced messages about alcohol, tobacco, and drugs in the media. Specifically, while the tobacco and alcohol industries spend billions of dollars each year promoting the use of their products with advertising increasingly directed toward young people, and while movies and music videos glamorize the use of alcohol, tobacco, and other drugs, there has been less political attention to and less media coverage of the negative consequences of tobacco, alcohol, and drug use. Waning public and political attention are likely to translate into less attention from parents, who may be less likely today to speak to their children about alcohol, tobacco, and drugs than they were 10 years ago.

Current Prevention Research

A comprehensive review of the published research on school-based drug abuse prevention from 1989 to 1994 provided the basis for identifying key elements in effective drug abuse prevention curricula (Dusenbury & Falco, 1995). In addition to this comprehensive review, wide-ranging interviews were conducted with the following leading prevention experts during 1994.

Dr. Gilbert J. Botvin, Director of the Institute of Prevention Research, Cornell University Medical College

Dr. Richard Clayton, Director of the Center for Prevention Research, University of Kentucky

Dr. Phyllis Ellickson, Senior Behavioral Scientist and Resident Scholar at RAND

Dr. Susan Ennett, Research Health Analyst at the Center for Social Research and Policy Analysis at the Research Triangle Institute

Dr. Brian Flay, Director of the Prevention Research Center at the University of Illinois at Chicago

Dr. William B. Hansen, Associate Professor at Bowman Gray Medical College

Dr. J. David Hawkins, Director of the Social Development Research Group at the University of Washington

Dr. Karol Kumpfer, Associate Professor in the Department of Health Education at the University of Utah

Dr. Joel Moskowitz, Associate Director of the Center for Family and Community Health at the University of California at Berkeley

Dr. Mary Ann Pentz, Associate Professor of Research, Institute for Health Promotion and Disease Prevention Research at the University of Southern California

Dr. Cheryl Perry, Professor in the Division of Epidemiology, School of Public Health at the University of Minnesota

Dr. Christopher Ringwalt, Research Health Analyst at the Center for Social Research and Policy Analysis at the Research Triangle Institute

Dr. Steven Schinke, Professor at the School of Social Work, Columbia University

Dr. Nancy Tobler, Research Associate Professor, School of Social Welfare, State University of New York in Albany

Dr. Roger Weissberg, Professor in the Department of Psychology at the University of Illinois at Chicago

The lengthy telephone interviews (30 to 60 minutes) were organized around two basic questions: "What do you think we currently know about what works in drug abuse prevention?" and "What would you say we know about the effective ingredients of drug abuse prevention programs?" Experts also were asked specific questions relating to their own research.

General Findings

Several recent literature reviews (Botvin & Botvin, 1992; Hansen, 1992, 1993; Mrazek & Haggerty, 1994; Perry & Kelder, 1992) as well as a series of meta-analyses (Bangert-Drowns, 1988; Bruvold, 1990, 1993; Bruvold & Rundall, 1988; Hansen, Rose, & Dryfoos, 1993; Rundall & Bruvold, 1988; Tobler, 1992, 1994, in press) conclude that certain types of school-based programs can achieve measurable reductions in adolescent drug use. There is also general agreement that some prevention programs are not effective, particularly those designed to increase knowledge about drugs rather than to change behavior (Botvin & Botvin, 1992).

Evaluations of drug abuse prevention programs have become increasingly rigorous in the past decade, with larger samples, longer follow-up periods, more complex research designs, and more thorough data analyses, as well as greater concern for implementation fidelity and the accuracy of assessment measures. Recently published studies are impressive in their size, scope, and methodological sophistication and for the replicability and consistency of findings across different research groups (Botvin, Baker, Dusenbury, Botvin, & Diaz, 1995; Botvin, Baker, Dusenbury, Tortu, & Botvin, 1990; Ellickson & Bell, 1990; Pentz et al., 1989; Pentz et al., 1990; Shope, Kloska, Dielman, & Maharg, 1994). Most important, these studies show that measurable reductions in adolescent drug, alcohol, and tobacco use can be sustained through high school and into young adulthood.

Specifically, M. A. Pentz (personal communication, 1994) and her colleagues at the University of Southern California and Botvin et al. (1995) at Cornell University Medical College have found persistence of behavioral effects 6 years after program administration. Although previous studies showed reductions in initial smoking, drinking, and marijuana use, these long-term follow-ups demonstrate an impact on other illicit drug use, as well. Pentz reports effects on stimulant use, including cocaine, whereas Botvin found effects on use of hashish, heroin, PCP, and inhalants, but not cocaine.

In addition, the follow-up by M. A. Pentz (personal communication, 1994) and her colleagues found less need for drug treatment among young adults who had participated in the drug abuse prevention program during junior high. G. J. Botvin (personal communication, 1994) and his colleagues found a reduction in risky driving among young people 6 years after participating in the drug abuse prevention program.

Key Elements of Effective Prevention Curricula

The research literature, as well as expert opinion, suggests that the following elements are critical for effective drug prevention curricula (Dusenbury & Falco, 1995).

1. *Programs should reflect proved prevention theory and research.* At present, the most effective curricula are based on three major theoretical approaches: social learning theory (Bandura, 1977), normative expectancy theory (Ajzen & Fishbein, 1980), and adolescent problem behavior theory (Jessor & Jessor, 1977), briefly described below.

A. *Social learning theory.* Behavior is generally learned from observing important role models, particularly as they are rewarded for their actions. Adolescents look to their friends, older peers, and media figures. Curricula based largely on this learning theory are *social resistance skills training programs* (Botvin & Botvin, 1992; Hansen, 1992, 1993; Mrazek & Haggerty, 1994; Perry & Kelder, 1992; Tobler, 1992, 1994, in press) that help young teens recognize influences to use drugs and teach them how to resist while still maintaining their friendships.

B. *Normative expectancy theory.* Normative expectancy theory recognizes the power perceptions about the actions and opinions of others have in shaping behavior. The programs based on normative expectancy theory are called *normative education.* Social resistance skills training programs usually include normative education, which teaches adolescents that drug use is not the norm. Normative education includes activities designed to correct overestimates about the prevalence of smoking, drinking, and drug use and/or activities designed to show adolescents that most peers and adults do not think tobacco, alcohol, and drug use is cool. In an experimental manipulation, Hansen and Graham (1991) found that normative education was a critical ingredient in reducing drug use. Some experts (e.g., W. B. Hansen, personal communication, 1994; J. D. Hawkins, personal communication, 1994) are convinced that normative education is essential to the long-term success of drug abuse prevention programs. G. J. Botvin (personal communication, 1994) and his colleagues, however, found that although normative education is important to drug prevention, it is not sufficient to reduce drug use and that resistance skills training continues to be necessary.

C. *Adolescent problem behavior theory.* Adolescent problem behavior theory views problem behaviors such as drug use, violence, and premature sexual activity as useful or functional to the adolescent. These behaviors serve a perceived purpose; adolescents may believe these behaviors will help them achieve personal goals such as gaining admission to a peer group, demonstrating independence from parents, or coping with boredom, stress, anxiety, or hopelessness. Programs based on adolescent problem behavior theory provide adolescents with *broader personal and social skills training.* They promote self-esteem and teach adolescents how to set and achieve realistic goals, make competent decisions, cope with stress and anxiety, communicate effectively, make friends, and be assertive. Social resistance skills training and normative education are often done within the context of broader personal and social skills training, and there is evidence that these broader-based programs produce slightly larger reductions in drug use than social resistance training alone (Tobler, in press).

2. *Programs should provide developmentally appropriate information about tobacco, alcohol, and drugs.* Children and adolescents are more interested in concrete information and here-and-now experience than they are in information about possibilities in the far-off future (Mussen, Conger, & Kagan, 1979). Effective curricula contain information about drugs that is accurate and relevant—information that emphasizes short-term and negative social consequences of use. Extensive information about the types and effects of drugs is not necessary and may be counterproductive (G. J. Botvin, personal communication, 1994). Effective prevention programs also recognize the importance of peers and acceptance by peers during adolescence (Lerner, Petersen, & Brooks-Gunn, 1991) and provide adolescents with training in how to make independent decisions and resist peer pressure while maintaining friendships.

3. *Interactive teaching techniques are most effective at promoting skill development.* Social resistance skills approaches and broader personal and social skills training rely on interactive teaching techniques such as discussions, small-group activities, and role playing; unlike more didactic techniques such as lecture, interactive techniques are designed to promote active participation of students

(Bosworth & Sailes, 1993; Tobler, in press). Unfortunately, some teachers are less comfortable using interactive teaching techniques (Bosworth & Sailes, 1993), and these teachers will be less likely to effectively implement promising prevention programs.

4. *Curricula should provide adequate coverage and sufficient follow-up.* Many drug abuse prevention programs tend to be short, with fewer than 10 sessions in the first year and fewer than 5 sessions in the second year. As B. Flay (personal communication, 1994) observed, "Realistically, the interventions we are doing are puny compared to the myriad of other influences kids are exposed to that are ongoing." The brevity of drug abuse prevention interventions may help explain recent findings that prevention effects decay through time (e.g., Bell, Ellickson, & Harrison, 1993). Given the brevity of interventions, none of the experts interviewed were surprised that effects would decay (e.g., B. Flay, personal communication, 1994; J. Moskowitz, personal communication, 1994). A critical element of effective prevention programming, then, is sufficient and continued follow-up.

5. *Programs should be culturally sensitive.* To be successful, drug abuse prevention strategies must be sensitive to the ethnic and cultural backgrounds of the youth they target. Studies by Botvin and his colleagues (Botvin, Batson, et al., 1989; Botvin, Dusenbury, Baker, James-Ortiz, & Kerner, 1989; Botvin, Schinke, Epstein, & Diaz, 1994; Botvin, Schinke, Epstein, Diaz, & Botvin, 1995) suggest that broader-based personal and social training approaches that include social resistance skills training can be adapted to make them more sensitive and appropriate to the experience of African American and Latino youth.

6. *Programs should provide teacher training and support.* Results from a series of studies (Botvin, Baker, Dusenbury, et al., 1990; Ross, Luepker, Nelson, Saavedra, & Hubbard, 1991; Smith, McCormick, Steckler, & McLeroy, 1993) reveal that drug prevention programs are most successful when teachers receive training and support from program developers or prevention experts. Much research remains to be done to determine the optimal length of teacher training, the most effective teacher training strategies, and

the most critical content areas to be covered in teacher training (e.g., the theory behind a prevention program, evaluation studies concerning prevention programs, classroom management issues, and guidelines for using a particular curriculum). A major emphasis of teacher training, however, should be interactive teaching techniques, given their apparent importance in promising prevention curricula (N. Tobler, personal communication, 1995). To help teachers become familiar with and comfortable using interactive teaching techniques, teacher trainers should model these behaviors during training sessions. In addition, teachers should be given ample opportunity to practice these new skills, as well as feedback and reinforcement during practice sessions. Ideally, initial training session should be followed by booster sessions.

7. *Additional components may enhance program effectiveness.* Although much research remains to be done, components designed for the family, the community, the media, and special populations are expected to enhance the effectiveness of drug abuse prevention. For example, large projects by three different research groups (Hawkins, Catalano, & Kent, 1991; Pentz et al., 1989; Pentz et al., 1990; Perry, Kelder, Murray, & Klepp, 1992; Perry et al., 1993) suggest that broadening school-based approaches to include family, community, and the media may be valuable. A definitive study of the relative contribution of additional components to the efficacy of drug abuse prevention curricula, however, has yet to be done. Indeed, the need for research on this issue was highlighted in *Healthy People 2000* (DHHS, 1991), which included a recommendation to test the effectiveness of combined interventions (e.g., school-based programs and mass media) on smoking initiation and determine which intervention elements are effective.

8. *Programs should demonstrate their effects in rigorous evaluation.* An important question for any drug abuse prevention curriculum is whether it can be demonstrated to have an impact on drug use behavior. The quality of evaluation studies must be assessed, as well, to know how confident one can be in the findings. At a minimum, evaluations should include pretest-posttest, control group design, and outcome measures of drug, alcohol, and tobacco use behavior. In addition, to confirm that research studies do not

have serious flaws, they should be published in peer-reviewed journals.

State of the Art in Practice

We recently completed a guide to drug abuse prevention curricula called *Making the Grade* (Drug Strategies, 1996). This guide reviews nationally available classroom-based drug abuse prevention programs, including curriculum materials and research reports of their evaluation, to assist educators in choosing programs that are most likely to be effective and appropriate for their students.

A total of 47 school-based curricula were identified (one program, Me-Me, declined to participate). Of these, 46 were assessed. One program (BABES) did not provide sufficient curriculum material for a complete assessment. See Table 3.1 for a list of these programs.

Of the 46 curricula, 14 are comprehensive health education programs that cover many of the following topics *in addition to drug prevention:* growth and development, disease prevention, nutrition, fitness, dental health, sexuality, AIDS, safety and injury prevention, child abuse, environmental concerns, and consumer health. Because a *Healthy People 2000* goal is to provide prevention education to students, preferably through quality comprehensive health education, these programs are particularly important. Unfortunately, only 3 of the 14 comprehensive curricula have been carefully evaluated. Indeed, a gap continues between the types of comprehensive health education educators are encouraged by policymakers to adopt and the state-of-the-art programs of limited scope and duration that have been evaluated (Weissberg & Elias, 1993).

Of the 46 programs reviewed, 43 include social resistance skills training, and 36 provide training in broader personal and social skills. Despite the importance of normative education, just over half (24) of the programs had well-developed normative education activities.

Most drug abuse prevention curricula currently available have not been evaluated in published, pretest-posttest control group design studies with measures of substance use behavior. Only 10 programs (22%) have been rigorously evaluated using sound research designs. On the basis of these evaluations, eight promising

Table 3.1 Listing of Drug Abuse Prevention Curricula Currently Available

	Grade Level	*Social Resistance Skills Training*	*Broader Personal and Social Skills*	*Normative Education*	*Adequate Evaluation*
Comprehensive Health Programs					
Actions for Health	K-6	X	X		
Comprehensive Health	5-9	X	X	X	
Discover: Decisions for Health	7-12	X	X		
Entering Adulthood	9-12	X	X		
Great Body Shop	K-6	X	X		
Growing Healthy	K-6	X	X		X
Health Skills for Life	K-12	X	X		
Know Your Body	K-6	X	X	X	X
Michigan Model	K-8	X	X	X	
Quest: Skills for Growing	K-5	X	X		
Quest: Skills for Adolescence	6-8	X	X	X	
Quest: Skills for Action	9-12	X	X	X	
Science for Life and Living	K-6	X	X		
Teenage Health Teaching Modules	6-12	X	X	X	X
K-12 Programs					
BABES	P-12	*	*	*	
Choosing for Yourself II	K-12	X	X		
DARE	K-12	X	X	X	X*
Discover Skills for Life	K-12	X	X	X	
Here's Looking at You, 2000	K-12	X	X	X	
Learning About Alcohol and Other Drugs	K-12	X	X	X	
Learning to Live Drug Free	K-12	X	X		
Project Oz	K-12	X	X	X	
That's Life	K-10	X	X		

Elementary and Middle School Programs					
CounterAct	4, 5, or 6	X			
Facts, Feelings, Family and Friends	K-6	X	X	X	
Growing Up Strong	P-6	X	X		
Growing Up Well	K-8	X	X		
I'm Special	3 or 4		X		
McGruff	P-6	X			
Paper People	P-3	X	X		
Positive Action	K-8	X	X	X	
Project Charlie	K-6	X	X		
Starting Early	K-6	X	X		
Middle and High School Programs					
Al-Co-Hol	7-9				
Alcohol Misuse Prevention Program	6-8	X		X	X
Drug Proof	6-8	X	X		
From Peer Pressure to Peer Support	7-12	X	X	X	
Healthy for Life	6-8	X	X	X	
Life Skills Training	6-8 or 7-9	X	X	X	X
Ombudsman	5-9	X	X		
Project Alert	6, 7 or 7, 8	X		X	X*
Project All-Stars	6, 7			X	
Project Northland	6-8	X		X	X
Setting Norms for Refusal	6, 7, or 8	X		X	
Social Competence Promotion Program	5, 6, or 7	X	X	X	X
STAR	5-8	X		X	X
Talking With Your Students About Alcohol	5-12	X		X	

* Insufficient curriculum materials provided to assess program content.
X* Effects disappear over time.

curricula include the Alcohol Misuse Prevention Program (Dielman, Kloska, Leech, Schulenberg, & Shope, 1992; Dielman, Shope, Leech, & Butchart, 1989; Shope, Dielman, Butchart, Campanelli, & Kloska, 1992), Growing Healthy (Connell & Turner, 1985; Connell, Turner, & Mason, 1985), Know Your Body (Walter, Vaughan, & Wynder, 1989), Life Skills Training (Botvin, Baker, Dusenbury, et al., 1990; Botvin, Baker, Filazzola, & Botvin, 1990; Botvin, Batson, et al., 1989; Botvin, Dusenbury, et al., 1992; Botvin et al., 1994; Botvin, Schinke, et al., 1995), Project Northland (Perry et al., 1996), the Social Competence Promotion Program (Caplan et al., 1992), STAR (Johnson et al., 1990; Pentz et al., 1989), and the Teenage Health Teaching Modules (Errecart et al., 1991). Growing Healthy, Know Your Body, and Teenage Health Teaching Modules are comprehensive health education programs. In addition, two programs have been rigorously evaluated, although long-term studies suggest that effects of these programs disappear over time: DARE (Clayton, Cattarello, & Walden, 1991; Ennett, Rosenbaum, et al., 1994; Harmon, 1993; Ringwalt, Ennett, & Holt, 1991) and Project Alert (Bell et al., 1993; Ellickson & Bell, 1990; Ellickson, Bell, & McGuigan, 1993). Results of the evaluations of these programs are summarized below.

These summaries report the number of studies that have evaluated each program, the number of students included in each evaluation, and outcome results in tobacco, alcohol, and drug use behavior. We have elected, where possible, to present results in percentage reductions of substance use. There is no standard way of presenting data in drug abuse prevention evaluations. Although it might be more appropriate to report an effect size for each study because an effect size standardizes the data, researchers do not always report the standard deviation of the control group, making it impossible to calculate effect sizes for every study. Moreover, because studies are often 5 or more years old, it is not an easy matter for many researchers to locate that information when asked.

The summaries also report the proportion of minority youth in each sample because relatively few studies have included significant samples of minority youth. Given space limitations, the summaries do not report findings relating to attitudes, intentions, other mediating variables, or implementation fidelity. For information concerning these issues, or for additional detail, the reader is referred to the original studies cited below.

Alcohol Misuse Prevention Project

There have been two separate studies of two versions of the Alcohol Misuse Prevention Program (Dielman et al., 1992; Dielman et al., 1989; Shope et al., 1992), which focuses on alcohol prevention; the strongest and most complete version is for students in grades 6 to 8. Evaluation of that program showed that among 121 high-risk sixth grade students (of 1,725 students in sample) who were already drinking at pretest (without parental supervision), there were significant reductions in misuse of alcohol. There were inconsistent results for students who had not been drinking at pretest. Minority students composed 5% of the sample (2% Black, 3% other ethnic group).

DARE

There have been four published studies of DARE (Clayton et al., 1991; Ennett, Rosenbaum, et al., 1994; Harmon, 1993; Ringwalt et al., 1991), the most widely used drug prevention approach in the United States. DARE is a K-12 program with a 17-session core curriculum in the fifth or sixth grade. DARE is implemented by uniformed police officers. Some studies show posttest reductions in tobacco, alcohol, and drug use that disappear shortly after the initial posttest. Other studies show no reductions in use. One of the most recent studies (Ennett, Rosenbaum, et al., 1994), a 2-year follow-up with 1,334 fifth and sixth graders, found 50% reduction in tobacco use for all students and 50% reductions in alcohol use for rural students at posttest, but effects disappeared by 1-year follow-up. Drug use was not measured. Minority students composed 46% of the sample of this study (22% Black, 9% Hispanic, 15% other ethnic group). Earlier studies also included substantial minority samples.

A major reason DARE may not have shown more consistent or lasting effects is that the core curriculum of DARE is usually delivered in fifth grade, when base rates of tobacco, alcohol, and drug use are low and effects hard to find. In addition, the DARE core curriculum has been revised to address criticisms concerning its content but has not yet been evaluated.

Growing Healthy

There has been one published evaluation study of Growing Healthy (Connell & Turner, 1985; Connell et al., 1985), a comprehensive health program consisting of 40 or more sessions per year for grades K-6. Approximately 30,000 fourth- to seventh-grade students were in the 2-year study, which looked at smoking behavior as an outcome. The program reduced smoking by 29% by ninth grade. Minority students composed 19% of the sample (15% Black, 2% Hispanic, 2% other ethnic group).

Know Your Body

There has been one published evaluation study of Know Your Body (Walter et al., 1989), a comprehensive health program with an average of 60 sessions per year for grades K-6. The sample included 1,105 fourth-grade students, who were followed 6 years. Evaluation results revealed smoking reductions of 73.3% at follow-up in ninth grade. There were greater reductions for males. No data were collected on alcohol or drugs. Minority students composed 19% of the sample (14% Black, 2% Hispanic, 5% other ethnic group).

Life Skills Training (LST)

The LST program, a broader personal and social skills training program for middle school students, designed to prevent tobacco, alcohol, and drug use, has been evaluated in 10 published studies (Botvin, Baker, Botvin, Filazzola, & Millman, 1984; Botvin, Baker, et al., 1995; Botvin, Baker, Dusenbury, et al., 1990; Botvin, Baker, Filazzola, & Botvin, 1990; Botvin, Batson, et al., 1989; Botvin, Dusenbury, et al., 1989; Botvin, Dusenbury, et al., 1992; Botvin & Eng, 1982; Botvin, Renick, & Baker, 1983; Botvin et al., 1994; Botvin, Schinke, et al., 1995). These studies have shown reductions of up to 50% to 75% in tobacco, alcohol, or marijuana use at seventh-grade posttest. A recent 6-year follow-up of 4,466 seventh-grade students showed that results erode only slightly by the end of high school, with 44% reductions in tobacco, alcohol, *or* marijuana use, and 66% reductions in use of all three: tobacco, alcohol, *and* marijuana use. Minority students composed at least 75% of the sample in 4 of 10 separate studies; in each of these 4 studies, there was a combination of Blacks (11% to 87%) and Hispanics (10% to 74%).

Project Alert

There has been one published, 6-year evaluation of Project Alert (Bell et al., 1993; Ellickson & Bell, 1990; Ellickson et al., 1993), a social resistance skills training program for students in grades 6 and 7 or 7 and 8. Project Alert consists of 11 sessions in the first year and 3 in the second. There were 3,852 seventh-grade students in the evaluation study sample. Results showed immediate posttest reductions in drinking of up to 50%. In the second year of the study (in the 8th grade), there were declines in marijuana use of 33% to 60% and smoking reductions of 17% to 55%. All positive effects disappeared after 15 months. In addition, there were some negative effects for high-risk youth. Minority students composed 30% of the sample (10% Asian, 9% Hispanic, 8% Black, 3% other ethnic group).

Project Northland

There has been one published 3-year evaluation study of Project Northland (Perry et al., 1996), a social resistance skills training approach to alcohol prevention. Project Northland consists of eight sessions per year for grades 6 through 8. There were 1,901 sixth-grade students in the evaluation study sample. The program reduced the use of both alcohol and tobacco in the past month by 27% for all students. Those who did not use alcohol before the program showed declines of 50% in marijuana use and 37% in tobacco use. Minority students composed 5% of the sample (4% Native American, 1% other ethnic group).

Social Competence Promotion Program

There has been one published pretest-posttest study of the Social Competence Promotion Program, a 27-session social problem-solving program with a 9-session drug abuse prevention module (Caplan et al., 1992). A total of 282 sixth- and seventh-grade students were in the evaluation sample. At posttest, there were reductions in frequent heavy alcohol use. Minority students composed 73% of the sample (66% Black, 6% Hispanic, 1% other ethnic group).

STAR

There has been one published 3-year study of Project STAR (Pentz et al., 1989; Pentz et al., 1990), an 18-session social resistance skills training approach for students in grades 5 through 8. There were 4,978 students in the evaluation study sample. Drinking, smoking, and marijuana use dropped 30% at 1-year follow-up; results persisted through the 3 years of the study. The evaluation study involved a multicomponent intervention (school curriculum, family program, and media spots), but variables were not manipulated to determine the contribution of each program component to overall effectiveness. The school-based program, however, did appear critical to success. Minority students composed 22% of the sample (17% Black, 2% Hispanic, 1% Asian, 2% other ethnic group).

Teenage Health Teaching Modules

There has been one published evaluation study of Teenage Health Teaching Modules (Errecart et al., 1991), a comprehensive health program with 40 to 70 sessions per year for grades 7 through 12. The evaluation, which included 4,806 junior and senior high school students in the sample, did not include follow-up beyond the posttest. Evaluation results revealed moderate reductions in alcohol, tobacco, and illegal drug use for senior high students. Minority students composed 26% of the sample (12% Hispanic, 10% Black, 3% Asian, 1% Native American).

Conclusion

On the basis of these evaluations, it appears that eight programs have been effective at reducing drug use, in at least some studies. At least one of the programs (LST) reviewed above has been shown in published reports to have effects into young adulthood. Six of these programs have been shown to have effects lasting for at least a year after the pretest. Two other programs have not been evaluated beyond the posttest, so it is impossible to know whether their effectiveness will be lasting. In addition, one program (Project Alert) produced declines in drug abuse early on, but these effects diminished and disappeared through time. This does not necessarily mean that this program might not make an important contribution to drug abuse prevention, if done within the context of continuing prevention efforts. As discussed earlier, prevention programming must have adequate coverage and sufficient follow-up, which may not have been true for Project Alert and DARE. In addition, as mentioned above, in the case of DARE, the core curriculum takes place in the fifth grade, when the rate of substance use may well be too low to show effects.

Dissemination of the Most Promising Approaches

Despite considerable agreement among experts and in the literature about the critical ingredients of promising prevention curricula, most of the money spent in this country on drug education has not been spent on what evaluation studies suggest are the most promising programs. DARE, QUEST, and Here's Looking at You, 2000 are the three most widely used programs (Hansen et al., 1993). Other aggressively marketed programs include BABES, Project Charlie, Ombudsman, and Project Adventure. Of the aggressively marketed curricula, only DARE has been adequately evaluated. Although DARE has been extremely successful at diffusion and dissemination (R. Clayton, personal communication, 1994), evaluations reviewed above, as well as a recent meta-analysis (Ennett, Tobler, Ringwalt, & Flewelling, 1994), suggest that DARE is not consistently effective at reducing substance use behavior (Ennett, Rosenbaum, et al., 1994; Ennett, Tobler, et al., 1994; Ringwalt et al., 1991; Ringwalt et al., 1994).

Why are the most promising programs not more widely used? A key reason is that schools have received little guidance about how to select the most effective prevention program. Indeed, although there is a strong consensus among researchers about the types of prevention approaches that work, this information is often buried in highly technical journals and is not readily available beyond the research community.

Another major reason that the most promising programs have not been more widely disseminated is that they were usually developed by researchers, who have not felt that it was appropriate in their role as evaluators of these programs to also promote them. Even when researchers may be motivated to disseminate their programs, they often lack necessary resources. In addition, when curricula are developed as part of research projects, researchers and universities both may claim an interest in these programs. Resolving these issues can delay dissemination indefinitely. Although tremendous energy and resources have gone into the development and evaluation of prevention programs, dissemination of these same programs has been largely neglected (Rohrbach, D'Onofrio, Backer, & Montgomery, 1996).

Policy Recommendations for *Healthy People 2010*

Research in drug abuse prevention is quite impressive, with a number of large field trials showing that prevention can have lasting effects. We now know quite a lot about what works in drug abuse prevention. *We therefore recommend that schools adopt curricula that include the key elements of effective drug abuse prevention; ideally, they should adopt curricula that have been rigorously evaluated.* Three major goals are related to this recommendation:

1. *All drug prevention curricula should be assessed to determine the extent to which each addresses the key elements of effective prevention, as in the guide* Making the Grade *(Drug Strategies, 1996).* Minimum criteria that should be considered when choosing a program include the following:

- Drug abuse prevention should provide students with social resistance skills training.
- Programs must also provide students with accurate information about drug-using norms. Almost half the programs we reviewed lacked a good normative education component. We encourage curriculum developers to address this weakness.
- Programs should include developmentally appropriate information about drugs.
- Interactive techniques promote the development of skills and are an important ingredient in drug abuse prevention.

- Programs should provide teachers with training and support. Because some teachers are less comfortable using interactive techniques than using didactic techniques, training in this area will be especially important.
- Programs should show a sensitivity to the culture(s) of students in the classroom. In our multiethnic society, virtually every classroom is a unique mix of ethnic and economic backgrounds. It is impossible for a nationally available curriculum to make itself culturally sensitive to every possible classroom. There are, however, ways in which curricula can help teachers make the best use of material. At a most basic level, curricula might use multiethnic names or models in materials, or they might be directly translated into another language. Programs need to go beyond this, however. They should provide teachers with detailed instructions in lessons about how to adapt curriculum material to make it most relevant and appropriate, depending on the culture(s) of students in their classes. Without such instruction, it is doubtful that all teachers will use curriculum materials to their best advantage for cultural sensitivity.
- To have any chance of being effective through time, programs should be sufficiently long and have adequate follow-up. Fewer than 10 sessions in a year and less than 3 years of follow-up may be too little, but there has not yet been much research to nail this down. Ideally, prevention programming should be continual. Students should receive prevention every year in school.
- Programs that provide training in broader personal and social skills are even more powerful in reducing drug use. Because these programs tend to be a bit longer, schools must consider how much time they can commit to drug abuse prevention. It is unwise to select any program if it is unlikely teachers will be able to teach all of it. Although some drug abuse prevention curricula acknowledge that teachers may choose to teach parts of their programs, we saw few that provided any real guidance about what parts are essential or nonessential. A program cannot be expected to work if teachers choose to teach different parts. If teachers or schools decide to start changing programs or leaving parts out, we have serious concerns about whether a curriculum would still be effective.
- School-based programs that include media, family, or community-based components are likely to be more effective than programs limited to classroom activities. Research will be needed to determine the relative contribution of different components to overall program effectiveness.

2. *All drug education curricula should be rigorously evaluated using pretest-posttest control group designs with measures of substance use behavior.* Program developers and marketers have a responsibility to determine the efficacy of the approaches they promote. *Healthy People 2000* includes as a service goal that all students receive prevention, preferably through quality comprehensive health education. Only three comprehensive health education programs had been rigorously evaluated, however, and only one included outcome measures of drug or alcohol use in addition to tobacco use. A future research objective of *Healthy People 2010* should be to adequately evaluate additional comprehensive health education programs.

3. *Drug prevention curricula demonstrated to be effective in research should be aggressively promoted.* Although there are questions about the lasting effectiveness of DARE, its success at dissemination deserves careful study to identify effective strategies. DARE provides a powerful example of how a curriculum can be effectively disseminated when community agencies and policymakers get behind a program and when mass marketing techniques are used. Part of the original success of DARE may be that it offered a concrete focus for the public and political energy generated by the Reagan administration's War on Drugs.

The staying power of DARE in the face of waning public attention, however, underscores the effectiveness of its dissemination strategy. The DARE example suggests important characteristics of programs that are likely to be used and institutionalized. DARE appears to have wide appeal for students and teachers (Ringwalt et al., 1994). Prevention coordinators report that curriculum materials such as videos, games, and even hand puppets can be particularly useful because they capture the attention of students. Programs that have been successfully mass-marketed tend to have developed more appealing curriculum materials, compared with programs that were developed in research laboratories. For example, in DARE, students enjoy the unusual opportunity to work with a police officer, and overworked teachers appreciate that someone else is responsible for delivering the program. The program also has many appealing extras, including a stuffed lion named DAREN, buttons, caps, bumper stickers, and so on.

We recommend that mechanisms be developed at the state and federal level to disseminate the most effective prevention programs. A simple step would be to identify interested curriculum publishers who can help researchers develop appealing program materials and who already have in place successful dissemination strategies such as presentations at education conferences and mass mailings. Researchers will also need help in resolving issues of ownership with their universities; federal clarification and guidelines concerning this issue would be helpful.

Conclusion

School-based drug education curricula represent one promising approach to the problem of adolescent drug abuse, although, by themselves, they are not enough. Public attention must be refocused on the problem of drug abuse to correct the current course toward increasing adolescent drug use. The family, the media, and the community as a whole must work with schools to promote anti-drug-using norms.

References

Ajzen, I., & Fishbein, M. (1980). *Understanding attitudes and predicting behavior.* Englewood Cliffs, NJ: Prentice Hall.

Bandura, A. (1977). *Social learning theory.* Englewood Cliffs, NJ: Prentice Hall.

Bangert-Drowns, R. L. (1988). The effects of school-based substance abuse education: A meta-analysis. *Journal of Drug Education, 18,* 243-264.

Bell, R. M., Ellickson, P. L., & Harrison, E. R. (1993). Do drug prevention effects persist into high school? How Project ALERT did with ninth graders. *Preventive Medicine, 22,* 463-483.

Bosworth, K., & Sailes, J. (1993). Content and teaching strategies in 10 selected drug abuse prevention curricula. *Journal of School Health, 63,* 247-253.

Botvin, G. J., Baker, E., Botvin, E. M., Filazzola, A. D., & Millman, R. B. (1984). Prevention of alcohol misuse through the development of personal and social competence: A pilot study. *Journal of Studies on Alcohol, 45,* 550-552.

Botvin, G. J., Baker, E., Dusenbury, L., Botvin, E. M., & Diaz, T. (1995). Long-term follow-up results of a randomized drug abuse prevention trial in a White middle-class population. *Journal of the American Medical Association, 273,* 1106-1112.

Botvin, G. J., Baker, E., Dusenbury, L., Tortu, S., & Botvin, E. M. (1990). Preventing adolescent drug abuse through a multimodal cognitive-behavioral approach:

Results of a 3-year study. *Journal of Consulting and Clinical Psychology, 58,* 437-446.

Botvin, G. J., Baker, E., Filazzola, A. D., & Botvin, E. M. (1990). A cognitive behavioral approach to substance abuse prevention: One-year follow-up. *Addictive Behaviors, 15,* 47-63.

Botvin, G. J., Batson, H. W., Witts-Vitale, S., Bess, V., Baker, E., & Dusenbury, L. (1989). A psychosocial approach to smoking prevention for urban Black youth. *Public Health Reports, 104,* 573-582.

Botvin, G. J., & Botvin, E. M. (1992). School-based and community-based prevention approaches. In J. Lowinson, P. Ruiz, & R. Millman (Eds.), *Comprehensive textbook of substance abuse* (pp. 910-927). Baltimore: Williams & Wilkins.

Botvin, G. J., Dusenbury, L., Baker, E., James-Ortiz, S., & Kerner, J. (1989). A skills training approach to smoking prevention among Hispanic youth. *Journal of Behavioral Medicine, 12,* 279-296.

Botvin, G. J., Dusenbury, L. D., Baker, E., Ortiz, S., Botvin, E. M., & Kerner, J. (1992). Smoking prevention among urban minority youth: Assessing effects on outcome and mediating variables. *Health Psychology, 11,* 290-299.

Botvin, G. J., & Eng, A. (1982). The efficacy of a multicomponent approach to the prevention of cigarette smoking. *Preventive Medicine, 11,* 199-211.

Botvin, G. J., Renick, N. L., & Baker, E. (1983). The effects of scheduling format and booster sessions on a broad-spectrum psychosocial smoking prevention program. *Journal of Behavioral Medicine, 5,* 359-379.

Botvin, G. J., Schinke, S. P., Epstein, J. A., & Diaz, T. (1994). Effectiveness of culturally focused and generic skills training approaches to alcohol and drug abuse prevention among minority youths. *Psychology of Addictive Behaviors, 8,* 116-127.

Botvin, G. J., Schinke, S. P., Epstein, J. A., Diaz, T., & Botvin, E. M. (1995). Effectiveness of culturally focused and generic skills training approaches to alcohol and drug abuse prevention among minority adolescents: Two-year follow-up results. *Psychology of Addictive Behaviors, 9,* 183-194,

Bruvold, W. H. (1990). A meta-analysis of the California school based risk reduction program. *Journal of Drug Education, 20,* 139-152.

Bruvold, W. H. (1993). A meta-analysis of adolescent smoking prevention programs. *American Journal of Public Health, 83,* 872-880.

Bruvold, W. H., & Rundall, T. G. (1988). A meta-analysis and theoretical review of school based tobacco and alcohol intervention programs. *Psychology and Health, 2,* 53-78.

Caplan, M., Weissberg, R. P., Grober, J. S., Sivo, P. J., Grady, K., & Jacoby, C. (1992). Social competence promotion with inner-city and suburban young adolescents: Effects on social adjustment and alcohol use. *Journal of Consulting and Clinical Psychology, 60,* 56-63.

Clayton, R. R., Cattarello, A., & Walden, K. P. (1991). Sensation seeking as a potential mediating variable for school-based intervention: A two-year follow-up of DARE. *Health Communications, 3,* 229-239.

Connell, D. B., & Turner, R. R. (1985). The impact of instructional experience and the effects of cumulative instruction. *Journal of School Health, 55,* 324-331.

Connell, D. B., Turner, R. R., & Mason, E. F. (1985). Summary of findings of the School Health Education Evaluation: Health promotion effectiveness, implementation and costs. *Journal of School Health, 55,* 316-321.

Dielman, T. E., Kloska, D. D., Leech, S. L., Schulenberg, J. E., & Shope, J. (1992). Susceptibility to peer pressure as an explanatory variable for the differential effectiveness of an alcohol misuse prevention program in elementary schools. *Journal of School Health, 62,* 233-237.

Dielman, T. E., Shope, J. T., Leech, S. L., & Butchart, A. T. (1989). Differential effectiveness of an elementary school-based alcohol misuse prevention program. *Journal of School Health, 59,* 255-263.

Drug Strategies. (1996). *Making the grade: A guide to school drug prevention programs.* Washington, DC: Author.

Dusenbury, L., & Falco, M. (1995). Eleven components of effective drug abuse prevention curricula. *Journal of School Health, 65,* 420-425.

Ellickson, P. L., & Bell, R. M. (1990). Drug prevention in junior high: A multi-site longitudinal test. *Science, 247,* 1299-1305.

Ellickson, P. L., Bell, R. M., & McGuigan, K. (1993). Preventing adolescent drug use: Long-term results of a junior high program. *American Journal of Public Health, 83,* 856-861.

Ennett, S., Rosenbaum, D. P., Flewelling, R. L., Bieler, G. S., Ringwalt, C. L., & Bailey, S. L. (1994). Long-term evaluation of drug abuse resistance education. *Addictive Behaviors, 19,* 113-125.

Ennett, S., Tobler, N. S., Ringwalt, C. L., & Flewelling, R. L. (1994). How effective is Project DARE? A meta-analysis of outcome evaluations. *American Journal of Public Health, 84,* 1394-1401.

Errecart, M. T., Walberg, H. J., Ross, J. G., Gold, R. S., Fiedler, J. L., & Kolbe, L. J. (1991). Effectiveness of Teenage Health Teaching Modules. *Journal of School Health, 61,* 26-30.

Fleming, M. (1996). *Healthy youth 2000: A mid-decade review.* Chicago: American Medical Association, Department of Adolescent Health.

Hansen, W. B. (1992). School-based substance abuse prevention: A review of the state of the art in curriculum, 1980-1990. *Health Education Research, 7,* 403-430.

Hansen, W. B. (1993). School-based alcohol prevention programs. *Alcohol Health and Research World, 17,* 54-60.

Hansen, W. B., & Graham, J. W. (1991). Preventing alcohol, marijuana, and cigarette use among adolescents: Peer pressure resistance training versus establishing conservative norms. *Preventive Medicine, 20,* 414-430.

Hansen, W. B., Rose, L. A., & Dryfoos, J. G. (1993, May 26). *Causal factors, interventions and policy considerations in school-based substance abuse prevention.* Report submitted to the U.S. Congress, Office of Technology Assessment, Washington, DC.

Harmon, M. A. (1993). Reducing the risk of drug involvement among early adolescents: An evaluation of Drug Abuse Resistance Education (DARE). *Evaluation Review, 17,* 221-239.

Hawkins, J. D., Catalano, R. F., & Kent, L. A. (1991). Combining broadcast media and parent education to prevent teenage drug abuse. In L. Donohew, H. E.

Sypher, & W. J. Bukoski (Eds.), *Persuasive communication and drug abuse prevention* (pp. 283-294). Hillsdale, NJ: Lawrence Erlbaum.

Jessor, R., & Jessor, S. L. (1977). *Problem behavior and psychosocial development: A longitudinal study of youth.* New York: Academic Press.

Johnson, C. A., MacKinnon, D. P., & Pentz, M. A. (1996). Breadth of program and outcome effectiveness in drug abuse prevention. *American Behavioral Scientist, 39,* 884-896.

Johnson, C. A., Pentz, M. A., Weber, M. D., Dwyer, J. H., Baer, N., MacKinnon, D. P., Hansen, W. B., & Flay, B. R. (1990). Relative effectiveness of comprehensive community programming for drug abuse prevention with high-risk and low-risk adolescents. *Journal of Consulting and Clinical Psychology, 58,* 447-456.

Johnston, L. D., O'Malley, P. M., & Bachman, J. G. (1995). *National survey results on drug use from the Monitoring the Future Study, 1975-1994: Vol. 1. Secondary school students.* Washington, DC: U.S. Department of Health and Human Services, Public Health Service.

Lerner, R. M., Petersen, A. C., & Brooks-Gunn, J. (Eds.). (1991). *Encyclopedia of adolescence* (Vols. 1 & 2). New York: Garland.

Mrazek, P. J., & Haggerty, R. J. (Eds). (1994). *Reducing risk for mental disorders: Frontiers for preventive intervention research.* Washington, DC: Institute of Medicine, National Academy Press.

Mussen, P. H., Conger, J. J., & Kagan, J. (1979). *Child development and personality* (5th ed.). New York: Harper & Row.

National Institute on Drug Abuse. (1991-1996). *Survey results from the Monitoring the Future Study.* Bethesda, MD: Author.

Pentz, M. A., Dwyer, J. H., MacKinnon, D. P., Flay, B. R., Hansen, W. B., Wang, E. Y. I., & Johnson, C. A. (1989). Multicommunity trial for primary prevention of adolescent drug abuse. *Journal of the American Medical Association, 261,* 3259-3266.

Pentz, M. A., Trebow, E. A., Hansen, W. B., MacKinnon, D. P., Dwyer, J. H., Johnson, C. A., Flay, B. R., Daniels, S., & Cormack, C. C. (1990). Effects of program implementation on adolescent drug use behavior: The Midwestern Prevention Project (MPP). *Evaluation Review, 14,* 264-289.

Perry, C. L., & Kelder, S. H. (1992). Models for effective prevention. *Journal of Adolescent Health, 13,* 355-363.

Perry, C. L., Kelder, S. H., Murray, D. M., & Klepp, K. (1992). Community wide smoking prevention: Long term outcomes of the Minnesota Heart Health Program and the Class of 1989 Study. *American Journal of Public Health, 82,* 1210-1216.

Perry, C. L., Williams, C. L., Forster, J. L., Wolfson, M., Wagenaar, A. C., Finnegan, J. R., McGovern, P. G., Veblen-Mortenson, S., Komro, K. A., & Anstine, P. S. (1993). Background, conceptualization and design of a community-wide research program on adolescent alcohol use: Project Northland. *Health Education Research, 8,* 125-136.

Perry, C. L., Williams, C. L., Veblen-Mortenson, S., Toomey, T. L., Komro, K. A., Anstine, P. S., McGovern, P. G., Finnegan, J. R., Forster, J. L., Wagenaar, A. C., & Wolfson, M. (1996). Project Northland: Outcomes of a communitywide alcohol use prevention program during early adolescence. *American Journal of Public Health, 86,* 956-965.

Ringwalt, C., Ennett, S. T., & Holt, K. D. (1991). An outcome evaluation of Project DARE (Drug Abuse Resistance Education). *Health Education Research, 6,* 327-337.

Ringwalt, C., Greene, J. M., Ennett, S. T., Iachan, R., Clayton, R. R., & Leukefeld, C. G. (1994, September). *Past and future directions of the DARE program: An evaluation report.* Draft final report prepared for the U.S. Department of Justice, National Institute of Justice, Office of Justice Programs, Washington, DC.

Rohrbach, L. A., D'Onofrio, C. N., Backer, T. E., & Montgomery, S. B. (1996). Diffusion of school-based substance abuse prevention programs. *American Behavioral Scientist, 39,* 919-934.

Ross, J. G., Luepker, R. V., Nelson, G. D., Saavedra, P., & Hubbard, B. (1991). Teenage Health Teaching Modules: Impact of teacher training on implementation and student outcomes. *Journal of School Health, 61,* 31-34.

Rundall, T. G., & Bruvold, W. H. (1988). A meta-analysis of school-based smoking and alcohol use prevention programs. *Health Education Quarterly, 15,* 317-334.

Shope, J. T., Dielman, T. E., Butchart, A. T., Campanelli, P. C., & Kloska, D. D. (1992). An elementary school-based alcohol misuse prevention program: A follow-up evaluation. *Journal of Studies on Alcohol, 53,* 106-121.

Shope, J. T., Kloska, D. D., Dielman, T. E., & Maharg, R. (1994). Longitudinal evaluation of an enhanced alcohol misuse prevention study (AMPS): Curriculum for grades six-eight. *Journal of School Health, 64,* 160-166.

Smith, D. W., McCormick, L. K., Steckler, A. B., & McLeroy, K. R. (1993). Teachers' use of health curricula: Implementation of Growing Healthy, Project SMART and the Teenage Health Teaching Modules. *Journal of School Health, 63,* 349-354.

Tobler, N. S. (1992). Drug prevention programs can work: Research findings. *Journal of Addictive Diseases, 11,* 1-28.

Tobler, N. S. (1994). *Meta-analysis of adolescent drug prevention programs.* Doctoral dissertation submitted to the State University of New York at Albany, School of Social Welfare.

Tobler, N. S. (in press). Meta-analytical issues for prevention intervention research. In L. Seitz & L. Collins (Eds.), *Advances in data analysis for prevention intervention research.* Bethesda, MD: National Institute on Drug Abuse.

U.S. Department of Health and Human Services, Public Health Service. (1991). *Healthy people 2000: National health promotion and disease prevention objectives* (DHHS Publication No. PHS 91-50212). Washington, DC: U.S. Government Printing Office.

U.S. Department of Health and Human Services, Public Health Service. (1993). *National household survey on drug abuse.* Washington, DC: Author.

U.S. Department of Health and Human Services, Public Health Service. (1995). *Healthy people 2000: Midcourse review and 1995 revisions.* Washington, DC: U.S. Government Printing Office.

Walter, H. J., Vaughan, R. D., & Wynder, E. L. (1989). Primary prevention of cancer among children: Changes in cigarette smoking and diet after six years of intervention. *Journal of the National Cancer Institute, 81,* 995-998.

Weissberg, R. P., & Elias, M. J. (1993). Enhancing young people's social competence and health behavior: An important challenge for educators, scientists, policy makers, and funders. *Applied & Preventive Psychology, 2,* 179-190.

• *CHAPTER 4* •

Preventing High-Risk Sexual Behavior, Sexually Transmitted Diseases, and Pregnancy Among Adolescents

LYNDA M. SAGRESTANO
ROBERTA L. PAIKOFF

Adolescent sexual activity and the resulting pregnancy and transmission of sexually transmitted diseases (STDs) have been on the rise during the past several decades, with large increases in the 1980s and early 1990s (Moore, Sugland, Blumenthal, Glei, & Snyder, 1995). In an effort to promote the health of America's youth, the U.S. Department of Health and Human Services, Public Health Service (DHHS; 1991) established goals for healthy behavior change, including goals for reducing teen pregnancy and STD transmission. These guidelines were clear with respect to adolescent sexual behavior: (a) Reduce early sexual behavior, (b) reduce adolescent pregnancy, and (c) increase adoles-

---

AUTHORS' NOTE: We gratefully acknowledge the generous support of the National Institute of Mental Health for grant support to the second author through the Office on AIDS (MH50423; MH55701) and the Services Research Branch (MH54212), postdoctoral funding to the first author through the NIMH Prevention Research Training Program in Urban Children's Mental Health and AIDS Prevention at the University of Illinois at Chicago (MH19933), as well as support from a William T. Grant Foundation Faculty Award to the second author.

cent use of contraceptives for pregnancy and STD/HIV prevention. At the midcourse review, however, these goals had only partially been reached (DHHS, 1995). Specifically, national surveys reveal that since *Healthy People 2000* (DHHS, 1991) was released, the proportion of sexually active adolescents has increased, sexual initiation is occurring at younger ages, and the rates of adolescent pregnancy have increased, especially among minority youth. Among adolescents who have been sexually active in their lifetime, however, the proportion of adolescents who later choose abstinence and who use contraceptives has increased (DHHS, 1995).

In addition to the objectives outlined above, *Healthy People 2000* (DHHS, 1991) identified minority youth as a group at high risk for unintended pregnancy, early sexual behavior, and sexually transmitted diseases, and thus targeted minority youth for risk reduction programs. Urban minority youth pose a particularly important area of concern because urban minority adolescents are overrepresented among adolescents at risk for exposure to STDs and HIV (Centers for Disease Control and Prevention [CDC], 1995; Parfenoff, Paikoff, Brooks-Gunn, Holmbeck, & Jarrett, 1995). Children growing up in urban settings are more likely than suburban youth to be living in poverty and to experience increased stress due to growing up in such contexts (Jarrett, 1995; McLoyd, 1990). The impact of this context also may have short- and long-term effects on the negotiation of healthy behavior and the prevention of sexual risk taking. Little is known about the normative behavior of urban minority youth living in poverty. Much of the research conducted on normative development has focused on middle-class White children growing up in suburban areas, whereas research on urban minority youth has focused on problem behavior (Paikoff, 1995; Spencer & Dornbusch, 1990). More recently, however, urban minority youth are the focus of primary preventive interventions designed to prevent pregnancy and HIV, with data relevant to normative behavior embedded in these contexts (Paikoff, 1995). The development of more effective programming would likely benefit substantially from more baseline information on the normative development of sexuality in urban and minority youth.

In this chapter, we will address each of the three objectives regarding sexual behavior outlined in *Healthy People 2000* (DHHS, 1991). We will first consider background data and trends in adolescent sexual behavior for each of the three target areas (early sex, adolescent pregnancy, and contraceptive use). Second, we will discuss prevention efforts aimed at reducing high-risk sexual behavior, highlighting both limitations and strengths of existing programs. Specifically, we will distinguish between primary prevention efforts that are designed to reduce early initiation of sexual behavior and secondary prevention efforts that are designed to promote safer sex practices among sexually active adolescents. Finally, we will make recommendations for improving preventive interventions and thus reducing high-risk sexual behavior among America's youth.

Trends in Adolescent Sexual Behavior

Early Initiation of Sexual Behavior

One objective of *Healthy People 2000* (DHHS, 1991) is to reduce early sexual behavior through delaying onset of sexual intercourse and encouraging abstinence. More specifically, the guidelines specified reducing the proportion of adolescents who have engaged in sexual intercourse to 15% by age 15 and to 40% by age 17, and increasing to 40% the proportion of ever sexually active adolescents age 17 and younger who have abstained in the past 3 months. Midcourse revisions called for a focus on ages 15 through 17 and, in particular, on African American boys and girls (Fleming, 1996). According to the 1988 baseline statistics, 27% of girls and 33% of boys were sexually active by age 15, and 50% of girls and 66% of boys were active by age 17 (DHHS, 1991). Data from a 1990 national survey (Leigh, Morrison, Trocki, & Temple, 1994), 1991 statistics provided in the midcourse review (DHHS, 1995), and the 1993 Youth Risk Behavior Surveillance (YRBS; Kann et al., 1995) indicate even higher percentages of youth are active by these ages, and African American youth were more likely to report being active than were White or Hispanic youth (Kann et al., 1995; Leigh et al., 1994). Furthermore, research indicates that African American youth become sexually active at younger ages than their White counterparts, and boys at younger ages than girls (Brooks-Gunn & Furstenberg, 1989; Hayes, 1987; Keller et al., 1991). One multicultural sample indicated that African Americans reported earliest onset, followed by Hispanics, Whites, and Asians (Moore & Erickson, 1985). These gaps are narrowing, however, as White youth and girls become active at younger ages (Brooks-Gunn & Furstenberg, 1989; Hayes, 1987). Studies of urban minority youth indicate that the median age of onset of sexual activity may be as low as 12 to 14 (Keller et al., 1991; Levy, Handler, Weeks, et al., 1995; Levy, Lampman, Handler, Flay, & Weeks, 1993; Stanton et al., 1994).

Earlier onset of sexual behavior places adolescents at higher risk for pregnancy and sexually transmitted diseases; earlier initiation increases the probability of pregnancy and STDs because of the increased period in which an adolescent is engaged in sexual activity, and increased number of lifetime partners (Brooks-Gunn & Furstenberg, 1989). In addition, research indicates that young adolescent girls are likely to be having sex with older boys and men (Males & Chew, 1996), which places them at higher risk for STDs and HIV. Older adolescents and young men are more likely to have had exposure to multiple partners and intravenous drug use (Hein, 1989), and having sex with a partner more than 5 years older is associated with not using condoms (Weisman et al., 1989).

Adolescent Pregnancy

The second objective set out by *Healthy People 2000* (DHHS, 1991) was to reduce early pregnancies among girls aged 17 and younger to no more than 50 per 1,000 adolescents. Baseline data from 1985 indicated an overall rate of 71.1 per 1,000. By 1990, pregnancy rates had increased to 74.3 (DHHS, 1995). The birthrate decreased between 1991 and 1993, however, to 59.6 (Children's Defense Fund, 1996). The guidelines also targeted reducing adolescent pregnancies in African American and Hispanic adolescents aged 15 to 19 to 120 and 105 per 1,000, respectively, on the basis of baseline data of 186 and 158. The midcourse review reported increased pregnancy rates in African American girls aged 15 to 17 from 134 to 140 per 1,000 between 1985 and 1988 (no data were presented for changes in Hispanic birthrates). The baseline statistics reflect the number of pregnancies per 1,000 adolescents, including those who are not currently sexually active. Among sexually experienced adolescents only, the numbers are obviously higher. On the basis of 1990 data (Alan Guttmacher Institute, 1994), among sexually experienced teenagers, 9% of 14-year-olds, 18% of 15- to 17-year-olds, and 22% of 18- to 19-year-olds become pregnant each year, which reflects both higher rates of reproductive maturity (fecundity) and higher frequency of intercourse in older teens. Furthermore, among adolescents aged 15 to 19, 19% of African American, 13% of Hispanic, and 8% of White teens become pregnant each year. These ethnic differences reflect differences in rates of sexual experience among ethnic groups.

The rates of adolescent pregnancy in the United States are much higher than rates in other developed countries, despite similar rates of adolescent sexual activity. This difference has been attributed to greater acceptance of adolescent sexuality in other countries, resulting in more effective education and use of contraception (Jones, Forrest, Henshaw, Silverman, & Torres, 1988), and suggests that increased education and availability of birth control could decrease the pregnancy rate in this country, to the extent that this reflects a larger cultural shift.

Although most data on adolescent pregnancy have been collected on women, from the perspective of prevention it is critical to consider adolescent fathers as well. National studies find that the partners of pregnant teens, that is, the babies' fathers, are 5 years older on average than the mothers (Males & Chew, 1996). For pregnancies in young women under age 18, only 26% of the fathers are under age 18, whereas 35% are 18 to 19, and 39% are 20 and older (Alan Guttmacher Institute, 1994; Henshaw, 1992). In terms of pregnancy rates, only 4% of sexually experienced adolescent males aged 15 to 17 impregnate their partners, compared with the female pregnancy rate of 18% for this age range (Alan Guttmacher Institute, 1994; Henshaw, 1992; Sonenstein, Pleck, & Ku, 1989). This suggests that adolescent boys may be having sex with younger girls who have not yet reached reproductive maturity, older girls who "initiate" them, or that they may not be having sex as frequently as their female peers (Alan Guttmacher Institute, 1994).

The resolution of teenage pregnancies depends in part on whether the pregnancy was intended. Approximately 85% of teenage pregnancies are unintended; intention, however, is influenced by socioeconomic status, race/ethnicity, and marital status. Higher-income teens are less likely to intend to become pregnant than lower-income teens, and African American and White teens are less likely to intend to become pregnant than Hispanic teens (although the majority of Hispanic teens also do not intend to get pregnant). Among married pregnant teens, most did not intend to become pregnant (67%; Alan Guttmacher Institute, 1994; Henshaw, 1992).

When pregnancies do occur, they are resolved through miscarriages (14%), abortion (35%), or giving birth (50%). Among adolescents who give birth, 14% of pregnancies were intended, and 37% were unintended. Among White teens giving birth following an unintended pregnancy, the adoption rate has declined substantially to a rate of 3% in the late 1980s. This trend reflects, in part, the increased acceptability of teens having children outside marriage (Bachrach, Stolley, & London, 1992; Henshaw, 1992).

The outcomes associated with adolescent pregnancy are variable and can be seen in both the short and the long term. In general, teenage pregnancy and childbearing result in increased health and developmental risks to the offspring (Ketterlinus, Henderson, & Lamb, 1990; Rosenthal, 1993), interruption or discontinuation of the teenager's education (Upchurch & McCarthy, 1990), reduced employment opportunities (Hayes, 1987; Hofferth & Moore, 1979), and unstable or nonexistent marriages. These outcomes, however, are highly associated with the level of poverty and lack of adequate health care experienced by many pregnant adolescents (Hayes, 1987). Furthermore, in the long term, many pregnant adolescents return to school, and by 10 years postpregnancy, differences in educational attainment and workplace participation are reduced (Furstenberg & Brooks-Gunn, 1985). Finally, the outcomes associated with adolescent pregnancy likely emotionally affect the lives of the adolescents, their families, and their extended social networks, although the emotional ramifications of adolescent pregnancy have not been well researched.

Contraceptive Use

The third objective set out by *Healthy People 2000* (DHHS, 1991) was to increase to at least 90% the proportion of sexually active, unmarried people aged 19 and younger who use contraception. In particular, combined methods of contraception that effectively prevent pregnancy and provide barrier protection against sexually transmitted diseases are preferred. According to 1988 baseline reports, 78% of youth used contraceptives at most recent intercourse, and 63% at first intercourse. Only 2% of women aged 15 to 19 used both oral contraceptives and condoms at most recent intercourse. Furthermore, only one third of youth report using contraceptives all the time, and low-income teens are the least likely to use contraceptives consistently (DHHS, 1991). In 1991, reported contraceptive use at last intercourse had increased to more than 80% (DHHS, 1995). Only 52.8% of students surveyed in the 1993 YRBS, however, reported using condoms at last intercourse (Kann et al., 1995).

Reported rates of condom use among urban minority youth vary considerably, depending on how the question is asked. Most frequently, researchers ask about most recent intercourse or intercourse within the past 6 to 12 months. Results indicate that 30% to 60% of African American and Hispanic adolescents report using condoms (Kegeles, Adler, & Irwin, 1988; Millstein, Moscicki, & Broering, 1994; Stanton et al., 1994; St. Lawrence, 1993), with inner-city youth reporting lower rates of use than national samples (Ford, Rubinstein, & Norris, 1994). When asked if they always use condoms, smaller percentages (2% to 37%) report consistent use of condoms (DiClemente et al., 1992; Kegeles et al., 1988; Keller et al., 1991; Millstein et al., 1994). When asked about intentions to use condoms in the future, 60% to 70% of sexually active youth report that they plan to use condoms (Stanton et al., 1994; Walter, Vaughan, Ragin, Cohall, & Kasen, 1994).

Results of comparisons of condom use among inner-city ethnic groups are mixed (CDC, 1992; Durant, Seymore, Pendergrast, & Beckman, 1990; Ford et al., 1994; Levy, Handler, et al., 1995). Females report using contraceptives more than do males (Moore & Erickson, 1985), but males report using condoms more than do females (CDC, 1992; DiClemente, 1992). This may reflect women's use of birth control pills or other female methods without the knowledge of their partners. Age comparisons yield mixed results, with some studies indicating that older adolescents are more likely to use contraceptives, including condoms, than are younger adolescents (Moore & Erickson, 1985; Levy, Handler, et al., 1995), whereas others conclude either that age differences do not exist (DiClemente et al., 1992) or that younger adolescents are more likely to use contraceptives (DiClemente, 1992).

Interventions Designed to Reduce Early Sexual Behavior, Adolescent Pregnancy, and Unprotected Sexual Intercourse

During the past several decades, many programs have been designed to reduce early sexual behavior, adolescent pregnancy, and unprotected sexual intercourse. Interventions range from comprehensive, multifaceted programs that focus on multiple goals to enhance life options (including delaying parenting), to targeted programs that focus specifically on adolescent sexual behavior (Dryfoos, 1990). Programs take place in a variety of settings, including schools, churches, family planning clinics, and the larger community (Dryfoos, 1990; Miller, Card, Paikoff, & Peterson, 1992). Although earlier programs were aimed at reducing adolescent pregnancy, often through abstinence, the rise of the AIDS epidemic has changed the nature of programming. The newest generation of programs emphasize delaying sexual debut, and for those who are sexually active, practicing effective contraception to prevent both pregnancy and the transmission of STDs (Kirby, Barth, Leland, & Fetro, 1991; Kirby & DiClemente, 1994).

Broad-based programs represent a more sociological approach to prevention in which pregnancy and other risky behaviors (e.g., substance use, school dropout, and delinquency) are seen as embedded in problematic contexts that require comprehensive treatment. Programs are designed to meet multiple goals through changing the social environment. By enhancing opportunities for a positive future, the programs aim to provide impetus to delay parenting (Dryfoos, 1990). Programs include skills training in areas such as academic achievement (Jollah & Alston, 1988; Sipe, Grossman, & Milliner, 1988), life planning and goal setting (Philliber & Allen, 1992), career planning (Hunter-Geboy, Peterson, Casey, Hardy, & Renner, 1985; Jollah & Alston, 1988), and job placement (Jollah & Alston, 1988; Sipe et al., 1988). In addition, many programs include personal counseling (Philliber & Allen, 1992; Sipe et al., 1988), family communication (Nicholson & Postrado, 1992), and sexual and reproductive development and decision making (Jollah & Alston, 1988; Sipe et al., 1988).

Evaluations of such programs are not always comprehensive or rigorous by research standards (Card, Peterson, & Greeno, 1992; Dryfoos, 1990; Kelly, Murphy, Sikkema, & Kalichman, 1993; Moore et al., 1995; Oakley, Fullerton, & Holland, 1995; Zabin & Hirsch, 1987), in part because their broad-based approach does not allow for targeted programming subject to targeted evaluation and in part because the outcomes of such programming are also broad based and longer term. Such programs, however, have been found to reduce the rate of teen pregnancy (Berrueta-Clement, Schweinhart, Barnett, Weikart, & Epstein, 1984; Jollah & Alston, 1988; Nicholson & Postrado, 1992; Philliber & Allen, 1992) and increase the effective use of contraception (Jollah & Alston, 1988; Nicholson & Postrado, 1992; Sipe et al., 1988).

In contrast to the broad-based, life options programs, targeted programs focus primarily on sexual behavior and on changing the individual factors presumed to be linked to sexual behavior. Targeted programs include school-based interventions and sex education, counseling programs, school-based clinics, and multicomponent community-based programs. Programs usually provide information and knowledge, as well as training to increase problem-solving, decision-making, and behavioral skills (Howard & McCabe, 1992; Kirby et al., 1991; Levy et al., 1994; Levy, Perhats, et al., 1995; Pittman & Govan, 1986; Schinke & Gilchrist, 1984; St. Lawrence et al., 1995; Walter & Vaughan, 1993). Various formats are used, including small group discussions (Stern, 1988), individual counseling (Stern, 1988; Zabin, Hirsch, Smith, Streett, & Hardy, 1986), role playing (Schinke & Gilchrist, 1984), and provision of family planning services in a clinic setting (Edwards, Steinman, Arnold, & Hakanson, 1980; Galavotti & Lovick, 1989; Zabin et al., 1986).

Programs report change in the areas of increased knowledge and positive attitudes (Jemmott, Jemmott, & Fong, 1992; Stern, 1988; Walter & Vaughan, 1993), postponing the onset of sexual intercourse (Howard & McCabe, 1992; Pittman & Govan, 1986; Zabin et al., 1986); increased intentions to use condoms (Jemmott et al., 1992; Levy, Perhats, et al., 1995), increased use of contraception

(Galavotti & Lovick, 1989; Stern, 1988; St. Lawrence et al., 1995; Zabin et al., 1986), fewer partners (Jemmott et al., 1992), and decreased pregnancy rates (Zabin et al., 1986).

Methodological Considerations: Program Evaluation, Developmental Appropriateness, and Contextual Appropriateness

Program Evaluation

Although many interventions have been shown to be effective in changing behavior, at least in the short term, serious methodological constraints need to be considered. Recent reviews of behavioral interventions to prevent pregnancy and HIV reveal that few programs are methodologically strong enough to generate reliable conclusions concerning effectiveness (Moore et al., 1995; Oakley et al., 1995). Oakley et al. identified core criteria, including using control groups, providing pre- and postintervention data, and reporting on all targeted outcomes, and found only nine adolescent HIV prevention interventions that met such standards. Of those nine, four were judged to be effective. Oakley et al. call for the increased use of randomized trials, increased reporting of the intervention's impact on health outcomes, and raising journal publication standards to meet more stringent methodological criteria.

Similarly, Moore et al. (1995) note that programs often do not demonstrate significant impact because of weak programming, weak evaluation, or both. Their comprehensive evaluation of pregnancy prevention programs led them to conclude that programs need to be grounded in theory, ecologically sound, and multicomponent oriented. Furthermore, they outline essential steps in designing a program, including defining the purpose, setting clear and attainable goals, identifying the target population, specifying the nature of the treatment, systematically documenting service delivery, establishing the duration of the study and follow-ups, collaborating with program implementers during the design phase, and using control groups.

Developmental Appropriateness

Although improvements in methodological and evaluative aspects of interventions are necessary, they are insufficient to increase the effectiveness of interventions. Programs must also be designed to fit the developmental maturity of the target population. The transition to adolescence is marked by changes in multiple domains, including biological, cognitive, and emotional maturation; family communication; and peer influence. The developmental challenges associated with each of these domains may have important implications for early sexual behavior. Indeed, research indicates that the correlates of early sexual behavior include complex interrelations among individual and contextual factors (Brooks-Gunn & Paikoff, 1993; Chase-Lansdale & Brooks-Gunn, in press), and given the complex relations among these factors, the task of behavior change is a complicated problem likely requiring multifaceted approaches.

For example, the timing of pubertal development (early, on-time, or late with respect to peers) is associated with the timing of onset of sexual behavior, with earlier-developing boys and girls initiating sexual activity earlier than later maturers (Stattin & Magnusson, 1990; Zabin et al., 1986). Research indicates that early-maturing girls may begin sexual activity earlier, in part because of their increased social ties with older girls, linking them to interactions with older boys and men (Hofferth & Hayes, 1987; Irwin, Shafer, & Millstein, 1985). From a social cognitive development perspective, however, early-maturing adolescents may not have the skills needed to understand and make decisions about sexual behavior because they may not yet systematically consider abstract or hypothetical events related to intimate relationships or risk taking (Brooks-Gunn, Boyer, & Hein, 1988; Brooks-Gunn & Paikoff, 1993; Chase-Lansdale & Brooks-Gunn, in press; Fischoff, Bostrom, & Quadrel, 1993; Furby & Beyth-Marom, 1992).

Furthermore, large numbers of adolescents experience emotional difficulties such as depression, low self-esteem, negative self-image, and substance abuse, which have implications for early sexual behavior. As such, interventions must be designed to help adolescents, and in particular, early-developing adolescents, manage risk while also being sensitive to cognitive and emotional developmental issues (Brooks-Gunn & Paikoff, 1993). Ideally, adolescents would be provided not only with sufficient knowledge and understanding of the problem but also with the skills and capacity to act on the knowledge when confronted with a risky situation (Schinke & Gilchrist, 1984).

The transition to adolescence is also accompanied by developmental changes in family and peer relationships that influence the onset of sexual behavior. Adolescents place increasing importance on peer relationships (Brown, 1990), and younger adolescents may be more susceptible to peer pressure than older adolescents (Hill & Holmbeck, 1986; Lewis & Lewis, 1984). Perhaps the greatest source of adolescents' information about sex comes from peers (Hayes, 1987; Thornburg, 1978), allowing for a great deal of misinformation (Brooks-Gunn & Paikoff, 1993). Furthermore, adolescent perceptions of peer attitudes and behavior may not be accurate; these perceptions, however, predict individual sexual behavior (Fisher, 1988).

Communication with parents regarding sexuality also influences sexual behavior, although little is known about the process in which parents influence their teenagers' sexual attitudes and behavior (Brooks-Gunn & Furstenberg, 1989; Brooks-Gunn & Paikoff, 1993). Recent research indicates that adolescents who report discussing sexuality with their parents, including how pregnancy occurs, birth control, and protection from STDs, are more likely to attempt to avoid AIDS through using condoms and having fewer partners (Leland & Barth, 1993). Teenagers who perceive their communication with their parents as poor, however, are likely to initiate sex earlier than those who do not (Christopherson, Miller, & Norton, 1994; Jessor & Jessor, 1977). Perceptions of a close relationship with parents, including feelings of connectedness and supportiveness, have been associated with later intercourse and use of contraceptives (Inazu & Fox, 1980; Leland & Barth, 1993), as have consistency of values between parents and adolescents (Christopherson et al., 1994; Jessor & Jessor, 1977). As such, family communication is an important area for intervention, especially in light of the changing nature of the parent-child relationship at this point in development. More specifically, the transition to adolescence is accompanied by child attempts to increase autonomy, and parental attempts at supervising and monitoring their children become more difficult. Yet increased monitoring may be necessary because it has been linked to later initiation of sexual behavior (Newcomer & Udry, 1985; Paikoff, 1995; Steinberg, 1990) by limiting children's experiences in private, unsupervised, mixed-sex groups (Paikoff, 1995). Working with parents to increase positive communication while effectively monitoring their children could be one aspect of a multicomponent intervention approach.

Contextual Appropriateness

Preventionists also need to consider the effects of contextual factors such as ethnicity, socioeconomic status, and the community because the correlates and patterns of early sexual behavior may differ among different groups. Specifically, differences in cultural and community values and norms, as well as available financial resources, may result in differentially socializing environments. For example, characteristics of the community such as poverty and high proportions of single-parent households are associated with early sexual behavior and adolescent pregnancy (Chase-Lansdale & Brooks-Gunn, in press; McCormick & Brooks-Gunn, 1989). For many adolescents growing up in contexts of urban poverty, pregnancy may be seen as acceptable and in keeping with community age norms for behavior. In addition, parents may want to protect their children from early pregnancy and HIV but, in the context of urban poverty, may not perceive themselves as efficacious in changing their children's behavior. As such, interventions must be designed with sensitivity to contextual factors. A particularly intriguing and worrisome issue to be faced by those designing interventions aimed at reducing high-risk sexual behavior is how best to structure programs for a context that is developmentally inappropriate (e.g., filled with risks and dangers to be negotiated that are beyond the abilities of children or young adolescents).

Primary Versus Secondary Prevention

Similar to other developmental transitions, the development of sexuality can be seen as a series of transitions, and interventions can be designed to target different stages of the sexual transition (Moore et al., 1995). For example, an intervention designed to delay the onset of sexual intercourse (primary prevention) would be different from an intervention designed to increase the use of contraception (secondary prevention). *Primary prevention,* as defined by the Institute of Medicine Committee on Prevention of Mental Disorders (Mrazek & Haggerty, 1994), "seeks to decrease the number of new cases of a disorder or illness (incidence)" (p. 20). Within the context of sexual risk behavior, primary prevention refers to delaying the initiation of sexual behavior among adolescents who have not yet had sexual intercourse. In contrast, *secondary prevention* "seeks to lower the rate of established cases of the disorder or illness in the population (prevalence)" (p. 20). With respect to sexual risk behavior, secondary prevention refers to reducing sexual risk taking among sexually active adolescents, including encouraging abstinence, reducing number of partners, and using effective contraception. Therefore, although both primary and secondary preventive programs have the goal of reducing adolescent pregnancy and STDs through reducing sexual risk taking, the curriculum used for each type of program should differ substantially. Unfortunately, most interventions do not make this distinction, instead including both primary and secondary preventive measures with all participants, regardless of their sexual experience.

Attending to the distinction between primary and secondary prevention facilitates the process of designing a developmentally sensitive intervention by reducing the types of issues to be addressed and restricting the age range and experience of the targeted participants. Next, we describe four programs that attend to the methodological and developmental issues raised in this section, within the context of primary or secondary prevention.

Primary Prevention Programs

Because of the young age at which adolescents are initiating sexual behavior, primary preventive interventions must target *preadolescents.* As mentioned above, programs targeting preadolescents must be sensitive to their level of developmental maturity, as well as the contextual and cultural needs of the target population. Preadolescents, in particular, may not have the developmental maturity to understand the long-term implications of their sexual behavior, and therefore curriculums must be designed with much attention to the cognitive level at which the program is pitched. Furthermore, such programs can help preadolescents identify risk situations and learn to manage them *before* being confronted by them (Brooks-Gunn & Paikoff, 1993), thus heading off the process of behavior change.

Two examples of primary preventive interventions that are methodologically rigorous and developmentally sensitive are the Postponing Sexual Involvement Program (PSIP; Howard & McCabe, 1990, 1992) and Teen Outreach (Philliber & Allen, 1992). The PSIP is a targeted intervention designed to provide information and decision-making skills to help 8th graders resist peer pressure to have sex. The program is a hospital-based outreach educational program implemented in the public school system in Atlanta. Participants in the program are low-income African American boys and girls in the 8th grade (age 13 to 14). Youth are assigned to the program or a comparison group by school. Students in the comparison school receive a basic sexuality education program. Pretest data indicate that the treatment groups do not differ. Follow-up data are collected by telephone interview through the 12th grade (5 years), including students who have dropped out of school, and medical records are used to verify reported pregnancies (Howard & McCabe, 1990, 1992; Moore et al., 1995).

The program has two components. The first component, Human Sexuality, is a 5-class-period curriculum designed to provide basic factual information, decision-making skills, and information about proper use of contraceptives. This component is administered by nurses and counselors. The second component, Postponing Sexual Involvement, is designed to build on the first component by building skills to deal with social and peer pressures to engage in sexual behavior (Howard & McCabe, 1990, 1992). More specifically, this component is designed to help young people (a) understand the societal pressures that influence teen sexual behavior, (b) learn where to go for information regarding sexuality, (c) understand their personal rights in relationships, (d) deal assertively with pressure situations, and (e) postpone sexual involvement (Howard & Mitchell, 1990). This component is presented by older teen leaders in 11th and 12th grades, who serve as role models and illustrate that teens who postpone sexual involvement can still be admired leaders in their peer group. The teen leaders are trained and supervised by nurses and counselors.

Program evaluation results indicate that students in the combined 10-session program were significantly more likely to postpone sexual involvement than students not in the program. For those youth who did initiate sex during the program year, students in the program reported having sex fewer times and being more likely to use contraceptives than those not in the program, which was reflected in their decreased rate of pregnancy relative to controls. Among those youth sexually active prior to the program, however, there were no changes in sexual involvement or pregnancy rates (Howard & McCabe, 1990, 1992).

The second primary prevention program, Teen Outreach (Allen, Philliber, & Hoggson, 1990; Philliber & Allen, 1992), is a school-based program designed to promote school progress and prevent pregnancy by promoting other life options. The program has been implemented nationally, and although certain aspects remain similar across sites, other aspects are more variable. Participants in Teen Outreach are students in 7th through 12th grade, ranging in age from 11 to 19. Nationwide, 75% of participants are women, 40% are African American, 40% are White, and 13% are Hispanic. Some sites recruit through announcements and posters, whereas others seek out students identified by school counselors as "high risk" for school dropout or pregnancy. Matched comparison groups are recruited through participants and school counselors, and both participants and controls complete pretest evaluations as well as follow-ups conducted at the end of the 9-month program. Recently, the program was implemented at 25 sites using random assignment to allow for experimental evaluation of outcomes. The similar findings of the experimental trial suggest that the nonrandom sampling procedure does not bias program outcome evaluation (Allen, Philliber, Herrling, & Kuperminc, 1996).

The program includes two main components: (a) weekly small group discussions led by a facilitator and (b) community service volunteering (Philliber & Allen, 1992). The small group discussions meet at least once weekly for 1 hour. The curriculum emphasizes life planning and goal setting through discussion of developmental tasks faced by adolescents, such as understanding themselves and their values, communication skills, human growth and development, issues related to parenting, family relationships, and community resources. The facilitators serve not as teachers but as friends and mentors, creating a support group-like environment. The community service volunteering projects, usually coordinated by the Junior League, vary according to the needs of the area and the ages of the participants. Typical service projects include working in hospitals and nursing homes, participating in walkathons, working at the school, and tutoring younger students. Students perform a minimum of 1 hour per week of community service volunteering.

The Teen Outreach program was evaluated on four dimensions: pregnancy, school suspension, course failure, and school dropout (Philliber & Allen, 1992). Analyses during several program years indicate that students in the program had lower pregnancy rates and lower rates of school dropout than did the comparison students. With respect to school suspension and course failure, program participants in 4 of the 5 years had lower rates than did control students. Furthermore, participation in Teen Outreach was related to not getting arrested, having reduced rates of truancy, getting on the honor roll, and using contraception more consistently. Teen Outreach participation was not significantly related to reducing substance use or increasing aspirations to finish high school, however, although a trend in this direction was detected for both outcomes.

In-depth analyses examining the process by which the program effects change indicate that two components of Teen Outreach, the classroom program promotion of autonomy and relatedness and the quality of volunteer work performed, predicted lower levels of problem behaviors in middle school students but not in high school students. This suggests that the autonomy component of the classroom program and volunteer work are developmentally appropriate for middle school students, but aspects of the program that best affect outcomes for high school students are not captured by these program components or evaluation measures. Further research is needed to identify the process by which the program effects change for high school students (Allen, Kuperminc, Philliber, & Herre, 1994), or if the primary prevention battle is not already "lost" at this later age.

Secondary Prevention Programs

Although primary prevention efforts show promising outcomes, many adolescents will still become involved in sexual activity. Therefore, secondary prevention programs, designed to reduce sexual risk taking among sexually active adolescents, are also needed. Secondary prevention programs recognize that many adolescents are sexually active and that rather than stressing abstinence as the only solution to preventing pregnancy and STDs, sexually active adolescents need skills with which to manage their sexuality safely, within the context of their level of developmental maturity. For example, a program that emphasizes the use of birth control pills or Norplant as a means of reducing pregnancy may be counterproductive to the prevention of STDs through condom use because adolescents may be less able to appreciate the immediacy of the risk of STDs and therefore may be less likely to use condoms. Two examples of secondary preventive interventions that are methodologically sound and developmentally sensitive are Reducing the Risk (Barth, Leland, Kirby, & Fetro, 1992; Kirby et al., 1991) and Be Proud, Be Responsible (Jemmott et al., 1992).

Reducing the Risk is a targeted sexuality education curriculum that uses a social and cognitive approach to prevent pregnancy by increasing resistance to social pressures and encouraging parental discussions of abstinence, pregnancy, and STDs (Barth et al., 1992; Kirby et al., 1991). The 15-class-period, 3-week program was implemented by specially trained high school teachers as part of the 10th-grade health education course in 13 schools in California. Classrooms were randomly assigned to either the Reducing the Risk curriculum or the control curriculum (i.e., the sex education already offered by the school). All participants and controls completed pre- and posttest evaluations, as well as follow-ups at 6 and 18 months. Through peer modeling and role playing, the program, based on social learning theory, social inoculation theory, and cognitive behavior theory, stressed increasing knowledge about pregnancy and contraception, efficacy of contraception and one's ability to use it, and the anticipated benefits of avoiding pregnancy. Through role playing, the students become familiar with various forms of social pressure and build cognitive and behavior skills rendering them better able to resist such pressures. Explicit norms against unprotected sexual intercourse are established and reinforced through such role playing. Students are also given assignments in which they practice certain skills, such as buying condoms or discussing sex with parents.

Evaluation of outcomes indicated that students in the program were less likely to initiate sexual intercourse within the 18-month follow-up than were controls. Among those who did initiate intercourse during the follow-up, students in the intervention condition were more likely to have protected intercourse than those in the control condition. Furthermore, among already sexually active students in the intervention condition, lower-risk students and females were more likely to have protected intercourse than higher-risk students and males. Students in the intervention condition were more likely to discuss abstinence and birth control than were students in the control group. Discussions of pregnancy were increased for females in the intervention condition, and discussions of STDs were not increased for any group.

A second example of a secondary prevention program, Be Proud, Be Responsible, is an intervention designed to reduce the frequency of HIV-risk-associated sexual behaviors among inner-city African American adolescent males in Philadelphia (Jemmott et al., 1992). Participants in this targeted intervention were either recruited from an outpatient medical clinic, students participating in 10th- through 12th-grade assemblies at a high school, or adolescents at a YMCA. Most of the participants were still in school, and their major source of risk for HIV was through heterosexual activities. Participants were randomly assigned to either the AIDS risk reduction intervention or to a control (career opportunities intervention). All participants completed pre- and posttests on the day of the intervention, as well as a 3-month follow-up. The AIDS intervention was a 1-day, 5-hour program designed to increase knowledge about HIV/AIDS and to change attitudes toward risky sexual behavior. Information was provided concerning the risks associated with specific sexual activities via videotapes, games, and small group exercises that were culturally (i.e., videotapes had multiethnic casts) and developmentally appropriate and encouraged active participation. The correct use of condoms was demonstrated, and participants practiced role-playing situations in which they implemented safer sex practices including abstinence and condom use. Evaluation of outcomes indicated that 3 months following the intervention, participants in the AIDS condition reported more AIDS knowledge and stronger intentions to avoid risky sexual behavior in the next 3 months than participants in the control condition. In addition, they reported engaging in less risky behavior in the 3 months following the intervention, including having sexual intercourse on fewer occasions, with fewer partners, and with fewer partners who were also having sexual relations with others. Furthermore, they were less likely to have intercourse without a condom and less likely to have anal intercourse with a woman.

These short-term gains, however, have not been assessed in longitudinal follow-ups.

Recommendations for Designing Interventions to Reduce Early Sexual Behavior, Adolescent Pregnancy, and Unprotected Sexual Intercourse

In this chapter, we have reviewed current trends in adolescent sexual behavior as well as approaches to preventive interventions. Methodological, developmental, and contextual considerations were raised, and four programs that dealt effectively with such issues were described. In the last section, we outline our recommendations, based on the literature and our own experiences, for designing preventive interventions. Within this context, we note the strengths of the programs described above with respect to these issues.

First, interventions based on empirical research are better able to address the issues most relevant to the target population (Kirby & DiClemente, 1994). Interventions designed for adolescents should be designed for the developmental level of the target group, which may mean different approaches for preadolescents, early adolescents, and late adolescents. Early interventions, with children as young as 9 to 10 years of age, will best facilitate primary prevention of adolescent pregnancy and HIV through a focus on delaying the onset of sexual behavior (Choi & Coates, 1994). Thus far, none have really done this with the preadolescent age group. Both Teen Outreach and PSIP focus on abstinence within a developmental model. Teen Outreach, in particular, accomplishes this by identifying the developmental tasks faced by early adolescents and designing programming that facilitates developmental maturity around such tasks. Secondary prevention, in contrast, is more appropriate for older teens who are more likely to be sexually active and should focus more on reducing number of partners and effective use of contraception to prevent pregnancy and HIV. Both Reducing the Risk and Be Proud, Be Responsible accomplish this through targeted programming. One caveat of distinguishing between primary and secondary prevention, however, is the difficulty in forming groups that are at the same stage of sexual experience. Given that many programs take place in school settings, age is used as a proxy for experience. Therefore, within a framework of either primary or secondary prevention, it may be important to include messages of abstinence as well as safe sexual practices.

The process of designing an intervention would also benefit from an interdisciplinary approach in which multiple perspectives (i.e., anthropology, public health, and education) inform the development of goals and programming (Kelly et al., 1993). Furthermore, collaboration within the community (Choi & Coates, 1994; Kelly et al., 1993) can serve to better define the problem, identify the most vulnerable populations and the issues most important to address, and the best approaches for addressing sensitive topics, with a mind toward cultural sensitivity. Be Proud, Be Responsible uses culturally sensitive materials such as videotapes with multiethnic casts to achieve this goal. Involvement of the community will also aid in implementation, to the extent that researchers rely on community members for recruitment and retainment. In doing so, development of a sense of community ownership can lead to future community implementation when the research team is no longer present. Although the extent of community involvement is unclear from the reports of the four programs presented here, Teen Outreach tailors its volunteer program to the needs of the particular community to ensure greater sensitivity to community needs.

The use of multiple formats and methods (e.g., small group exercises and peer educators) that will keep the attention of adolescents will likely increase effectiveness (Kirby & DiClemente, 1994). Basic knowledge and information training, in combination with problem solving, decision making, and behavioral skills training, can be combined to provide the tools for change on multiple levels (Kirby & DiClemente, 1994). Furthermore, time-intensive interventions (Choi & Coates, 1994) are most likely to be effective, especially when combined with periodic booster sessions. Reducing the Risk, Teen Outreach, and PSIP each use time-intensive, multiple-component approaches to increase effectiveness, although none use periodic booster sessions.

The importance of family influences during early adolescence suggests that a family-based intervention would be most effective for primary prevention because individual factors can be addressed within the context of the family. An approach that fosters family communication both in general and with respect to sex will allow parents to reinforce their own values concerning sexuality and pass these values on to their children, as well as addressing issues of parental monitoring, supervision, and social support. Reducing the Risk attempts to include family by encouraging increased communication about sexuality with parents, although family members are not an integral part of the program. Recent initiatives funded by the National Institute of Mental Health (NIMH) will address these issues of family-based interventions and primary prevention in early and middle adolescents as well as other age groups with the NIMH Consortium of Family Grantees (W. Pequegnat, personal communication, July 23, 1996).

Peer influence is also a key concern to be addressed. Given the misperceptions that teens have about their peers' behavior, increasing awareness of actual attitudes and behaviors can serve to change community and peer norms for sexual behavior, including when and with whom it is appropriate to have sex and decreasing fears that teens may have about the consequences of suggesting condom use to their partners (Kelly et al., 1993). Reducing the Risk and PSIP are especially sensitive to peer influence. The latter uses older teen leaders as friends and mentors to illustrate that teens can postpone sex and still be respected in their peer group, whereas Reducing the Risk builds skills to resist peer influence and resets peer norms for sexual behavior.

Finally, evaluation of programming is of utmost importance to establishing which approaches and components are most effective in changing outcomes (Card et al., 1992; Choi & Coates, 1994; Kelly et al., 1993; Miller & Paikoff, 1992). All four of the programs described use some form of evaluation, but each has strengths and weaknesses. All four include control groups and pre- and posttest evaluations, although only Be Proud, Be Responsible and one trial of Teen Outreach are true experimental studies. To prevent the Hawthorne effect, Reducing the Risk and Be Proud, Be Responsible include alternative interventions for their control groups. Furthermore, only PSIP follows participants through the end of adolescence and uses external verification of outcomes.

In conclusion, if it is really the goal of *Healthy People 2000* (DHHS, 1991) to reduce the risk for adolescent pregnancy and HIV transmission, several criteria must be followed. First, prevention efforts must focus on reducing sexual risk taking through primary prevention (delaying the onset of sexual behavior) because preventive interventions have been much less successful with nonvirgins.

The only way to delay the onset of sexual intercourse is to start intervening early and focus on a broad range of variables. It is not sufficient to implement a program with 9- or 10-year-olds. Long-term follow-ups and booster sessions are required to address the changing nature of risk factors as youth progress developmentally through adolescence. Teen Outreach has demonstrated the specificity of intervention components at different ages, underscoring the need for developmental sensitivity in programming.

Second, primary prevention is not sufficient to reduce sexual risk taking. Secondary prevention efforts are also needed to ensure that sexually active adolescents are engaging in safer sex. Secondary preventive interventions need to focus on the contexts in which adolescents engage in risky behavior, and to address the barriers to safer sex. Cultural sensitivity is especially important in identifying such contexts and facilitating change. Finally, both primary and secondary prevention efforts need to be more methodologically rigorous. Experimental studies, including random assignment, pre- and posttest evaluation, and control groups who receive alternative programming, are imperative for valid evaluation. Only through carefully designed primary and secondary preventive intervention efforts can we hope to reach the goals of *Healthy People 2000*.

References

Alan Guttmacher Institute. (1994). *Sex and America's teenagers.* Washington, DC: Author.

Allen, J. P., Kuperminc, G., Philliber, S., & Herre, K. (1994). Programmatic prevention of adolescent problem behaviors: The role of autonomy, relatedness, and volunteer service in the Teen Outreach Program. *American Journal of Community Psychology, 22*, 617-638.

Allen, J. P., Philliber, S., Herrling, S., & Kuperminc, G. P. (1996). *Preventing teen pregnancy and academic failure: Experimental evaluation of a developmentally-based approach.* Manuscript submitted for publication.

Allen, J. P., Philliber, S., & Hoggson, N. (1990). School-based prevention of teen-age pregnancy and school dropout: Process evaluation of the national replication of the Teen Outreach Program. *American Journal of Community Psychology, 18*, 505-524.

Bachrach, C. A., Stolley, K. S., & London, K. A. (1992). Relinquishment of premarital births: Evidence from national survey data. *Family Planning Perspectives, 24*, 27-32.

Barth, R. P., Leland, N., Kirby, D., & Fetro, J. V. (1992). Enhancing social and cognitive skills. In B. C. Miller, J. J. Card, R. L. Paikoff, & J. L. Peterson (Eds.), *Preventing adolescent pregnancy* (pp. 53-82). Newbury Park, CA: Sage.

Berrueta-Clement, J., Schweinhart, L., Barnett, W., Weikart, D., & Epstein, A. (1984). *Changed lives: The effects of the Perry Preschool Programs on youths through age 19*. Ypsilanti, MI: High-Scope Educational Research Foundation.

Brooks-Gunn, J., Boyer, C. B., & Hein, K. (1988). Preventing HIV infection in children and adolescents: Behavioral research and intervention strategies. *American Psychologist, 43,* 958-964.

Brooks-Gunn, J., & Furstenberg, F. F. (1989). Adolescent sexual behavior. *American Psychologist, 44,* 249-257.

Brooks-Gunn, J., & Paikoff, R. L. (1993). "Sex is a gamble, kissing is a game": Adolescent sexuality and health promotion. In S. G. Millstein, A. C. Petersen, & E. O. Nightingale (Eds.), *Promoting the health of adolescents: New directions for the 21st century* (pp. 180-208). New York: Oxford University Press.

Brown, B. B. (1990). Peer groups and peer cultures. In S. Feldman & G. Elliott (Eds.), *At the threshold: The developing adolescent* (pp. 171-196). Cambridge, MA: Harvard University Press.

Card, J. J., Peterson, J. L., & Greeno, C. G. (1992). Adolescent pregnancy prevention programs: Design, monitoring, and evaluation. In B. C. Miller, J. J. Card, R. L. Paikoff, & J. L. Peterson (Eds.), *Preventing adolescent pregnancy* (pp. 1-27). Newbury Park, CA: Sage.

Centers for Disease Control and Prevention. (1992). Sexual behavior among high school students: United States, 1990. *Morbidity and Mortality Weekly Review, 40,* 885-888.

Centers for Disease Control and Prevention. (1995). *HIV/AIDS surveillance report* (Vol. 6). Atlanta, GA: Author.

Chase-Lansdale, P. L., & Brooks-Gunn, J. (in press). Correlates of adolescent pregnancy and parenthood. In C. B. Fisher & R. M. Lerner (Eds.), *Applied developmental psychology*. Cambridge, MA: McGraw-Hill.

Children's Defense Fund. (1996). *The state of America's children: Yearbook 1996*. Washington, DC: Author.

Choi, K., & Coates, T. J. (1994). Prevention of HIV infection. *AIDS, 8,* 1371-1389.

Christopherson, C. R., Miller, B. C., & Norton, M. C. (1994, February). *Pubertal development, parent/teen communication, and sexual values as predictors of adolescent sexual intentions and sexually related behaviors*. Paper presented at the Society for Research on Adolescence, San Diego.

DiClemente, R. J. (1992). Psychosocial determinants of condom use among adolescents. In R. J. DiClemente (Ed.), *Adolescents and AIDS: A generation in jeopardy* (pp. 34-51). Newbury Park, CA: Sage.

DiClemente, R. J., Durbin, M., Siegel, D., Krasnovsky, F., Lazarus, N., & Comacho, T. (1992). Determinants of condom use among junior high school students in a minority, inner-city school district. *Pediatrics, 89,* 197-202.

Dryfoos, J. G. (1990). *Adolescents at risk: Prevalence and prevention*. New York: Oxford University Press.

Durant, R. H., Seymore, C., Pendergrast, R., & Beckman, R. (1990). Contraceptive behavior among sexually active Hispanic adolescents. *Journal of Adolescent Health Care, 11,* 490-496.

Edwards, L., Steinman, M., Arnold, K., & Hakanson, E. (1980). Adolescent pregnancy prevention services in high school clinics. *Family Planning Perspectives, 12,* 6-14.

Fischoff, B., Bostrom, A., & Quadrel, M. J. (1993). Risk perception and communication. *Annual Review of Public Health, 14,* 183-203.

Fisher, J. D. (1988). Possible effects of reference group-based social influence on AIDS-risk behavior and AIDS prevention. *American Psychologist, 43,* 914-920.

Fleming, M. (1996). *Healthy youth 2000: A mid-decade review.* Chicago: American Medical Association, Department of Adolescent Health.

Ford, K., Rubinstein, S., & Norris, A. (1994). Sexual behavior and condom use among urban, low-income, African-American and Hispanic youth. *AIDS Education and Prevention, 6,* 219-229.

Furby, L., & Beyth-Marom, R. (1992). Risk taking in adolescence: A decision making perspective. *Developmental Review, 12,* 1-44.

Furstenberg, F. F., Jr., & Brooks-Gunn, J. (1985). Adolescent fertility: Causes, consequences, and remedies. In L. Aiken & D. Mechanic (Eds.), *Applications of social science to clinical medicine and health policy.* New Brunswick, NJ: Rutgers University Press.

Galavotti, C., & Lovick, C. (1989). School-based clinic use and other factors affecting adolescent contraceptive behavior. *Journal of Adolescent Health Care, 10,* 506-512.

Hayes, C. D. (Ed.). (1987). *Risking the future: Adolescent sexuality, pregnancy, and childbearing* (Vol. 1). Washington, DC: National Academy Press.

Hein, K. (1989). AIDS in adolescence: Exploring the challenge. *Journal of Adolescent Health Care, 10,* 10S-35S.

Henshaw, S. K. (1992). Abortion trends in 1987 and 1988: Age and race. *Family Planning Perspectives, 24,* 85-86.

Hill, J. P., & Holmbeck, G. N. (1986). Attachment and autonomy during adolescence. *Annals of Child Development, 3,* 145-189.

Hofferth, S. L., & Hayes, C. D. (Eds.). (1987). *Risking the future: Adolescent sexuality, pregnancy, and childbearing* (Vol. 2). Washington, DC: National Academy Press.

Hofferth, S. L., & Moore, K. A. (1979). Early childbearing and later economic well-being. *American Sociological Review, 44,* 784-815.

Howard, M., & McCabe, J. A. (1990). Helping teenagers postpone sexual involvement. *Family Planning Perspectives, 22,* 21-26.

Howard, M., & McCabe, J. A. (1992). An information skills approach for younger teens: Postponing sexual involvement program. In B. C. Miller, J. J. Card, R. L. Paikoff, & J. L. Peterson (Eds.), *Preventing adolescent pregnancy* (pp. 83-109). Newbury Park, CA: Sage.

Howard, M., & Mitchell, M. E. (1990). *Postponing sexual involvement: An educational series for preteens.* Atlanta, GA: Grady Memorial Hospital, Emory/Grady Teen Services Program.

Hunter-Geboy, C., Peterson, L., Casey, S., Hardy, L., & Renner, S. (1985). *Life planning education: A youth development program.* Washington, DC: Center for Population Options.

Inazu, J. K., & Fox, G. L. (1980). Maternal influences on the sexual behavior of teenage daughters. *Journal of Family Issues, 1,* 81-102.

Irwin, C. E., Jr., Shafer, M. A., & Millstein, S. G. (1985). Pubertal development in adolescent females: A marker for early sexual debut [Abstract]. *Pediatric Research, 19,* 112A.

Jarrett, R. L. (1995). Growing up poor: The family experiences of socially mobile youth in low-income African American neighborhoods. *Journal of Adolescent Research, 10,* 111-135.

Jemmott, J. B., III, Jemmott, L. S., & Fong, G. T. (1992). Reductions in HIV risk-associated sexual behaviors among Black male adolescents: Effects of an AIDS prevention intervention. *American Journal of Public Health, 82,* 372-377.

Jessor, R., & Jessor, S. L. (1977). *Problem behavior and psychosocial development.* New York: Academy Press.

Jollah, M., & Alston, S. (1988, November). *Mantalk: A pregnancy prevention program for teen males.* Paper presented at the annual meeting of the American Public Health Association, Boston.

Jones, E., Forrest, J. D., Henshaw, S., Silverman, J., & Torres, A. (1988). Unintended pregnancy, contraceptive practice and family planning services in developed countries. *Family Planning Perspectives, 20,* 53-67.

Kann, L., Warren, C. W., Harris, W. A., Collins, J. L., Douglas, K. A., Collins, M. E., Williams, B. I., Ross, J. G., Kolbe, L. J., & State & Local YRBSS Coordinators. (1995). Youth risk behavior surveillance: United States, 1993. *Morbidity and Mortality Weekly Review, 44,* 1-55.

Kegeles, S. M., Adler, N. E., & Irwin, C. E., Jr. (1988). Sexually active adolescents and condoms: Changes over one year in knowledge, attitudes and use. *American Journal of Public Health, 78,* 460-461.

Keller, S. E., Bartlett, J. A., Schleifer, S. J., Johnson, R. L., Pinner, E. & Delaney, B. (1991). HIV-relevant sexual behavior among a healthy inner-city heterosexual population in an endemic area of HIV. *Journal of Adolescent Health, 12,* 44-48.

Kelly, J. A., Murphy, D. A., Sikkema, K. J., & Kalichman, S. C. (1993). Psychological interventions to prevent HIV infection are urgently needed: New priorities for behavioral research in the second decade of AIDS. *American Psychologist, 48,* 1023-1034.

Ketterlinus, R. D., Henderson, S. H., & Lamb, M. E. (1990). Maternal age, sociodemographics, prenatal health and behavior: Influences on neonatal risk status. *Journal of Adolescent Health Care, 11,* 423-431.

Kirby, D., Barth, R. P., Leland, N., & Fetro, J. V. (1991). Reducing the risk: Impact of a new curriculum on sexual risk-taking. *Family Planning Perspectives, 23,* 253-263.

Kirby, D., & DiClemente, R. J. (1994). School-based interventions to prevent unprotected sex and HIV among adolescents. In R. J. DiClemente & J. L. Peterson (Eds.), *Preventing AIDS: Theories and methods of behavioral interventions* (pp. 117-139). New York: Plenum.

Leigh, B. C., Morrison, D. M., Trocki, K., & Temple, M. T. (1994). Sexual behavior of American adolescents: Results from a U.S. national survey. *Journal of Adolescent Health, 15,* 117-125.

Leland, N. L., & Barth, R. P. (1993). Characteristics of adolescents who have attempted to avoid HIV and who have communicated with parents about sex. *Journal of Adolescent Research, 8,* 58-76.

Levy, S. R., Handler, A. S., Weeks, K., Lampman, C., Flay, B. R., & Rashid, J. (1994). Adolescent risk for HIV as viewed by youth and their parents. *Family Community Health, 17,* 30-41.

Levy, S. R., Handler, A. S., Weeks, K., Lampman, C., Perhats, C., Miller, T. Q., & Flay, B. R. (1995). Correlates of HIV risk among young adolescents in a metropolitan midwestern center. *Journal of School Health, 65,* 28-32.

Levy, S. R., Lampman, C., Handler, A., Flay, B. R., & Weeks, K. (1993). Young adolescent attitudes towards sex and substance use: Implications for AIDS prevention. *AIDS Education and Prevention, 5,* 340-351.

Levy, S. R., Perhats, C., Weeks, K., Handler, A. S., Zhu, C., & Flay, B. R. (1995). Impact of a school-based AIDS prevention program on risk and protective behavior on newly sexually active students. *Journal of School Health, 65,* 145-151.

Lewis, C. E., & Lewis, M. A. (1984). Peer pressure and risk taking behaviors in children. *American Journal of Public Health, 74,* 580-584.

Males, M. A., & Chew, K. S. Y. (1996). The ages of fathers in California adolescent births, 1993. *American Journal of Public Health, 86,* 565-568.

McCormick, M. C., & Brooks-Gunn, J. (1989). The health of children and adolescents. In H. E. Freeman & S. Levine (Eds.), *Handbook of medical sociology* (pp. 347-380). Englewood Cliffs, NJ: Prentice Hall.

McLoyd, V. C. (1990). The impact of economic hardship on black families and their children: Psychological distress, parenting, and socioemotional development. *Child Development, 61,* 311-346.

Miller, B. C., & Paikoff, R. L. (1992). Comparing adolescent pregnancy prevention programs: Methods and results. In B. C. Miller, J. J. Card, R. L. Paikoff, & J. L. Peterson (Eds.), *Preventing adolescent pregnancy* (pp. 265-284). Newbury Park, CA: Sage.

Miller, B. C., Card, J. J., Paikoff, R. L., & Peterson, J. L. (Eds.). (1992). *Preventing adolescent pregnancy.* Newbury Park, CA: Sage.

Millstein, S. G., Moscicki, A. B., & Broering, J. M. (1994). Female adolescents at high, moderate, and low risk for exposure to HIV: Differences in knowledge, beliefs, and behavior. *Journal of Adolescent Health, 15,* 133-142.

Moore, D. S., & Erickson, P. I. (1985). Age, gender, and ethnic differences in sexual and contraceptive knowledge, attitudes, and behavior. *Family and Community Health, 8,* 38-51.

Moore, K. A., Sugland, B. W., Blumenthal, C., Glei, D., & Snyder, N. (1995). *Adolescent pregnancy prevention programs: Interventions and evaluations.* Washington, DC: Child Trends.

Mrazek, P. J., & Haggerty, R. J. (Eds). (1994). *Reducing risks for mental disorders: Frontiers for preventive intervention research.* Washington, DC: National Academy Press.

Newcomer, S. F., & Udry, J. R. (1985). Parent child communication and adolescent sexual behavior. *Family Planning Perspectives, 17,* 169-174.

Nicholson, H. J., & Postrado, L. T. (1992). A comprehensive age-phased approach: Girls Incorporated. In B. C. Miller, J. J. Card, R. L. Paikoff, & J. L. Peterson (Eds.), *Preventing adolescent pregnancy* (pp. 110-138). Newbury Park, CA: Sage.

Oakley, A., Fullerton, D., & Holland, J. (1995). Behavioural interventions for HIV/AIDS prevention. *AIDS, 9,* 479-486.

Paikoff, R. L. (1995). Early heterosexual debut: Situations of sexual possibility during the transition to adolescence. *American Journal of Orthopsychiatry, 65,* 389-401.

Parfenoff, S. H., Paikoff, R. L., Brooks-Gunn, J., Holmbeck, G. N., & Jarrett, R. L. (1995). *Early sexual behavior and the risk for HIV/AIDS in early adolescence: The contribution of family and contextual factors.* Manuscript submitted for publication.

Philliber, S., & Allen, J. P. (1992). Life options and community service: Teen outreach program. In B. C. Miller, J. J. Card, R. L. Paikoff, & J. L. Peterson (Eds.), *Preventing adolescent pregnancy* (pp. 139-155). Newbury Park, CA: Sage.

Pittman, K., & Govan, C. (1986). *Model programs: Preventing adolescent pregnancy and building youth self-sufficiency.* Washington, DC: Children's Defense Fund.

Rosenthal, M. B. (1993). Adolescent pregnancy. In D. E. Stewart & N. L. Stotland (Eds.), *Psychological aspects of women's health care: The interface between psychiatry and obstetrics and gynecology.* Washington, DC: American Psychiatric Press.

Schinke, S., & Gilchrist, L. (1984). *Life skills counseling with adolescents.* Baltimore: University Park Press.

Sipe, C., Grossman, J., & Milliner, J. (1988). *Summer training and education program (STEP): Report on the 1987 experience.* Philadelphia: Public/Private Ventures.

Sonenstein, F. L., Pleck, J. H., & Ku, L. C. (1989). Sexual activity, condom use and AIDS awareness among adolescent males. *Family Planning Perspectives, 21,* 151-158.

Spencer, M. B., & Dornbusch, S. M. (1990). Challenges in studying minority youth. In S. Feldman & G. Elliott (Eds.), *At the threshold: The developing adolescent* (pp. 123-146). Cambridge, MA: Harvard University Press.

Stanton, B., Li, X., Black, M., Ricardo, I., Galbraith, J., Kaljee, L., & Feigelman, S. (1994). Sexual practices and intentions among preadolescent and early adolescent low-income urban African-Americans. *Pediatrics, 93,* 966-973.

Stattin, H., & Magnusson, D. (1990). *Pubertal maturation in female development.* Hillsdale, NJ: Lawrence Erlbaum.

Steinberg, L. D. (1990). Autonomy, conflict, and harmony in the family relationship. In S. Feldman & G. Elliott (Eds.), *At the threshold: The developing adolescent* (pp. 255-276). Cambridge, MA: Harvard University Press.

Stern, M. (1988). Evaluation of a school-based pregnancy prevention program. *TEC Newsletter, 19,* 5-8.

St. Lawrence, J. S. (1993). African American adolescents' knowledge, health-related attitudes, sexual behavior, and contraceptive decisions: Implications for the prevention of adolescent HIV. *Journal of Consulting and Clinical Psychology, 61,* 104-112.

St. Lawrence, J. S., Brasfield, T. L., Jefferson, K. W., Alleyne, E., O'Bannon, R. E., & Shirley, A. (1995). Cognitive-behavioral intervention to reduce African American adolescents' risk for HIV infection. *Journal of Consulting and Clinical Psychology, 63,* 221-237.

Thornburg, H. D. (1978). Adolescents sources of initial sex information. *Psychiatric Annals, 8,* 419-423.

U. S. Department of Health and Human Services, Public Health Service. (1991). *Healthy people 2000: National health promotion and disease prevention objectives* (DHHS Publication No. PHS 91-50212). Washington, DC: U.S. Government Printing Office.

U. S. Department of Health and Human Services, Public Health Service. (1995). *Healthy people 2000: Midcourse review and 1995 revisions.* Washington, DC: U.S. Government Printing Office.

Upchurch, D. M., & McCarthy, J. (1990). The timing of a first birth and high school completion. *American Sociological Review, 55,* 224-234.

Walter, H. J., & Vaughan, R. D. (1993). AIDS risk reduction among a multiethnic sample of urban high school students. *Journal of the American Medical Association, 270,* 725-730.

Walter, H. J., Vaughan, R. D., Ragin, D. F., Cohall, A. T., & Kasen, S. (1994). Prevalence and correlates of AIDS-related behavioral intentions among urban minority high school students. *AIDS Education and Prevention, 6,* 339-350.

Weisman, C. S., Nathanson, C. A., Ensminger, M., Teitelbaum, M. A., Robinson, J. C., & Plichta, S. (1989). AIDS knowledge, perceived risk and prevention among adolescent clients of a family planning clinic. *Family Planning Perspectives, 21,* 213-217.

Zabin, L., & Hirsch, M. (1987). *Evaluation of pregnancy prevention programs in the school context.* Lexington, MA: Lexington.

Zabin, L., Hirsch, M., Smith, E., Streett, R., & Hardy, J. (1986). Evaluation of a pregnancy prevention program for urban teenagers. *Family Planning Perspectives, 18,* 119-126.

• *CHAPTER 5* •

Violence Prevention for the 21st Century

MARY E. MURRAY
NANCY G. GUERRA
KIRK R. WILLIAMS

Although the United States is recognized for leading the world in public health and other scientific advances, it is also known for leading the industrialized world in violent death rates, with homicide and suicide accounting for more than 50,000 deaths annually. In addition, 2.2 million people are injured each year by violent assaults (U.S. Department of Health and Human Services, Public Health Service [DHHS], 1995). These rates serve as indicators of a public health crisis that affects all segments of the population, with recent violent crime rates hovering at the highest levels of the past three decades. Of particular concern are the escalating rates of youth violence. For example, from 1985 to 1994, the homicide rates of youth ages 14 to 17 increased by 172% (Fox, 1996).

The increase in youth violence is primarily attributable to an increase in the *lethality* and not the *frequency* of violent acts. Indeed, about the same proportion of youth is committing violent offenses today as in 1980, and the frequency of offending is quite comparable (Elliott, 1994). Changed is the lethality of these crimes. A much larger proportion of these crimes involves handguns and results in serious injury or death. If current trends continue, the death rate from firearms will surpass that of motor crashes by the year 2003 (DHHS, 1995). Furthermore, rates of serious violent crimes have risen sharply for both African American and White males, but not for females. Given that the population of teenage males is projected to increase by approximately 20% during the next decade, these trends can be expected only to worsen.

It is clear that the challenge for the future is how best to prevent violence, particularly lethal violence, among teenage males. *Healthy People 2000* objectives list six broad areas of concern for reduction of violence related to (a) homicide and assaultive violence, (b) domestic violence, (c) maltreatment of children under age 18, (d) rape and attempted rape, (e) suicide, and (f) firearm injury (DHHS, 1991). In addition, specific risk reduction and services and protection objectives that relate to these broad goals are detailed. For example, these objectives include calls for (a) the reduction of physical fighting among adolescents aged 14 through 17, (b) the reduction of weapon carrying by adolescents aged 14 through 17, and (c) an increase in health education curricula that address conflict resolution and related skills intended to decrease violent and abusive behavior. Many of the objectives of *Healthy People 2000* relate directly to the issue of youth violence and the need for an effective prevention response aimed at the most lethal forms of violence.

To date, there has been a proliferation of prevention programs but relatively little conclusive data regarding their impact, particularly in broad-based strategies for communitywide programming. Efforts also have been hampered by a number of pertinent issues. These include how to determine the "clinical" or real-world significance of changes in correlates of violence, including age-typical antisocial behaviors; the lack of specificity of program impact for specific types of violence (e.g., relationship violence versus predatory violence); the extent to which intervention effects are moderated by other microlevel and macrolevel factors; and limitations of evaluation measures and methods. Of particular importance are the shortcomings of risk-focused approaches to prevention that have virtually dominated the field during the last decade and the need to situate comprehensive violence prevention strategies in an interdisciplinary framework that is sensitive to the dynamics of human development in multiple social settings through time.

In this chapter, we first review the existing literature on violence prevention programs for children and youth. This review is intended not to be comprehensive but rather to provide a perch from which to assess how best to define and accomplish violence prevention goals for the 21st century.[1] Because most previous efforts have been directed at preventing or reducing identified risk factors for aggression and violence, we review outcomes studies that relate to specific areas of risk across major developmental periods. We highlight issues of clinical significance (in other words, will programs likely affect serious and/or lethal violence), outcome specificity, moderator effects, and evaluation concerns, followed by a more in-depth discussion of these issues as they relate to future directions.

Following this programmatic review, we revisit the strengths and limitations of a risk-focused approach to violence prevention. We propose an alternative model that builds on the contributions of the risk-focused framework but goes beyond its limitations. This model emphasizes life course development and situates violence in a broader, dynamic framework of human development. By casting violence as a negative developmental outcome, prevention efforts can be geared toward promoting healthy human development via direct services to individuals as well as by reforming the systems and settings in which development unfolds. Finally, we review and critique the violence prevention goals of *Healthy People 2000* as they relate to the empirical and theoretical perspectives presented and make recommendations for linking goals and strategies within a broader developmental model.

Overview of Preventive Interventions

During the past several decades, a variety of preventive interventions have been implemented and evaluated. These interventions range from prenatal attempts to decrease risk factors such as low birth weight to interventions that teach incarcerated youth alternative thinking strategies in an attempt to reduce recidivism. In many cases, pertinent data have been garnered from interventions that were not originally designed as violence prevention programs but that addressed relevant risk factors and later have been evaluated for impact on youth violence. Because risk factors and contexts vary by age, the review is organized developmentally.

Pre- and Postnatal Service to Families

Pre- and postnatal interventions address the earliest stages of a child's development. These interventions frequently involve the prevention of childhood problems associated with poor maternal health (such as low birth weight and birth trauma) and inadequate pre- and postnatal care (including a variety of early childhood disorders). At these earliest stages of development, a child's risk is inextricably linked to the mother's or caretaker's behavior and well-being. Thus, these interventions provide educational and support services to mothers with known risk factors such as poverty, young age, or single-parent status.

One frequently cited example of this type of program is the University of Rochester Nurse-Home Visitation Program (Olds, Henderson, Tatelbaum, & Chamberlin, 1986), which provided expectant mothers with home visits from a nurse during the prenatal period until the child's second birthday. The intervention and its immediate aims varied at different points in the child's development. Early home visits included parent education about basic health and nutrition during pregnancy. After the child's birth, parent education focused more on infant development and also included assistance in building support networks and using other health and human service programs.

The intervention had significant short-term effects on maternal and child health. When compared with a similar group of mothers who received only minimal services, mothers in the intervention group experienced more positive health-related outcomes, higher levels of employment, and fewer verifiable cases of child abuse and neglect. Reducing child maltreatment is a goal of *Healthy People 2000* and should be affected by this type of program. In addition, because early maltreatment is a risk factor for later violence and delinquency, such programs may be useful preventive strategies for adolescent violence. This project, however, was primarily concerned with decreasing reliance on welfare, and no long-term outcome data on serious youth violence are available.

A similar program for mothers raising children in high-risk environments, the Yale Child Welfare Research Program, was carried out by Provence and Naylor (1983). This intervention provided prenatal and early infancy home visits by a social worker, who offered a range of medical, financial, and support services. These services were based on the premise that parental stress can impede family functioning, in turn hindering the development of socially adjusted behaviors in children. Ten years after receiving services, intervention mothers were more likely to report a positive emotional atmosphere in the family and were more involved in their children's education than were mothers in a control group. In addition, intervention children were rated less aggressive and less disruptive in class by teachers. These results point toward the positive impact of infant programs on family functioning and the long-term consequences of early intervention in the prevention of aggression. Still, the impact of such programs on serious and/or lethal youth violence has not been established, and it is unlikely that such early programs alone will be sufficient.

Preschool Enrichment Programs

A number of interventions have attempted to provide preschool enrichment, particularly to economically disadvantaged and minority children. The most well known of these enrichment programs is Head Start. In its original form, Head Start consisted of a brief summer preschool experience just prior to kindergarten. The program has since evolved to include family services and now lasts longer. This intervention has resulted in short-term intellectual and social gains for participants (Darlington, Royce, Snipper, Murray, & Lazar, 1980; Lee, Brooks-Gunn, Schnur, & Liaw, 1990).

Two landmark preschool enrichment studies, the Perry Preschool Project and the Houston Parent-Child Development Center, have reported encouraging results using an intensive, well-articulated preschool program. Both projects used random assignment to condition and collected extensive follow-up data. The Perry Preschool Project provided 1 to 2 years of academically oriented preschool education accompanied by frequent home visits and parent meetings. When compared with a nonintervention control group, intervention children displayed lower levels of mental retardation, dropping out of school, and reliance on welfare. In addition, they received better grades; scored better on standardized achievement tests; and had better high school graduation rates, higher employment, fewer acts of misconduct, and lower arrest rates (Berrueta-Clement, Schweinhart, Barnett, Epstein, & Weikart, 1984; Schweinhart & Weikart, 1988).

Similarly, follow-up studies of children in the Houston Parent-Child Development Program have indicated sustained behavior improvements as measured by reductions in aggression in elementary school (Johnson, 1988; Johnson & Walker, 1987). Still, even these promising results are clouded by concerns such as small sample size and high attrition rates. Although short-term academic gains can be established, their relation to long-term changes in serious adolescent violence is unclear, particularly given the multiple developmental influences that affect children during the early and middle school years.

Another approach to preschool intervention emphasizes building social competencies. For example, the Interpersonal Cognitive Problem-Solving Skills training program designed by Spivack, Shure, and their colleagues (Spivack, Platt, & Shure, 1976; Spivack & Shure, 1974) consists of a series of lessons that focuses primarily on teaching children to generate and evaluate multiple solutions to everyday social problems. Two-year follow-up studies revealed a resulting improvement in cognitive skills and classroom behavior. Replication studies, however, failed to find the same impact on behavioral outcomes (Rickel & Burgio, 1982; Rickel & Lampi, 1981). Thus, these data suggest that through appropriate intervention, preschool skills associated with nondelinquent behavior, such as the ability to generate various solutions to social problems, can be taught. It is unclear, however, if this produces long-term changes in relevant behavioral outcomes, particularly as related to more serious violent behavior later in development.

Interventions During the Elementary School Years

As children grow older, their exposure to multiple contexts increases, and the etiology of violence becomes more complex. Although the family continues to play a key role in development, the school now becomes a primary socialization context, and the influence of the peer group increases. Relevant variables for this age group include academic and social development, relations with family members and peers, and the ability to behave appropriately in an increasing number of contexts. This diversity of risk factors and salient contexts is reflected in the diversity of interventions used with this age group. Some interventions are predominantly child centered and skill based, addressing the skills and competencies directly through instructional interventions. Other programs address these skills indirectly by educating teachers and parents about how to manage children's behavior and enhance relationships. Although some programs have demonstrated modest gains in targeted competencies, others have been less successful, and results have been discouraging in the most disadvantaged urban settings.

For example, in a study comparing the effects of social problem-solving training for suburban versus inner-city children, Weissberg, Gesten, Rapkin, et al. (1981) provided both groups of children with a 52-session social problem-solving training program. In addition, 6 parent training sessions were offered to reinforce children's skills. Although the suburban middle-class children outperformed control children on a number of cognitive and behavioral skills, the inner-city children actually got worse on some measures and displayed increased aggression. In a second study (Weissberg, Gesten, Carnrike, et al., 1981), a modified social problem-solving training program found uniformly positive effects for both suburban and urban children. The authors attributed these differential results to an improved curriculum, a more timely implementation (earlier in the school year), and an increased emphasis on teacher reinforcement of the curriculum in the handling of everyday conflicts.

A more recent study compared the impact of a similar social development training program for elementary school children in inner-city schools rated as adequate or distressed (Guerra, Eron, Huesmann, Tolan, & Van Acker, 1996). The program was also comprehensive and involved teacher training, classroom instruction, peer relations training, and family intervention. Significant reductions in aggression and increases in prosocial behavior were noted only in the schools rated adequate, with no effects in the most distressed schools (Guerra, Henry, Tolan, Huesmann, & Eron, 1996).

These studies point to the importance of setting as a moderator of intervention effects. Several studies that have examined intervention effects as a function of location, social class, and/or ethnicity suggest that program impact is not uniform. Elementary school interventions designed to build social competencies tend to be least effective for lower-class, urban minority children in the most disadvantaged environments (Coie, Underwood, & Lochman, 1991; DuBow, Huesmann, & Eron, 1987; Hawkins, Von Cleve, & Catalano, 1991). Thus, it seems that no one intervention is ideal for all populations in all contexts. It may be that prevention programs are most difficult to develop and implement in the most disorganized settings and that repeated implementations with appropriate modifications are needed to increase effectiveness (Coie et al., 1991; Weissberg, Caplan, & Harwood, 1991).

In addition to child-centered intervention strategies aimed at altering cognitive, social, and academic skills (that may include training parents to help in the process), a number of interventions have focused primarily on training parents of elementary school children in child management and family relations. Perhaps the most well known approach is behavioral parent training aimed at reducing negative parenting and coercive interactions. Several studies have reported decreases in children's antisocial behavior following intervention (Patterson, 1986; Patterson, Reid, & Dishion, 1992; Wahler & Dumas, 1987). More recent studies have also examined how environmental constraints modify or limit intervention effects. For example, Wahler and Dumas (1989) report that the overwhelming demands single mothers face can produce quicker relapses to old child-rearing methods, even after successful completion of parent training. Thus, external stress can limit the effectiveness of family interventions.

An additional issue that surfaces during the elementary school years is whether and how to identify selected children for targeted preventive interventions. One strategy is to provide a *universal* intervention for all children in a classroom or school. Although populations can be selected on the basis of certain risk factors (e.g., poverty), this method cannot be sensitive to differences in individual factors and/or potential differential effects of the intervention. Overall, it is assumed that what is provided is likely to help everyone and not hurt anyone. It is unlikely, however, that such programs will produce dramatic change or affect the more extremely aggressive children, and evaluations of universal interventions have paid little attention to their differential effects.

An alternate approach has been to identify children on the basis of some marker of at-risk status, often concurrent level of aggression. *Selected* programs attempt to reduce prevalence at a given time to prevent future involvement, and *indicated* programs target youth already involved in serious antisocial behavior (Gordon, 1983). This strategy has the advantage of allowing for more intensive and focused services for youth who are more troubled. Although behavior during the elementary years is among the best predictors of later behavior, it is still only a weak predictor, however, and many children desist on their own. Therefore, interventions are provided for children who may not need them. This clearly points to the need to be quite vigilant about examining any possible iatrogenic or harmful effects of particular programs.

In summary, research has not suggested a single best approach to identifying and intervening with elementary school children to prevent youth violence. Many different approaches have displayed some success, however. Programs that directly teach specific social and cognitive skills while including parents and teachers as participants in this process have proved successful for some populations. Improving relationships between parents and children has also proved promising. Concerns about clinical significance for more disruptive children, iatrogenic effects, and potential moderators of intervention impact must be addressed for this age group.

Programs for Adolescents

Although some universal programs have been provided for adolescents, prevention efforts for this age group tend to become more targeted because of the marked increase in identified problem behavior incidents (e.g., arrests for delinquent acts). Most interventions for adolescents have been carried out as treatment programs, often involving adjudicated or incarcerated youth (for a review, see Guerra, Tolan, & Hammond, 1994). Unfortunately, as children get older, the magnitude of effects found for such preventive interventions decreases, with evidence suggesting mean effect sizes of about 0.2 (see Tremblay & Craig, 1995).

Universal interventions most frequently involve either skill training programs or efforts to modify the classroom or school environment. In one example of a skill-training program, Sarason and Sarason (1981) implemented a 13-week social problem-solving training program as part of the curriculum in an urban high school. When compared with no-treatment controls, students who received the intervention exhibited fewer absences and decreases in office referrals for inappropriate behavior along with increased social problem-solving skills. The impact on serious violent behavior was not assessed, however, and long-term follow-up evaluations were not conducted. To date, there is little conclusive evidence to support the use of classroom-based curricula for prevention of serious adolescent violence.

Other attempts have focused on modifying school environment. For example, the School Transitional Environmental Program (STEP) involved reorganizing the school social system in the first year of high school to involve students in a stable peer group (Felner & Adan, 1988). Homeroom teachers were then assigned to act as primary administrators and counselors for particular groups of students. In one set of follow-up studies, students in the STEP program showed lower dropout rates and fewer placements into programs for failing students. They also showed higher grades and fewer absences than did a control group during the first 2 years of high school. Replication studies demonstrated impact on behavioral dysfunction and delinquent behavior.

Gottfredson (1986, 1987) and colleagues have engaged in systematic efforts to alter school organization and management structures in a number of middle schools and high schools. Such programs emphasized efforts to increase participation in school improvement efforts, develop clear disciplinary procedures, and provide activities to enhance students' success experiences and feelings of belonging. Several studies have shown improvements in school climate and decreases in delinquency, with programs being most effective at the high school level (Gottfredson, 1986; Gottfredson, Gottfredson, & Hybl, 1993).

Among the more well known school reform programs affecting adolescents are the efforts undertaken in Norway by Olweus (1994) and colleagues. On the basis of studies suggesting that a select group of adolescent bullies repeatedly target other teenagers, a program was developed to alter environmental norms about bullying. The program included a large-scale campaign and efforts to change school practices. Because the campaign was nationwide, investigators were able to compare only pretest and posttest data, although dosage was available as a variable. Results indicated that reductions in bullying did occur and were directly related to intervention dosage.

Although there is some evidence for the effectiveness of schoolwide or communitywide programming on problem behavior, research designs are weaker than studies of individual behavior, and effects on serious violence have not been established. These programs may be useful in establishing a normative structure for behavior, but youth with more serious behavior problems may warrant more intensive, individualized programs.

Modest success has also been demonstrated with targeted programs for more serious offenders. For example, Guerra and Slaby (1990) conducted a controlled evaluation study with juveniles incarcerated for violent crimes. Small groups that focused on changing the beliefs and attitudes about the legitimacy of violent responses to conflict were conducted. Participants in the treatment group exhibited decreases in aggression after the intervention, when compared with no-treatment and attention-only control groups.

A growing body of evidence supports the effectiveness of intensive family interventions. The work of Patterson (1982, 1986) and colleagues (Patterson, Chamberlain, & Reid, 1982), discussed previously, has also been extended to adolescents. More recently, Henggeler (1989) and associates (Henggeler & Borduin, 1990) have developed a comprehensive family intervention for serious juvenile offenders. This program, Multisystemic Family Therapy (MST), focuses on improving parent practices and family cohesion as well as helping the family develop skills to address external demands. In several experimental studies using random assignment to condition, MST participants reported less delinquent behavior and had fewer subsequent arrests and fewer weeks of subsequent incarceration.

Of course, it would be shortsighted to discuss current status and future directions for prevention of serious youth violence without addressing the influence of the antisocial peer group and, in particular, juvenile gangs. Because of the well-documented influence of antisocial peers on youth violence, a number of interventions have targeted directly these peer group influences. Such programs frequently provide some type of group therapy or structured group program, often with the goal of restructuring peer interactions to increase conformity to prosocial norms. Many programs have been modeled on the Guided Group Interaction technique. Many of these programs have demonstrated no effects or negative effects on antisocial behavior when groups were composed of only problem youth; some decreases in antisocial behavior have been reported, however, when delinquent and nondelinquent youth were in mixed groups (Feldman, 1992; Gottfredson, 1987). As this suggests, the impact of group interventions may be related directly to moderating factors such as the composition of the treatment group.

Given the magnitude of the juvenile gang problem and its association with the most lethal forms of youth violence, the paucity of effective strategies in this area is alarming. Gang prevention programs have been implemented and evaluated since the 1930s, with few positive outcomes. In particular, single-component programs such as "detached street worker" models or suppression programs have not been successful. Rather, the most promising recent efforts are multicomponent, combining prevention, social intervention, treatment, suppression, and community mobilization in a coordinated effort conducted by community collaborations (Spergel, 1986).

Although not directly related to peer group influences, a number of youth involvement programs have been designed to provide youth with positive role models. Among the most promising programs are mentoring programs. In most such programs, the goals are to assist youth in developing skills and to provide sustained relationships with more experienced persons who serve as mentors. A recent comprehensive evaluation of the Big Brothers/Big Sisters mentoring program conducted by Public/Private Ventures (1995) suggests that a positive mentoring relationship relates to reductions in self-reported behaviors such as hitting and substance use. The most successful programs are also those that provide positive real-life experiences including training to help youth find and keep regular jobs.

Summary of Research on Preventive Interventions

In summary, youth violence prevention programs cover a broad range of activities at different developmental stages. There is little evidence to support striking effects for any one program or type of program. Rather, this review points to the questions researchers should be asking as we evaluate preventive interventions in the coming century and set directions for *Healthy People 2010*. Several major areas of concern were noted in this review and are again discussed briefly.

Key Issues in Evaluating Preventive Interventions

As mentioned earlier, our ability to draw conclusions about the impact of preventive interventions on serious youth violence is limited by several concerns. First, it is important to consider the issue of clinical significance of effects vis-à-vis the ultimate goal of preventing serious and lethal violence. Because some types of aggression are both frequent and age-typical, it is unlikely that reductions in this behavior, (i.e., for the less seriously aggressive children) will have any bearing on more lethal forms of violence. Clearly, aggressive behavior correlates with and predicts later violent behavior, but most aggressive children do not become involved in serious violence. Rather, we must distinguish the impact of prevention programs on the most extremely aggressive children, even if programs are implemented as universal interventions for all children.

A related issue concerns timing of interventions. As the previous review illustrates, violence prevention programs have ranged from postnatal to adolescent interventions. Given limited community resources, however, it is unclear where best to direct efforts. Because serious violent behavior peaks during adolescence and is usually short-lived (between 1 and 3 years), it is difficult to establish long-term benefits on this serious violence of programs offered during infancy and early childhood. Clearly, such programs are important from a youth development perspective, but their long-term impact, if not followed by other preventive strategies, is unclear.

In addition to addressing issues of timing, we must also distinguish intervention effects for different types of violence. Previous reviews of interventions have distinguished between four major types of violence: situational, relationship, predatory, and psychopathological (Tolan & Guerra, 1994b). Situational violence occurs in response to temporary events, such as extreme heat and riots, and reflects situational factors that increase an individual's willingness to use violence or increase the seriousness of the violence that occurs. Relationship violence arises from disputes between persons in relationships. Predatory violence is perpetrated intentionally to obtain personal gain, such as muggings and robbery. A more extreme form of violence, psychopathological violence, is characterized by extreme violence and is most likely the result of individual pathology.

Certain interventions should affect certain types of violence but not necessarily affect other types of violence. For example, conflict resolution training should have the greatest effect on interpersonal violence because such behavior arises from conflicts or disputes between individuals. It is unlikely to affect predatory violence, however, because such violence is not related to any preexisting conflict; it is unlikely that the perpetrator even knows his or her victim. Rather than treating *violence* as a global term encompassing any and all forms, future directions should aim at specifying types of violence and likely impact of related interventions.

Even if we were to focus specifically on one type of violence, in any case it is also naive to think that one program would work equally well for all participants. It is critical that intervention evaluations begin to examine carefully the proposed moderators of impact. As discussed previously, several studies have examined these effects and have illuminated conditions under which programs fare best. A compelling example can be found in comparisons of impact for a number of prevention programs in urban versus suburban schools. In almost all cases, skill-based interventions worked better in middle-class suburban schools than in lower-class urban schools, with some programs in the most disadvantaged settings actually causing harm to children. Thus, rather than searching for main effects, we must evaluate the impact of an intervention on different participants on the basis of potential moderators such as income, gender, ethnicity, and setting characteristics. The question is not "what works" but rather "what works for whom and under what conditions."

A continuing concern involves how best to evaluate violence prevention efforts, particularly for their ultimate impact on lethal youth violence. The most carefully evaluated preventive interventions typically have involved university-affiliated investigators who apply their models of behavior and behavior change to a school or community setting. Intervention implementation, however, is often compromised in a number of ways according to the unique features of the setting. In the most disadvantaged communities, problems such as high staff turnover, high student attrition, scarce resources, and other "interventions" that come and go quickly often make evaluation a challenging task. Furthermore, ecological programs that try to affect whole systems (e.g., schools) are plagued by concerns over how to achieve random assignment to condition and how to account for multilevel or nested effects of context.

In contrast, a myriad of violence prevention programs exist at the community level, with little or no evaluation of any type. These programs usually are quite sensitive to local concerns and community needs but are not necessarily based on a theory of violent behavior or how to effect behavior change. Needed is a blending of theory and practice—programs should be evaluated that are sensitive to both theories of violence and local community needs. Evaluation models such as FORECAST (Goodman & Wandersman, 1994) that involve collaborative efforts and assess both processes and impacts should be considered.

Beyond these issues, it is important to build on past responses to violence and to establish a framework that can effectively guide prevention activities in the 21st century. During the past decade, most violence prevention efforts have evolved from a risk-focused approach involving identification of risk and protective factors and development of related interventions. Clearly, the use of this framework has advanced the science and practice of violence prevention by emphasizing the importance of empirical findings, evaluation, and integration of programs with community efforts.

Still, this approach has a number of limitations. First, the risk-focused approach has led to the specification of "laundry lists" of risk and protective factors. The notion is that they are independent of each other and of equal value so that selecting any two is better than one, and so forth. Relatively little emphasis has been placed on the relative weighing of risk factors in specific populations and communities, although addressing a single strong cause in a given setting may be much more effective than targeting several weak factors. In addition, predicting risk is quite different from predicting behavior change. Longitudinal relations among variables still do not necessarily mean that changing the identified risk marker will result in corresponding changes in behavior.

Second, risk-focused approaches have resulted in a rush to plug in "programs" to influence risk factors, rather than emphasizing changing contexts or systems. Violence becomes an isolated problem, leading to a focus on the selected factors associated with that problem. Prevention plans become strategies to affect identified risk factors. The emphasis is usually on developing interventions for individuals within social contexts, rather than addressing the dynamics of how individuals navigate multiple and diverse contexts. Unfortunately, the particular risk factors addressed or programs identified often relate to program visibility (for example, the current popularity of peer mediation and conflict resolution programs) rather than an awareness of sets of risk factors and how they interact in a given setting.

Third, applications of the public health framework have successfully identified risk and protective factors in various social contexts, but they have not clearly described how these influences are interconnected through time. As the epidemiological data on youth violence indicate, the onset, desistance, continuity, and types of violence vary by age and are influenced by context. In other words, violence takes different forms during the life course. To develop comprehensive violence prevention responses and strategies that consider these changes through time, a model is needed that situates lethal violence in a broader, dynamic framework of human development.

Life Course Development and Violence Prevention

Rather than focus exclusively on sets of risk or protective factors that contribute to violence in its various forms, an ecological model of life course development model has been proposed and applied to violence prevention (Williams, Guerra, & Elliott, 1996). This model emphasizes factors that support or impede healthy human development during the life course. This approach does not lead to the development of new "programs" but rather to prevention strategies that remove *barriers* and buttress *supports* to prosocial and health-enhancing behavior. These strategies may involve developing new programs, altering social contexts, or reforming systems.

This model is described in depth elsewhere (see Williams et al., 1996). Briefly, it emphasizes how individuals meet developmental needs at each stage in multiple contexts. A careful review of risk and protective factors associated with youth violence indicates that most major risk factors for violence can easily be recast as unmet developmental needs. For example, the lack of a secure infant-caregiver attachment has been linked with risk for early aggression.

From the perspective of the life course model, this attachment is a developmental need of infancy. If unmet, it may predict later aggression and violence as well as a number of other related emotional and behavior problems.

"Risk factors" can thus be understood as barriers for successful human development. An understanding of developmental barriers leads to a focus on prevention as providing developmental supports, in other words, resources, activities, and system changes that help individuals meet developmental needs and/or reduce identified barriers. Supports can be stage-specific or remedial, in that they help meet unmet needs of earlier developmental stages specifically on the basis of the problems of the current developmental stage. For example, an impaired infant-caregiver bond may be manifest during adolescence in difficulties with intimate relationships. Remedial supports would not address directly the infant-caregiver bond but could strengthen family connections and/or relationship skills to address this unmet need.

Another important concept of the life course model centers on transitions and pathways. *Transitions* refer to entry into new developmental stages, and *pathways* refer to the sequencing of transitions and experiences within stages during the life course. Data on the stability of aggression and violence as well as "career" patterns of offending suggest that serious and lethal violence is often the result of difficulties in making transitions to new developmental stages and/or engaging deviant pathways. Timing is also important, in that age-graded transitions that are "off-time" can have negative behavioral consequences. Thus, the life course model provides a dynamic framework from which behavior through time can be understood.

Prevention strategies must also be sensitive to the multiple contexts of development. Not only do individuals develop in multiple contexts, but the relative importance of contexts varies through time. For example, in infancy, the family is the dominant context. During early childhood, the influence of school and peers increases, and during adolescence, the peer group becomes one of the most dominant developmental contexts. In addition, the life course model stresses the importance of the person-in-context interaction. That is, behavior is seen as influenced by both social contexts and the attributes individuals bring to these contexts. Rather than addressing only a set of individual and/or contextual attributes, we must understand the dynamic interaction between individuals and settings and develop prevention strategies accordingly.

The ecological model of life course development provides a broad framework for understanding violence and developing prevention strategies. It can be applied to program development by focusing on specific developmental needs and related programs to meet these needs. It is suggested, however, primarily as a tool for understanding the development of violent behavior through time and across contexts and for building prevention strategies that are comprehensive and provide for integrating and implementing services to prevent violence by supporting healthy human development.

Violence Prevention for the 21st Century: Reviewing *Healthy People 2000* Goals and Setting New Directions for 2010

Healthy People 2000 sets forth three types of objectives for each area of health-related outcomes: (a) health status objectives, (b) risk reduction objectives, and (c) services and protection objectives. In applying these to violence prevention, it is important to examine the relevance and viability of this categorization and the adequacy of the stated objectives. In addition, there is an urgent need to link any proposed objectives with specific strategies, programs, and activities known to be effective and to detail future research needs. Again, the need for an organizing framework that stresses healthy human development and that can link objectives across outcomes must be considered carefully.

As applied to violence prevention, health status objectives have been translated into a set of *target rates* for different types of violent and abusive behavior. These target rates represent significant reductions from previously reported levels of incidence or prevalence. For example, the first objective is to reduce homicides to no more than 7.2 per 100,000 people from an age-adjusted 1987 baseline of 8.5 per 100,000. A mid-decade review indicates that trends are actually heading in the wrong direction. In 1995, the rate had increased to 10.3 per 100,000 (DHHS, 1995). Given this trend, a critical evaluation of the objectives regarding youth violence is in order.

From the standpoint of patterns and trends in violent behavior, these objectives do not discriminate among types of violence, despite the differing etiologies and prevention strategies associated with differing types. These objectives also do not reflect the need to focus on *serious* and *lethal* violence, particularly among adolescents. The objectives do include, however, reductions in weapon possession, weapon carrying, and firearm-related deaths, as well as enhanced firearm storage laws. This focus on the direct relation of firearms to lethal violence is extremely important and is often neglected in the field of violence prevention programming. Given the high rates of firearms use and violence tied to juvenile gangs, it is surprising that no mention of juvenile gangs appears in the objectives, and this should be addressed. Even more puzzling is the rather arbitrary nature of the recommended reductions and the extent to which the goals have been revised by changing target rates, rather than linking goals with specific strategies and actions that address the multiple causes and pathways to violence.

Within a risk-focused public health framework, delineation of risk reduction objectives linked to violence should be useful. As previously detailed, however, at a minimum, targeted risk factors should reflect the changing nature of violence during the life course and in a given setting. Yet the risk factors targeted in the stated objectives focus only on fighting and weapon carrying by adolescents and improper weapon storage. No mention is made of even the most robust risk factors, and no attempts to detail age-specific risk factors have been made, although an expansive literature details risk for violence and other problem behaviors across the life course.

Services and protection objectives cover a range of system-level responses, including changes in firearm storage laws; extensions of assessment and review systems related to suicide, child maltreatment, and child death; and an increase in emergency housing for battered women. Programmatic goals directly related to youth violence call for an increase to at least 50% in the proportion of schools teaching conflict resolution skills and an extension of comprehensive violence prevention programs to at least 80% of local jurisdictions with populations more than 100,000. This emphasis on the extension of violence prevention programs is an important goal. The weakest link in the violence prevention objectives of *Healthy People 2000,* however, is the failure to integrate empirical data on effective programs, ineffective programs, and programs in need of more research into a set of recommended strategies and activities that are, in turn, directly linked to stated violence reduction goals, particularly for lethal violence. For instance, blanket endorsement of conflict resolution programs as one of the key violence prevention services objectives is not supported by empirical data. As discussed in this chapter, even when interventions have included conflict resolution training, their effectiveness in reducing serious violence has been limited, and impact has been moderated by factors such as community setting.

Rather than deal in general statements about increasing violence prevention programs, *Healthy People 2010* must focus on the link between goals and strategies and their relation to the changing patterns of violence across the life course. One approach would be first to differentiate categories of violence addressed (i.e., suicide, homicide and serious assaults, child maltreatment, domestic violence, and rape). From a risk-focused perspective, a next step would be to provide epidemiological data to identify those most at risk and to delineate age-specific risk factors that are modifiable through intervention. Recommended interventions that have been empirically supported (including conditions that maximize impact) can then be linked to specific populations and age groups, and a set of developmentally appropriate strategies and activities can be described.

As we have asserted in this chapter, however, risk factors can also be recast as barriers and supports to healthy development, and a broader ecological framework can be applied to the promotion of healthy human development including violence prevention. Many risk factors for violence are common to a range of problems including mental health disorders, substance use, and teenage pregnancy. A comprehensive response should focus on how schools, communities, and service systems can foster social, emotional, and physical health through strategies and activities that help individuals meet their developmental needs across the life course.

Note

1. Several comprehensive reviews are available focusing specifically on violence prevention (e.g., Guerra, Tolan, & Hammond, 1994; Tate, Reppucci, & Mulvey,

1995; Tolan & Guerra, 1994a). Other reviews cover a broader range of antisocial and delinquent behaviors (e.g., Kazdin, 1987; Lipsey, 1992; Tolan & Guerra, 1994b).

References

Berrueta-Clement, J. R., Schweinhart, L. J., Barnett, W. S., Epstein, A. S., & Weikart, D. P. (1984). *Changed lives: The effects of the Perry Preschool Program on youths through age 19* (Monographs of the High-Scope Educational Research Foundation, No. 8). Ypsilanti, MI: High-Scope Press.

Coie, J. D., Underwood, M., & Lochman, J. E. (1991). Programmatic intervention with aggressive children in the school setting. In D. J. Pepler & K. H. Rubin (Eds.), *The development and treatment of childhood aggression* (pp. 387-410). Hillsdale, NJ: Lawrence Erlbaum.

Darlington, R. B., Royce, J. M., Snipper, A. S., Murray, H. W., & Lazar, I. (1980). Preschool programs and later school competence of children from low-income families. *Science, 208,* 202-204.

DuBow, E. F., Huesmann, L. R., & Eron, L. D. (1987). Mitigating aggression promoting pro-social behavior in aggressive elementary school boys. *Behavior and Research Therapy, 25,* 257-531.

Elliott, D. S. (1994). *Youth violence: An overview.* Boulder, CO: Center for the Study and Prevention of Violence.

Feldman, R. A. (1992). The St. Louis experiment: Effective treatment of antisocial youths in prosocial peer groups. In J. McCord & R. Tremblay (Eds.), *Preventing antisocial behavior: Interventions from birth through adolescence* (pp. 233-252). New York: Guilford.

Felner, R. D., & Adan, A. M. (1988). The school transition environment project: An ecological intervention and evaluation. In R. H. Price, E. L. Cowen, R. P. Lorian, & J. Ramos-McKay (Eds.), *14 ounces of prevention: A casebook for practitioners* (pp. 111-122). Washington, DC: American Psychological Association.

Fox, J. A. (1996). *Trends in juvenile violence.* Washington, DC: U.S. Bureau of Justice Statistics.

Goodman, R. M., & Wandersman, A. (1994). FORECAST: A formative approach to evaluating community coalitions and community-based initiatives. *Journal of Community Psychology*(CSAP Special Issue), 6-24.

Gottfredson, D. C. (1986). An empirical test of school-based environmental and individual interventions to reduce the risk of delinquent behavior. *Criminology, 24,* 705-731.

Gottfredson, D. C. (1987). An evaluation of an organization development approach to reducing school disorder. *Evaluation Review, 11,* 739-763.

Gottfredson, D. C., Gottfredson, G. D., & Hybl, L. G. (1993). Managing adolescent behavior: A multiyear, multischool study. *American Educational Research Journal, 30,* 179-215.

Gordon, R. (1983). An operational definition of prevention. *Public Health Reports, 98,* 107-109.

Guerra, N. G., Eron, L. D., Huesmann, L. R., Tolan, P., & Van Acker, R. (1996). A cognitive-ecological approach to the prevention and mitigation of violence and aggression in inner-city youth. In P. Fry & K. Bjorkvist (Eds.), *Cultural variation in conflict resolution: Alternatives for reducing violence* (pp. 199-213). New York: Plenum.

Guerra, N. G., Henry, D., Tolan, P. H., Huesmann, L. R., & Eron, L. D. (1996). *A multi-component, multi-context program to prevent the emergence of aggressive and antisocial behavior.* Manuscript submitted for publication.

Guerra, N. G., & Slaby, R. G. (1990). Cognitive mediators of aggression in adolescent offenders: 2. Intervention. *Developmental Psychology, 26,* 269-277.

Guerra, N. G., Tolan, P. H., & Hammond, R. (1994). Prevention and treatment of adolescent violence. In L. D., Eron, J. Gentry, & P. Schlegel (Eds.), *Reason to hope: A psychological perspective on violence and youth.* Washington, DC: American Psychological Association.

Hawkins, J. D., Von Cleve, E., & Catalano, R. F. (1991). Reducing early childhood aggression: Results of a primary prevention program. *Journal of the American Academy of Child and Adolescent Psychiatry, 30,* 208-217.

Henggeler, S. W. (1989). *Delinquency in adolescence.* New York: Grune & Stratton.

Henggeler, S. W., & Borduin, C. M. (1990). *Family therapy and beyond: A multisystemic approach to treating the behavior problems of children and adolescents.* Pacific Grove, CA: Brooks/Cole.

Johnson, D. L. (1988). Primary prevention of behavior problems in young children: The Houston parent-child development center. In R. H. Price, E. L. Cowen, R. P. Lorian, & J. Ramos-McKay (Eds.), *14 ounces of prevention: A casebook for practitioners* (pp. 44-52). Washington, DC: American Psychological Association.

Johnson, D. L., & Walker, T. (1987). The primary prevention of behavior problems in Mexican-American children. *American Journal of Community Psychology, 15,* 375-385.

Kazdin, A. E. (1987). Treatment of antisocial behavior in children: Current status and future directions. *American Psychologist, 102,* 187-203.

Lee, V. E., Brooks-Gunn, J., Schnur, E., & Liaw, F. (1990). Are Head Start effects sustained? A longitudinal follow-up comparison of disadvantaged children attending Head Start, no preschool, and other preschool programs. *Child Development, 61,* 495-507.

Lipsey, M. W. (1992). Juvenile delinquency treatment: A meta-analytic inquiry into the variability of effects. In T. D. Cook (Ed.), *Meta-analysis for explanation* (pp. 83-127). Newbury Park, CA: Sage.

Olds, D., Henderson, C., Tatelbaum, R., & Chamberlin, R. (1986). Improving the delivery of prenatal care and outcomes of pregnancy: A randomized trial of nurse-home visitation. *Pediatrics, 77,* 16-28.

Olweus, D. (1994). Bullying at school: Basic facts and effects of a school-based intervention program. *Journal of Child Psychology and Psychiatry and Allied Disciplines,* 35, 1171-1190.

Patterson, G. R. (1982). *Coercive family processes.* Eugene, OR: Castalia.

Patterson, G. R. (1986). Performance models for antisocial boys. *American Psychologist, 41,* 432-444.

Patterson, G. R., Chamberlain, P., & Reid, J. B. (1982). A comparative evaluation of a parent-training program. *Behavioral Therapy, 13,* 638-650.

Patterson, G. R., Reid, J. R., & Dishion, T. (1992). *Antisocial boys*. Eugene, OR: Castalia.

Provence, S., & Naylor, A. (1983). Psychological first aid and treatment approach to children exposed to community violence: Research implications. *Journal of Traumatic Stress, 4*, 445-473.

Public/Private Ventures. (1995). *Evaluation of the Big Brothers/Big Sisters Program*. Philadelphia: Author.

Rickel, A. U., & Burgio, J. C. (1982). Assessing social competencies in lower income preschool children. *American Journal of Community Psychology, 10*, 635-645.

Rickel, A. U., & Lampi, L. (1981). A two-year follow-up study of a preventive mental health program for preschoolers. *Journal of Abnormal Child Psychology, 9*, 455-464.

Sarason, I. G., & Sarason, B. R. (1981). Teaching cognitive and social skills to high school students. *Journal of Consulting and Clinical Psychology, 49*, 908-918.

Schweinhart, L. J., & Weikart, D. P. (1988). The High/Scope Perry Preschool Program. In R. H. Price, E. L. Cowen, R. P. Lorian, & J. Ramos-McKay (Eds.), *14 ounces of prevention: A casebook for practitioners* (pp. 53-65). Washington, DC: American Psychological Association.

Spergel, I. A. (1986). The violent youth gang in Chicago: A local community approach. *Social Service Review, 60*, 94-131.

Spivack, G., Platt, J. J., & Shure, M. B. (1976). *The problem-solving approach to adjustment*. San Francisco: Jossey-Bass.

Spivack, G., & Shure, M. B. (1974). *Social adjustment of young children: A cognitive approach to solving real-life problems*. San Francisco: Jossey-Bass.

Tate, D. C., Reppucci, N. D., & Mulvey, E. P. (1995). Violent juvenile delinquents: Treatment effectiveness and implications for future action. *American Psychologist, 50*, 777-781.

Tolan, P. H., & Guerra, N. G. (1994a). Prevention of delinquency: Current status and issues. *Applied & Preventive Psychology, 3*, 251-273.

Tolan, P. H., & Guerra, N. G. (1994b). *What works in reducing adolescent violence: An empirical review of the field*. Boulder, CO: Center for the Study and Prevention of Violence.

Tremblay, R. E., & Craig, W. M. (1995). Developmental crime prevention. In M. Tonry & D. P. Farrington (Eds.), *Building a safer society: Strategic approaches to crime prevention*. Chicago: University of Chicago Press.

U.S. Department of Health and Human Services, Public Health Service. (1991). *Healthy people 2000: National health promotion and disease prevention objectives* (DHHS Publication No. PHS 91-50212). Washington, DC: U.S. Government Printing Office.

U.S. Department of Health and Human Services, Public Health Service. (1995). *Healthy people 2000: Midcourse review and 1995 revisions*. Washington, DC: U.S. Government Printing Office.

Wahler, R. G., & Dumas, J. E. (1987). Family factors in childhood psychology: Toward a coercion-neglect model. In T. Jacob (Ed.), *Family interaction and psychopathology: Theories, methods, and findings* (pp. 581-627). New York: Plenum.

Wahler, R. G., & Dumas, J. E. (1989). Attentional problems in dysfunctional mother-child interactions: An interbehavioral model. *Psychological Bulletin, 105,* 116-130.

Weissberg, R. P., Caplan, M., & Harwood, R. L. (1991). Promoting competent young people in competence-enhancing environments: A systems-based perspective on primary prevention. *Journal of Consulting and Clinical Psychology, 59,* 830-841.

Weissberg, R. P., Gesten, E. L., Carnrike, C. L., Toro, P. A., Rapkin, B. D., Davidson, E., & Cowen, E. L. (1981). Social problem-solving skills training: A competence-building intervention with second- to fourth- grade children. *American Journal of Community Psychology, 9,* 411-423.

Weissberg, R. P., Gesten, E. L., Rapkin, B. D., Cowen, E. L., Davidson, E., de Apodaca, R. F., & McKim, B. J. (1981). The evaluation of a social problem-solving training program for suburban and inner-city third grade children. *Journal of Consulting and Clinical Psychology, 49,* 251-261.

Williams, K. W., Guerra, N. G., & Elliott, D. S. (1996). *Human development and violence prevention: A focus on youth.* Paper prepared for the Annie E. Casey Foundation.

• *CHAPTER 6* •

Prevention of Depression

BRUCE E. COMPAS
JENNIFER CONNOR
MARTHA WADSWORTH

Depression is widely recognized as a serious mental health concern among children and youth. After decades of misunderstanding of the fundamental nature of this disorder in young people, researchers have generated increased knowledge of the characteristics, prevalence, course, and etiology of depression during the 1980s and 1990s (Hammen & Rudolph, in press; Petersen et al., 1993). It is now clear that substantial numbers of children and adolescents experience symptoms of sadness, dysphoria, and other characteristics associated with depression, whereas a smaller but still significant number of young people experience depression as a disorder as manifested in adults. The consequences of depressive symptoms and disorder during childhood and adolescence are significant as well, including greatly increased risk for depression later in life, as well as concurrent disruption in functioning in childhood and greatly increased risk for suicidal ideation and attempts. Finally, the importance of depression in young people is reflected in the pernicious tendency for depression to co-occur with a wide range of other problems and disorders, including anxiety, disruptive behavior disorders, and substance abuse (Angold & Costello, 1993; Compas & Hammen, 1994). Depression that co-occurs with other problems or disorders greatly increases the level of associated social problems and impairment.

Despite the significance of depression as a mental health problem during childhood and adolescence, it received relatively little attention in *Healthy People 2000* (U.S. Department of Health and Human Services, Public Health Service [DHHS], 1991) or in the subsequent review of these national health objectives in *Healthy Youth 2000* (Fleming, 1996). Risk reduction objectives in *Healthy People 2000* that specifically target depression and those concerned with stress as a risk factor for depression are limited to goals for adults. The absence of attention to depression in young people is especially noteworthy in light of the emphasis that is given to youth suicide as a major health problem in both these documents because depression is one of the major risk factors for suicide in adolescence. Moreover, the goals for prevention that are outlined in *Healthy People 2000* underscore the need to prevent depression early in development to reduce its recurrence in adulthood.

The emerging knowledge base on the nature of depression in young people has set the stage for systematic efforts to prevent depression during childhood and adolescence. Although the field is poised to develop and evaluate the effects of preventive interventions, surprisingly little research has emerged on the prevention of depression (W. T. Grant Foundation Consortium, 1996). We will review research on depression in children and adolescents, including prior studies of preventive interventions aimed at depressive symptoms and disorder in young people. This research is used as a basis for setting future directions for the development of programs to prevent depression during childhood and adolescence. The evidence is clear that prevention of depression in young people should be a high priority for *Healthy People 2010*.

Nature of Depression in Children and Adolescents

Defining Depression in Young People

Perhaps more than any other disorder in childhood and adolescence, depression has presented challenges in conceptualization and definition (Compas, Ey, & Grant, 1993; Hammen & Rudolph, in press). These struggles have been the result of several factors.

First, for decades, there was resistance to the idea that young people could experience serious depression because psychoanalytic theory held that depression could not occur in childhood or adolescence as a consequence of inadequate development of the superego. Second, early conceptualizations of depression held that when this problem occurred, it was masked by other symptoms or disorders, especially externalizing disorders. Third, when the field finally came to recognize that depression does occur in young people, the criteria that were applied were a downward extension of adult criteria, with only minor exceptions, offering little or no acknowledgment of developmental differences.

Current conceptualizations of depression include recognition of depression as a symptom or mood, as a syndrome of intercorrelated symptoms, and as a psychiatric disorder (Angold, 1988; Cantwell & Baker, 1991; Compas et al., 1993; Kovacs, 1989). The first approach is concerned with *depressed mood* or affect and refers to the presence of sadness, unhappiness, or blue feelings for an unspecified time, as represented by the work of Petersen (e.g., Petersen, Sarigiani, & Kennedy, 1991), Kandel (e.g., Kandel & Davies, 1986), and others. The study of depressed mood during childhood and adolescence has emerged from developmental research in which depressive emotions are studied along with other features of biological, cognitive, and social development. No assumptions are made regarding the presence or absence of other symptoms that may reflect depression (e.g., poor appetite and insomnia).

The second approach is concerned with a *depressive syndrome,* a constellation of behaviors and emotions identified empirically through the reports of children/adolescents and other informants (e.g., parents and teachers). This strategy involves the use of multivariate statistical methods in the assessment and taxonomy of child and adolescent psychopathology, represented by the empirically based taxonomy of Achenbach (1985, 1993). Most pertinent here is the syndrome labeled *anxious/depressed,* composed of symptoms reflecting a mixture of anxiety and depression (see Table 6.1). The syndrome has been replicated in large samples in both the United States and the Netherlands (Achenbach, Verhulst, Baron, & Akkerhuis, 1987). A "pure" depressive (or anxious) syndrome did not emerge in this research in the reports of parents, teachers, and adolescents.

Table 6.1 Symptoms of the Anxious/Depressed Syndrome Based on Parent (CBCL) and Adolescent (YSR) Reports

Parent Report	*Adolescent Report*
Complains of loneliness	I feel lonely
Cries a lot	I cry a lot
Fears he or she might do something bad	I am afraid I might think or do something bad
Feels he or she has to be perfect	
Feels or complains that no one loves him or her	I feel that no one loves me
Feels others are out to get him or her	I feel that others are out to get me
Feels worthless or inferior	I feel worthless or inferior
Nervous, high-strung, or tense	I am nervous or tense
Too fearful or anxious	I am too fearful or anxious
Feels too guilty	I feel too guilty
Self-conscious or easily embarrassed	I am self-conscious or easily embarrassed
Suspicious	I am suspicious
Unhappy, sad, or depressed	I am unhappy, sad, or depressed
Worrying	I worry a lot
	I deliberately try to hurt or kill myself
	I think about killing myself

SOURCE: Achenbach (1991a, 1991b).

The third approach is based on a disease or disorder model of psychopathology and is currently reflected in the categorical diagnostic system of the *Diagnostic and Statistical Manual of Mental Disorders* (4th ed.; *DSM-IV*) of the American Psychiatric Association (1994) and the *International Classification of Diseases and Health Related Problems* (ICD-10) of the World Health Organization (1990). The *categorical diagnostic* approach assumes not only that depression includes the presence of an identifiable syndrome of associated symptoms but also that these symptoms are associated with significant levels of current distress or impairment in the individual's current functioning (American Psychiatric Association, 1994). With only a few exceptions, child or adolescent depression is diagnosed according to the same *DSM-IV* criteria as adult depression. Our focus is on major depressive disorder (MDD) and dysthymia (DY); readers are referred to the *DSM-IV* for more information regarding bipolar disorders (see also Carlson, 1994).

To meet the criteria for MDD, the child or adolescent must have experienced *five or more* of the specified symptoms for *at least a 2-week period* at a level that differs from prior functioning, and at least one of the symptoms includes either (a) depressed or irritable mood or (b) anhedonia (see Table 6.2). Irritable mood may be observed in lieu of depressed mood in children and adolescents and is believed to be more common in this age group than in adults. The criteria for diagnosis of DY in childhood and adolescence are that for at least 1 year (as compared with 2 years for adults), an individual must display depressed or irritable mood daily, without more than 2 months symptom-free, along with additional symptoms. There must be no evidence of an episode of MDD during the first year of DY.

Although these three conceptualizations of "depression" in childhood and adolescence differ considerably, it is best to view them as related and complementary perspectives on the same phenomenon (Compas et al., 1993). Depressed mood and a syndrome of mixed anxiety/depression are markers of increased risk for the development of MDD. Moreover, high levels of depressed mood and mixed anxiety/depression symptoms are associated with significant impairment and problems even in the absence of symptoms that meet criteria for major depression. All three of these levels of depressive phenomena are appropriate targets for preventive interventions in childhood and adolescence.

Prevalence of Depression in Young People

The rationale for any preventive intervention depends in part on the prevalence of the problem or disorder in question. The greater the prevalence of the problem, the greater the need to implement intervention efforts to reduce the incidence of new cases. Furthermore, the degree to which the onset of the problem or disorder occurs early in development determines the need to intervene in childhood or adolescence. Therefore, data on the onset and prevalence of depression as a function of age are important to consider in the prevention of this problem.

Table 6.2 *DSM-IV* Criteria for Major Depressive Episode and Dysthymic Disorder

Major Depressive Episode

A. Five (or more) of the following symptoms during the same 2-week period; at least one of the symptoms is depressed mood or loss of interest or pleasure.
   1. Depressed mood most of the day, nearly every day as indicated by subjective report or observation by others. (Note: In children and adolescents, can be irritable mood)
   2. Markedly diminished interest or pleasure in all or almost all activities most of the day, nearly every day, as indicated by subjective account or observation by others
   3. Significant weight loss when not dieting or weight gain (e.g., a change of more than 5% body weight in a month), or decrease or increase in appetite nearly every day. (Note: In children, consider failure to make expected weight gains)
   4. Insomnia or hypersomnia nearly every day
   5. Psychomotor agitation or retardation nearly everyday (observable by others)
   6. Fatigue or loss of energy nearly every day
   7. Feelings of worthlessness or excessive or inappropriate guilt nearly every day
   8. Diminished ability to think or concentrate, or indecisiveness, nearly every day (either subjective or observed by others)
   9. Recurrent thoughts of death (not just fear of dying), recurrent suicidal ideation without a specific plan, or a suicide attempt or a specific plan for committing suicide

SOURCE: *Diagnostic and Statistical Manual of Mental Disorders, Fourth Edition* (p. 327).

Although studies of depression in children and adolescents have reported widely varying prevalence rates, increasing evidence suggests that depressive disorders represent a serious difficulty faced by a sizeable and growing number of children and adolescents. Part of the difficulty in determining an accurate estimate of the prevalence of depression in children lies with the variety of ways in which depression has been conceptualized and measured (see above). Despite this problem, however, sufficient data are available on the prevalence of depressed mood, mixed anxiety/depression, and MDD and DY to indicate that they are targets worthy of preventive intervention.

In analyses of a single item reflecting unhappy, sad, or depressed mood, Achenbach (1991a, 1991b) found that parents reported 10%

Table 6.2 Continued

Major Depressive Episode (unipolar) can be further specified as mild, moderate, severe (based on functional impairment and severity of symptoms), with or without psychotic features, with or without melancholic features, whether or not recurrent, or chronic

Dysthymic Disorder

A. Depressed mood for most of the day, for more days than not, as indicated either by subjective account or observation by others, for at least 2 years. (Note: In children and adolescents, mood can be irritable and duration must be at least 1 year.)

B. Presence, while depressed, of two or more of the following:
   1. Poor appetite or overeating
   2. Insomnia or hypersomnia
   3. Low energy or fatigue
   4. Low self-esteem
   5. Poor concentration or difficulty making decisions

C. During period of depression, the person has never been without symptoms A or B for more than 2 months at a time; also, the disturbance must not be accounted for by chronic Major Depressive Disorder (or Major Depressive Disorder in partial remission)—i.e., no Major Depressive Disorder in the first 2 years of the disturbance (1 year for children and adolescents)

SOURCE: Adapted from *DSM-IV*, pp. 327 and 349, American Psychiatric Association (1994).

to 20% of boys and 15% to 20% of girls who had not been referred for mental health services experienced this symptom at least somewhat or sometimes during the previous 6 months. Adolescents' self-reports indicated that 20% to 35% of nonreferred boys and 25% to 40% of nonreferred girls reported feeling sad or depressed during the prior 6 months. Petersen et al. (1991) found that depressed mood increased during adolescence for girls but remained relatively stable for boys throughout adolescence. These authors also found that reports of significant episodes of depressed mood (lasting 2 weeks or longer) increased from early adolescence (i.e., episodes occurring between 6th and 8th grades) to late adolescence (i.e., episodes occurring between 9th and 12th grades) for both boys and girls. Girls reported more episodes of depressed mood than boys at all age levels, with this gender difference increasing from early to late adolescence.

The prevalence of an empirically derived syndrome of mixed anxiety/depression has been examined in a nationally representative sample of children and adolescents (Achenbach, 1991a). Using a cutoff that achieves optimal sensitivity and specificity in distinguishing between children and youth who have been referred for mental health services and those who have not been referred, it is estimated that between 5% and 6% of the population experience significant levels of mixed anxiety/depression (Compas et al., 1993).

Several reviews have examined the data on the prevalence of MDD and DY in young people (e.g., Angold & Costello, 1993; Fleming & Offord, 1990; Hammen & Rudolph, in press; Petersen et al., 1993). Ten studies of MDD in community samples of children/adolescents reported *lifetime prevalence* rates ranging from 0% to 31%, with a mean of 11% (Petersen et al., 1993). Hammen and Rudolph reviewed eight relevant epidemiological surveys of childhood depressive symptoms and reported an overall range of 6- to 12-month prevalence of 0.4% to 8.0% for *DSM-III*-diagnosed major depressive episode. In those studies that distinguished between DY and MDD, Hammen and Rudolph report the prevalence of DY ranged from 0.07% to 4.9%.

Point prevalence estimates have been provided by Lewinsohn and colleagues from a large community sample of adolescents (Lewinsohn, Rohde, Seeley, & Hops, 1991; Rohde, Lewinsohn, & Seeley, 1991). On the basis of diagnostic interviews, 2.9% of a sample of 1,710 adolescents received a current diagnosis of either MDD, DY, or comorbid MDD and DY (Lewinsohn et al., 1991). Lifetime prevalence of depressive disorders was 20% in this sample, a finding that is within the range of lifetime prevalence rates in the earlier studies reviewed by Fleming and Offord (1990).

Reporting prevalence rates for children and adolescents as a group disguises potential age and gender differences. It appears that depression is relatively rare in children under 6 years of age but that it increases during early to middle adolescence, for which the rates found are comparable with the rates of depression in adults (Compas et al., in press). In addition to age differences, there are gender differences in depression in young people, with more depressive problems occurring for girls than for boys. Early to middle adolescence is widely believed to be the developmental period when significant increases occur in depression and when girls begin to experience significantly more depression than boys (e.g., Angold & Rutter, 1992; Nolen-Hoeksema & Girgus, 1994; Petersen et al., 1991). Two recent reviews of the research on adolescent depression reveal that despite the increasing theoretical and empirical work devoted to explaining age and sex differences in depression during adolescence, these differences may not be as pervasive as is widely assumed (Leadbeater, Blatt, & Quinlan, 1995; Petersen, Compas, & Brooks-Gunn, 1992). Specifically, most studies of depression during adolescence have not examined age and gender differences, and among those that have, findings have been inconsistent with respect to the main effects of age and sex and, most important, the interaction of age and sex. More recently, Compas et al. (in press) found that gender differences in depressed mood, the anxious/depressed syndrome, and an analogue of MDD were more consistent and significantly larger in magnitude in a sample of adolescents who had been referred for mental health services than in a nonreferred sample. These findings suggest that the emergence of gender differences in depressive symptoms in adolescence may be limited to a subgroup of adolescent girls who represent an extreme of the distribution of depressive symptoms among the adolescent population.

Finally, it has been well documented that there has been a general increase in depression among youth in recent years (Cross-National Collaborative Group, 1992). In studies comparing older and younger siblings and peers during the past few years, a higher prevalence of depression has been found in the children born most recently (e.g., Kovacs & Gatsonis, 1994; Lewinsohn, Rohde, Seeley, & Fischer, 1993; Ryan et al., 1992). Similarly, studies have also found an increase in the anxious/depressed syndrome during a 3-year period (Achenbach & Howell, 1993). Such changes in prevalence rates, especially during such short periods, highlight the importance of environmental risk factors in childhood depression (Hammen & Rudolph, in press).

In summary, depressed mood, a syndrome of mixed anxiety/depression, and MDD and DY occur with considerable frequency in childhood and adolescence. Data on developmental differences highlight early adolescence as a time of moderate to substantial increases in the prevalence of depression, suggesting that late childhood and early adolescence may be important times for preventive interventions.

Persistence, Recurrence, and Continuity of Depression

The persistence, recurrence, and continuity of a problem or disorder are also important to consider in developing the rationale for preventive interventions. If problems are relatively transient and likely to remit on their own, the need for intervention may be much less than if problems persist through long periods. In contrast, problems that persist during extended periods of development may warrant intensive efforts to prevent their initial onset. There are three significant concerns about the course of depression in childhood and adolescence. First, studies suggest that depression is highly persistent during childhood and adolescence and into adulthood. Although most youngsters recover within a year, a sizable minority remain depressed—approximately 20% 1 year later and 10% at 2 years (Keller et al., 1988; McCauley et al., 1993; Strober, Lampert, Schmidt, & Morrell, 1993). Studies of youth scoring high on self-report measures of depressive symptoms also suggest considerable stability of depressive symptoms through repeated testing (e.g., Achenbach, Howell, McConaughy, & Stanger, 1995; Garrison, Jackson, Marstellar, McKeown, & Addy, 1990; Verhulst & van der Ende, 1992; Stanger, McConaughy, & Achenbach, 1992). For example, Verhulst and van der Ende found considerable stability in internalizing problems in a large community sample of children. Of children who were above the clinical cutoff for internalizing problems on the Child Behavior Checklist (CBCL), 36% remained above cutoff at each of three subsequent 2-year follow-ups. Similarly, Harrington, Fudge, Rutter, Pickles, and Hill (1990) found that individuals who were treated for a "depressive syndrome" during childhood were at increased risk for affective disorders in adulthood and were more likely than a control group to receive subsequent psychiatric hospitalizations and treatment.

Second, recurrence of episodes of major depression is common among children and adolescents. Lewinsohn et al. (1993) noted that 18% of their community sample had a recurrence of a major depressive episode within 1 year, and McCauley et al. (1993) reported 25% relapse within a year and 54% within 3 years. Kovacs, Feinberg, Crouse-Novak, Paulauskas, and Finkelstein (1984) reported that among an outpatient sample, 26% with MDD had a new episode within 1 year of recovery, 40% within 2 years, and 72% within 5 years.

A third issue is continuity between childhood/adolescent depression and adult depression. Although less information is available on this topic than on recurrence or chronicity during childhood and adolescence, available data do indeed indicate that those who have been depressed as youngsters are likely to have recurrent episodes or continuing symptoms in adulthood (Harrington et al., 1990; Lewinsohn, Hoberman, & Rosenbaum, 1988).

Comorbidity

Epidemiological data suggest that comorbidity of child and adolescent depression is the rule, rather than the exception (Angold & Costello, 1993; Compas & Hammen, 1994). *DSM* diagnoses of MDD and DY and a mixed anxiety/depression syndrome have been found to be highly comorbid with oppositional defiant and conduct disorders (21% to 83%), anxiety disorders (30% to 75%), substance use (53%), attention deficit/hyperactivity disorder (0% to 57%), suicide (27% to 40%), and a host of other internalizing and externalizing problems (Angold & Costello, 1993; Compas & Hammen, 1994; Lewinsohn, Rohde, & Seeley, 1995). The rates of comorbid disorders experienced by children who are depressed are much higher than the rates of depression experienced by children with other disorders (Angold & Costello, 1993).

Although the sheer rates of comorbidity are disturbing in themselves, the clinical consequences of comorbidity in children and adolescents are of even greater concern. Comorbid conditions have profound consequences for children in increased use of mental health services, increases in associated school problems, and poorer global functioning (Lewinsohn et al., 1995). For example, individuals who received diagnoses of both major depression and conduct disorder as adolescents were more likely as adults to be involved in criminal activity and receive a diagnosis of antisocial personality disorder than those who had major depression in absence of conduct problems (Harrington et al., 1990). A particularly disturbing pattern of comorbidity involves depression and substance abuse or conduct disorder as reflected in their increased risk for suicidal behavior (Wagner, Cole, & Schwartzman, in press; see below).

Comorbidity has clear implications for the prevention of depression in children and adolescents. Few interventions, however, provide guidelines for managing or including comorbid conditions. In addition, the majority of interventions have been developed using community samples of youth with elevated scores on measures of depressive symptoms, among whom comorbidity may be less of a problem than among youth who are at high risk for depression or have already manifested the disorder. Thus, comorbidity may be even more important to consider in indicated and targeted interventions than in universal interventions (see below).

Consequences of Depression

Researchers have examined both the short- and long-term sequelae of depressed affect, the anxious/depressed syndrome, and MDD. Among the outcomes that have been considered are impairment in academic and social functioning and suicide.

Social Impairment. Impairments in school behavior and academic functioning and in social and family functioning are apparent for youngsters with major depression and depressive symptoms (for reviews, see Hammen & Rudolph, in press; Kaslow & Racusin, 1990) and persist even after remission of a depressive episode (e.g., Puig-Antich et al., 1985). Elevated depressive symptoms not sufficient to meet diagnostic criteria are also associated with significant psychosocial impairment (Gotlib, Lewinsohn, & Seeley, 1995). In a longitudinal study of a large community sample of adolescents, Aseltine, Gore, and Colton (1994) examined emotional responsiveness to family and friend relations in previously depressed youth and nondepressed youth (on the basis of scores on the Center for Epidemiological Studies-Depression Scale [CES-D]). Adolescents who experienced chronically high levels of depressive symptoms were unresponsive to family problems but were highly reactive to peer relations. Among previously asymptomatic youth, family relations exerted greater effects on depressed mood than did relations with peers.

Achenbach and colleagues examined the 3- and 6-year consequences of symptoms on the anxious/depressed syndrome (Achenbach et al., 1995; Stanger, Achenbach, & McConaughy, 1993). The anxious/depressed syndrome generally was not a strong predictor of six "signs of disturbance" (e.g., academic problems, school behavior problems, suicidal behavior, and police contacts). Symptoms of anxiety/depression, however, predicted girls' referral for mental health services at the 3 year follow-up (Stanger et al., 1993) and predicted boys' referral for mental health services in the 6-year follow-up (Achenbach et al., 1995).

Impaired academic, family, and social functioning associated with depression may interfere with the mastery of important developmental tasks, leaving children with inadequate sources of self-esteem and low perceived competence to face challenges. To the extent that depression results, in part, from perceived lack of competence and diminished self-esteem (e.g., Cole, 1991), a recurring cycle of symptoms and failure may ensue. Moreover, to the extent that incompetence and impairment in developmentally important arenas contribute to depressive reactions, it may be possible to identify youngsters at risk for whom preventive interventions might forestall the development of the depressive cycle.

Adolescent Depression and Suicide. Because of the finality of suicide and heightened public concern about adolescent suicide, special attention must be given to the link between depressive symptoms and disorder and suicidal ideation, attempted suicide, and completed suicide in young people. Research has established a clear link between depression, whether measured as elevated symptoms or a diagnosis, and subsequent suicide attempts. As with research on the more general consequences of depression, risk for attempted suicide increases dramatically when co-occurring symptoms or comorbid disorders are taken into account.

Lewinsohn, Rohde, and Seeley (1996) have provided extensive data on the association between depression and attempted suicide from the Oregon longitudinal study. They examined comorbidity among adolescent suicide attempters in the community and found higher rates of suicide attempts among adolescents with comorbid major depression plus substance abuse, compared with the rates of suicide attempts among those with any single diagnosis alone. The percentages who had attempted suicide were 19% with pure MDD, 22.4% with MDD comorbid with anxiety, 34.6% with MDD comorbid with substance abuse, and 38.9% with MDD comorbid with disruptive behavior. Rates of attempted suicide for other pure disorders were 2% for anxiety, 9.3% for substance use, and 4.7% for disruptive behavior. Thus, a diagnosis of depression was a significant risk factor for attempted suicide, but the risk increased dramatically with the presence of a comorbid disruptive behavior disorder or substance abuse.

Similarly, in a study of a large community sample of adolescents, Wagner et al. (in press) found an association between depressive symptoms and attempted suicide. Of the sample, 14% responded affirmatively to the question, "Have you ever tried to take your own life?" Adolescents reporting high levels of depression along with either alcohol abuse or conduct problems were more likely to have made a suicide attempt than were adolescents reporting only one of these disorders. Adolescents reporting comorbid drug abuse plus either depression or conduct problems were more likely to have made a prior suicide attempt than those reporting only depression or conduct problems without drug abuse.

Risk Factors for Depression in Childhood and Adolescence

Many social, psychological, and biological factors have been examined as possible sources of risk for depressive symptoms and disorder in children and youth. Research has been guided by a wide range of theoretical perspectives, including psychodynamic, behavioral, cognitive, interpersonal, family, biological, and environmental models that vary in their comprehensiveness and in their level of empirical support. Although consensus has not been achieved on the risk factors and mechanisms that account for the occurrence of depression in young people, several research approaches show considerable promise. Each model can be used to identify factors that play an etiologic role in the development of depression and therefore may serve as a target in preventive interventions for children and adolescents. Integration of these various perspectives has led to a *developmental biopsychosocial* perspective on depression during childhood and adolescence (e.g., Cicchetti, Rogosch, & Toth, 1994; Gotlib & Hammen, 1992; Hammen & Rudolph, in press; Petersen et al., 1993). Integrative models have important implications for the prevention of depression in young people. First, they emphasize that developmental processes and children's developmental level must be taken into account in intervention process. Second, they highlight the need to consider a range of factors that may be associated with depression in children and adolescents. To the extent that depression is a heterogeneous disorder, it is not surprising that there may be a wide range of risk factors and a variety of etiological paths. These include both internal characteristics of the children as well as features of the children's social context. Third, integrative models recognize that the interplay among these factors and their salience may change with development.

Individual Factors

Biological Factors. Biological factors, including genetics, neurotransmitter processes, brain structure and functioning, and neuroendocrine processes play a central role in most current models of depression in adults. Research on biological processes in adults has led to the investigation of similar processes in children and adolescents. Enough evidence has been found to support the view that child and adolescent depression reflects biological dysregulation of multiple systems including the endocrine system, neurotransmitter functions, and basic body rhythms including sleep cycles. Many of the studies are preliminary, however, in that they have involved small sample sizes, and a number of contradictory results have been found. The most striking features of the child and adolescent research are that it is limited and has yielded inconsistent results (Brooks-Gunn, Petersen, & Compas, 1995).

For example, studies of depressed children and adolescents have not found consistent evidence of sleep disturbances similar to those of adults (e.g., Emslie, Rush, Weinberg, Rintelmann, & Roffwarg, 1994; Puig-Antich, 1987). In the area of growth hormone, most studies examining changes in growth hormone secretion in youngsters have shown changes as a function of depressive symptomatology similar to those in adults, but a few have not (for review, see Emslie et al., 1994). The same is true for cortisol hypersecretion (Weller, Weller, Fristad, Cantwell, & Preskorn, 1986). Overall, the evidence for clear-cut, well-defined biological abnormalities is less compelling in children and adolescents than in adults, but in each of the major areas there is some evidence that abnormalities are similar. Challenges to understanding the underlying biological changes in child and adolescent depression include biological changes during puberty and the lack of standardized normative data for many of the tests (Brooks-Gunn et al., 1995). The biological data suggest the need for continued investigation of possible subtypes of depression in children that may serve as markers of the need for early intervention or preventive efforts.

Cognitive Factors. On the basis of cognitive models of depression in adulthood, it has been established that depressed and nondepressed children and adolescents differ in most major cognitive processes associated with depression (for review, see Garber & Hilsman, 1992; Kaslow, Brown, & Mee, 1994). For example, depressed children and adolescents have low self-esteem (e.g., Altmann & Gotlib, 1988; King, Naylor, Segal, Evans, & Shain, 1993), and they often feel hopeless about their future, a risk factor for suicidal behavior in children and adolescents (e.g., Asarnow & Bates, 1988; McCauley, Mitchell, Burke, & Moss, 1988). Depressed children and adolescents report more negatively distorted cognitions (e.g., Kazdin, 1990; Kendall, Stark, & Adam, 1990), and depression particularly is associated with negative cognitions regarding loss and self-concept (Ambrose & Rholes, 1993; Jolly & Dykman, 1994). Depressed youngsters also display helpless or pessimistic styles of interpreting causes of negative and positive events (Gladstone & Kaslow, 1995; Hilsman & Garber, 1995; Nolen-Hoeksema, Girgus, & Seligman, 1986; Weisz, Sweeney, Proffitt, & Carr, 1993). An internal, stable, and global style of construing the causes of negative events is predictive of later depressive symptoms (e.g., Nolen-Hoeksema, Girgus, & Seligman, 1992), suggesting that this maladaptive attributional style may be a risk factor for depression.

Although it appears that for the most part depressed children and adolescents report negative cognitive patterns similar to those of depressed adults, it is unclear how these factors relate to broader environmental and developmental processes. For example, in a longitudinal investigation of the diathesis-stress version of the attributional style model of depression, Nolen-Hoeksema et al. (1992) examined the relations among stressful life events, attributional style, and depressive symptoms in school-age children from the third to the seventh grade. They found a developmental sequence in which stressful life events played a major role during the third grade, pessimistic explanatory styles began to have their impact during the fourth grade, and the two factors began to interact, as proposed by the diathesis-stress model, after the sixth grade. This study suggests that cognitive factors may interact with environmental stress, and their role may change with development.

Numerous questions about the development and function of children's cognitions remain to be answered, and their role in depression requires further clarification. Given the gaps in the knowledge of the significance and mechanisms in depression in children, it is surprising that cognitive factors have been given such heavy emphasis in current approaches to prevention (see below).

Social Problem-Solving and Coping Skills. Deficiencies in coping skills and social problem-solving strategies have also been examined as an individual source of vulnerability to depression. Various studies have indicated that depressed children are relatively impaired in various areas of social functioning. A few longitudinal studies further suggest that social deficiencies such as poorer quality of friendships (e.g., Goodyer, Wright, & Altham, 1990) and lower social competence (e.g., Cole, Martin, Powers, & Truglio, in press) increase the risk for future depression.

The ability to generate alternative solutions to hypothetical problems and the quality of interpersonal problem-solving strategies may distinguish depressed from nondepressed youngsters (e.g., Goodman, Gravitt, & Kaslow, 1995; Quiggle, Garber, Panak, & Dodge, 1992; Rudolph, Hammen, & Burge, 1994). Conversely, the use of strategies to cope with stress that focus on one's emotions and contribute to a process of rumination may increase the risk for depression (e.g., Grant & Compas, 1995; Nolen-Hoeksema & Girgus, 1994). Despite the promise of coping skills and problem-solving skills in clarifying risk and mechanisms of depression, many issues remain unresolved, including their etiological significance and their specificity to depression as opposed to other problems.

Contextual Factors

Social Context. As we have noted above, depression in young people has been increasing, and this increase is most likely associated with changes in the social environment of children and adolescents as opposed to increases in the reproductive rate of populations biologically at risk for depression. Poverty and economic hardship are broad contextual factors that may be associated with depression in young people. During the last 20 years, there has been a persistent increase in the poverty rate in the United States, both relatively and absolutely, especially for children (Huston, 1991).

The link between poverty or economic hardship and mental health is evident in a number of studies that have found higher levels of emotional and behavioral problems in poorer families (McLoyd, 1990). This association is mediated, however, by community and family factors that act on children, such as neighborhood violence, marital conflict, family disorganization, physical abuse, and child neglect (Conger et al., 1992). Most data on such effects have used child antisocial behavior as their mental health outcome measure (Dodge, Pettit, Gregory, & Bates, 1994). McLoyd, however, has proposed a pathway from poverty to parental depression that produced an increase in nonsupportive and punitive parenting and a subsequent increase in children's emotional problems, including higher levels of depressive symptoms. Following this theme, Conger and his colleagues (e.g., Conger et al., 1992; Ge, Conger, Lorenz, Shanahan, & Elder, 1995) found that economic pressure led to parental depressive symptoms and demoralization, producing marital problems and parenting disruption that contributed to depressive symptoms in adolescence.

Family. Several features of the family context constitute potential risk for depression in children: being the child of a depressed parent, dysfunctional relations between the parent and child, and parental discord and exposure to other adversities in the family context. Children of depressed parents have an increased risk for psychopathology and dysfunction, with some studies indicating that more than 70% of the offspring will experience diagnosable disorders (e.g., Fendrich, Warner, & Weissman, 1990; Hammen, Burge, Burney, & Adrian, 1990). Family studies have documented considerable impairments of functioning in infant, school-age, and adolescent children of depressed parents (e.g., Hammen et al., 1990; Keller et al., 1986; Weissman et al., 1987; Zahn-Waxler, Cummings, Iannotti, & Radke-Yarrow, 1984). Elevated rates of symptoms and diagnoses are found when children of depressed parents are compared both with normal families and with those with medical or other psychiatric illness (see review by Hammen, 1991).

The evidence of risk to children by virtue of having depressed parents is compelling and clearly calls for preventive interventions. Moreover, considerable evidence points to depression in youngsters as a frequent outcome of disrupted and dysfunctional family patterns. It is likely that rejecting, critical, or uninvolved parenting contributes to depression both directly by creating children's negative self-regard and indirectly by failing to provide skills and supports necessary to deal with life difficulties and challenges (Hammen, 1991). Moreover, dysfunctional families likely present children with exposure to high levels of stressors and continuing adversities, which in themselves may trigger depression. In view of the apparent impact of the family environment on children's depression, it is striking that some interventions for childhood depression attend rather minimally, and others not at all, to the family context. Interventions could be designed to target symptoms and disorder manifested in parental depression and/or to reduce marital conflict and discord (Downey & Coyne, 1990).

Stress. Whether measured as acute negative events or as continuing adversity, such as family disruption, studies of children and adolescents find a significant, moderately large association between stress and psychological symptoms (e.g., Compas, 1987; Jensen, Richters, Ussery, Bloedau, & Davis, 1991). The relation is not specific to depression, but both depressive symptoms and depressive disorders appear to result in part from psychosocial stressors (e.g., Compas, Grant, & Ey, 1994; Goodyer & Altham, 1991). Furthermore, relatively little research has clarified whether particular types of stressors are related to depressive symptoms. Family stressors, such as marital discord, abuse/neglect, aversive family climate, and parental illness, may certainly have a significant negative impact on children, but the effect is not specific to depression (e.g., Compas, Worsham, Epping-Jordan, & Grant, 1994).

Some studies have examined factors that mediate or moderate the effects of stress on depression in children (e.g., Robinson, Garber, & Hilsman, 1995). The role of dysfunctional cognitions, such as depressive attribution style or negative self-cognitions, has been examined, yielding mixed support (e.g., Hammen, 1988; Nolen-Hoeksema et al., 1992; Panak & Garber, 1992). A more specific version of the cognitive diathesis-stress model predicts that cognitive vulnerability in specific domains such as achievement or social relationships will trigger depression when negative life events match that domain; this model has received some support in the few studies that actually test it (Hammen & Goodman-Brown, 1990; Hilsman & Garber, 1995; Turner & Cole, 1994). Other research has focused on the moderating role of resources and social supports (including quality of relationship with the parent) in buffering the effects of stress on children's depression. Such studies generally have indicated that social and family resources exert a direct or buffering effect on stress outcomes (e.g., Forehand et al., 1991; Gore, Aseltine, & Colton, 1992; Hammen, Burge, & Adrian, 1991; Robinson & Garber, 1995).

Preventive Interventions

The conceptualization of preventive interventions has grown in its complexity and sophistication, as reflected in other chapters in this volume. We will consider the prevention of depression in young people in the context of recent broad conceptualizations of preventive interventions and "prevention science" (Coie et al., 1993). As a first step in understanding the current literature, it is essential to distinguish between treatment and prevention. *Treatment* is best viewed as the reduction in symptoms or the amelioration of disorder in already identified cases. Although treatment effects could manifest themselves through time, at least some effects are likely to be immediate. *Prevention* is commonly defined as a reduction in the occurrence of new cases or a delay in the onset of new cases or symptoms. For disorders such as depression, in which symptoms tend to fluctuate during the life span in number and severity, it is also possible to define prevention as a reduction in the recurrence of symptoms. It is, of course, possible for a single intervention to have both treatment and prevention effects. It seems likely that any intervention with the power to prevent future occurrences of depressive problems will also alleviate current symptoms.

Preventive interventions for psychopathology fall into three categories—universal, selective, and indicated (Institute of Medicine, 1994). A *universal preventive intervention* is one targeted to the general population, such as a social skills intervention provided to an entire school. Although the vast majority of individuals within the group are not at risk, universal interventions are typically nonintrusive and are likely to provide skills or information that will be helpful to a wide segment of the population, even if individuals are not at risk for a particular disorder. A *selective preventive intervention* is geared toward a group whose risk of developing a disorder is significantly higher than average because of the presence of biological and/or psychosocial risk factors. An example is a program delivered to children whose parents have a history of depression, regardless of the current distress levels of the individual children. Finally, an *indicated preventive intervention* is one targeted to high-risk individuals who are demonstrating early symptoms of mental disorder or who have biological and/or psychological markers indicating a predisposition for the disorder. Decisions about whether a universal, selective, or indicated prevention program is called for should be driven in part by a cost-benefit analysis of the effects of intervention. Ideally, prevention programs will address risk factors before they stabilize (Coie et al., 1993). This must be balanced, however, with careful consideration of whether an individual's or group's risk of developing a disorder outweighs the cost, time, and any possible harmful side effects (e.g., stigmatization or increased distress) of the proposed preventive intervention.

Although the distinctions between the three prevention categories may appear simple, it is often difficult to determine the level at which a preventive intervention is operating. In the case of depression, this is partly a consequence of the multiple levels of depressive phenomena described above. Because the overlap and predictive relationship of depressed mood, mixed anxiety/depression syndrome, and depressive disorders have not yet been fully established, it is unclear whether mild depressive symptoms represent risk factors for a major depressive episode, early signs of the onset of major depression, or a separate disorder entirely. Thus, for example, an attempt to prevent the onset of MDD in a sample of adolescents with high levels of depressive symptoms is a selective preventive intervention if depressive symptoms are viewed as risk factors for major depression or an indicated preventive intervention if they are considered early symptoms of the disorder itself. Further complicating matters, some interventions focus on the prevention of depressive symptoms rather than depressive disorder. Because the term *depression* has been used to refer to such a wide range of conditions, it is essential to carefully consider the operational definition of depression when comparing various prevention programs.

Outcome Studies

A small but growing body of research on the prevention of depression in children and adolescents has now appeared in the literature. Table 6.3 displays results from these studies, summarizing information about sample characteristics, research design, control groups, the nature of the targeted risk factors, characteristics of intervention, treatment effects, and prevention effects. These studies are quite varied with regard to the age of the participants, ranging from young children (Kellam, Rebok, Mayer, Ialongo, & Kalodner, 1994) to middle and older adolescents (Clarke et al., 1995). Sample sizes vary from moderate (*N* = 69) to large (*N* = 204); little attention has been given, however, to the statistical power generated by the size of these samples. Because the point prevalence of depressive disorder is often low, researchers will need either participants with a high likelihood of developing a depression or an extremely large sample. All the studies described here include a control group, with some form of random assignment to intervention and control conditions. All the studies include a measure of depressive symptoms as one of the outcomes (the Children's Depression Inventory [CDI] was used in three studies, and the CES-D in the other), whereas only one study includes a measure of MDD (Clarke et al., 1995). Three of the interventions are cognitive-behavioral in nature in that they are designed to reduce negative cognitions, enhance social problem-solving skills, and/or enhance skills for coping with stress.

Three of these studies use depressive symptoms as the primary risk factor in identifying their target groups for intervention, whereas the fourth uses reading delays as a risk factor (Kellam et al., 1994). The use of depressive symptoms as a risk factor reflects an indicated intervention approach for these programs. Elevated depressive symptoms have been used as a risk factor in part because they are one of the best predictors of subsequent depressive disorder. Only one study that included depressive symptoms as a risk factor, however, also specifically targeted the prevention of depressive disorders (Clarke et al., 1995). Unfortunately, the use of depressive symptoms as the primary risk factor leads to some

Table 6.3 Prevention of Depression Outcome Studies

Study	*Selection of Participants (N)*	*Control (N)*	*Mean Age*	*Risk Factors*	*Measures/ Source*	*Intervention*	*Treatment Effects*	*Prevention Effects*
Clarke et al. (1995)	High levels of depressive symptoms and no affective diagnosis (76)	Randomly assigned by individual (74)	15.5	Depressive symptoms; negative and irrational cognitions	CES-D/self; GAF/self; K-SADS-E/self; HDRS/ interviewer; parent interview	School-based; 11 hours during 5 weeks; master's+ leader taught identification and modification of negative thoughts	Decreased CES-D scores for prevention group	Fewer MDD and DY diagnoses in intervention group at 12 months
Jaycox et al. (1994)	High levels of depressive symptoms and parental conflict (69)	Randomly assigned by individual to wait-list control (24); no-treatent control from another school (50)	11.5	Depressive symptoms; cognitive distortions and deficiencies; pessimistic explanatory style; life stressors	CDI/self; CPQ/self; CASQ/self; RCDS/self; CBCL/parent; teacher report/teacher	Clinic based; 18 hours during 12 weeks; Graduate-level+ leader taught social problem-solving skills, skills for coping with family conflict, and/or modification of negative attributions	Decreased CDI scores for prevention groups, mediated by decrease in negative attributions and decreased externalizing behavior according to teacher report	Fewer children from intervention groups experienced "moderate depression" at 6 months
Gillham et al. (1995)	Same as above	Same as above	Same as above	Same as above	CDI/self; CPQ/self; CASQ/self; RCDS/self	Same as above	N/A	Prevention of symptom onset or recurrence in intervention groups at 24 months; effect mediated by explanatory style

(continued)

Table 6.3 Continued

Study	*Selection of Participants (N)*	*Control (N)*	*Mean Age*	*Risk Factors*	*Measures/ Source*	*Intervention*	*Treatment Effects*	*Prevention Effects*
Kellam et al. (1994)	General student population (204)	Randomly assigned by classrooms within schools (158) and across schools (226)	6.3	Reading delays; poor self-efficacy	CAT-Reading/self; CDI/self	Yearlong classroom reading enrichment program, with group-based approach to mastery and flexible correction routines	Reading achievement gains reduced continuity of depressive symptoms from fall to spring	No long-term follow-up
Petersen et al. (in press)	Student population oversampled for depressive symptoms (150+)	Randomly assigned by individuals (150+)	7th grade	Depressive symptoms; school, family, and social stressors; poor coping skills	SIQYA; mastery and coping, emotional tone/self; DISC/self; CDI/self; YSR/self	11 hours during 16 weeks; graduate-level+ leader taught skills for assessing events, problem solving, social skills	Improved coping and emotional tone, lower YSR internalizing and externalizing scores	All *ns* at 12 months.

NOTES: CASQ = Children's Attributional Style Questionnaire
CAT = California Achievement Test
CBCL = Child Behavior Checklist
CDI = Children's Depression Inventory
HDRS = Hamilton Depression Rating Scales
K-SADS-E = Schedule for Affective Disorders and Schizophrenia for School-Age Children-Epidemiological Version
RCDS = Reynolds Children's Depression Scale
SIQYA = Self-Image Questionnaire for Young Adolescents
YSR = Youth Self Report
CES-D = Center for Epidemiological Studies-Depression Scale
CPQ = Child's Perception Questionnaire
DISC = Diagnostic Interview Schedule for Children
GAF = Global Assessment of Functioning

difficulties because depressive symptoms are often both the risk factor and the target of prevention (Jaycox, Reivich, Gillham, & Seligman, 1994; Petersen, Leffert, Graham, Alwin, & Ding, in press). Thus, only prevention of symptom increase or recurrence can be studied, not prevention of symptom onset.

Because space does not permit a detailed description of each of the intervention protocols used in these prevention trials, we will focus on describing two of the interventions, each of which represents one of the main forms prevention trials have taken. The first study, the only trial to demonstrate a prevention effect for as long as 24 months post-intervention, is a school-based targeted prevention of depressive symptoms, based on the teaching of cognitive techniques (Gillham, Reivich, Jaycox, & Seligman, 1995; Jaycox et al., 1994). The prevention trials conducted by Clarke et al. (1995) and Petersen et al. (in press) are based on similar interventions. The second study described is a universal prevention program geared toward improving reading achievement (Kellam et al., 1994).

Seligman and colleagues (Gillham et al., 1995; Jaycox et al., 1994) focused on the prevention of depressive symptoms in 10- to 13-year-old children identified as "at-risk" on the basis of reports of parental conflict and current depressive symptoms. Participants were randomized to a control group, cognitive training group, social problem-solving group, or combined cognitive and social problem-solving group. The groups, consisting of 10 to 12 students, were conducted by doctoral students for 90 minutes weekly for 12 weeks during after-school hours. The cognitive component emphasized that beliefs about stressful events, rather than the events themselves, lead to distress. Students were taught to identify negative causal attributions and to challenge pessimistic explanations of events. The cognitive component also encouraged students to look for solutions to problems and to actively cope with negative feelings. The social problem-solving component specifically taught skills for dealing with problems, such as goal setting, information gathering, generation of multiple possible solutions, and decision making. Within the problem-solving component, coping with family conflict was emphasized, and students were taught to use distraction, relaxation skills, distancing, and social support in response to stressful family situations. Because there were no major differences among the three active intervention groups, intervention groups were collapsed for statistical analysis.

Although Kellam et al. (1994) also hypothesized that a pessimistic explanatory style is an important mechanism in the development and maintenance of depressive symptoms, they took a different approach to prevention, focusing on improving mastery rather than attempting to directly alter cognitions. On the basis of research suggesting that poor academic mastery may initiate and intensify depressive symptoms (Kellam, Werthamer-Larson, Dolan, & Brown, 1991), they designed a universal prevention program for first-grade students. First-grade teachers were trained in the use of an enriched curriculum, designed to improve reading achievement by using a group-based assessment of mastery and a flexible corrective process. Students did not progress to new material until 80% of the class had achieved at least 80% of the learning objectives of the current unit. Correction was tailored to individuals and was flexible in the timing and variety of corrective techniques. Within the prevention trial, students were randomized by classroom to receive either regular reading programs or the enriched curriculum throughout their first-grade year.

The initial outcomes of these studies are encouraging. Jaycox et al. (1994) demonstrated that brief training in modifying negative cognitions and social problem solving decreased the negative attributions made by young adolescents experiencing depressive symptoms and high levels of family conflict. This decrease in negative attributions mediated a decrease in depressive symptoms shown by the prevention group on a self-report measure. Teacher-reported externalizing behaviors also decreased in the prevention group; this effect, however, was not mediated by changes in attributions. Follow-up analyses with this sample (Gillham et al., 1995) found that differences in depressive symptoms between control and intervention groups grew through time. Children in the prevention group with initially high symptom levels showed some symptom decrease and were less likely than control group children to report symptoms in the moderate to severe range at the 6-month, 12-month, 18-month, and 24-month assessments, demonstrating maintenance of initial gains. Initially low-symptom children in the prevention group compared with the control group showed a significantly smaller increase in symptoms through time, indicating prevention of onset of depressive symptoms through the 24-month follow-up. Overall, at the 24-month follow-up, children in the intervention group were only half as likely as children in the control group to report depressive symptoms in the moderate to severe range. Gillham and colleagues also continued to explore the mechanism of prevention, demonstrating at all follow-up points that children in the prevention group demonstrated a significantly more optimistic explanatory style and that explanatory style mediated the program's effect of depressive symptoms. These effects are quite striking in light of the brief nature of the original intervention.

Kellam et al. (1994) demonstrated that children starting the year with high levels of depressive symptoms who made gains in reading achievement as a result of the intervention were less likely to have high levels of depressive symptoms at the end of the school year. The pattern was somewhat different for boys and girls, with the effect for girls based solely on achievement gains and the effect for boys also being related to placement in the reading intervention or nonintervention classroom, as well as achievement gains.

The problem-solving and social skills program implemented by Petersen et al. (in press) with seventh-grade students led to improvements in coping skills and decreases in self-reported internalizing and externalizing scores. The specific relationship between coping skills in leading to reduced depressive symptoms was not assessed. This study was one of the few to attempt to understand the impact of the intervention of subgroups, however, with data analyzed by sex and by high- or low-risk status. Improvements in emotional tone were most pronounced for high-risk girls in the intervention group.

In the Clarke et al. (1995) study of adolescents with depressive symptoms, on the basis of diagnostic interviews with adolescents at a 1-year follow-up, intervention participants had significantly fewer diagnoses of MDD or DY (14.5%) than did the control group (25.7%). There were no differences, however, between the control and intervention groups on questionnaire-rated levels of depressive symptoms, global functioning, or interviewer-rated depression.

All these studies have demonstrated some beneficial effects; they did not, however, all specifically assess the relationship between decreases in depressive symptoms and the hypothesized risk factors. For example, although Clarke et al. (1995) demonstrated a short-term reduction in CES-D scores for individuals who had been instructed in the identification and modification of negative thoughts, it is not clear whether this was due to participants' improved skills because coping with negative thoughts was not assessed.

Depression and Suicide Prevention

As we described above, there is a strong relationship between depressive disorders and suicide, particularly in individuals who also have substance abuse or conduct problems. Therefore, although suicide is addressed by Kalafat in the next chapter in this volume, it warrants some attention here. As rates of suicide have climbed in the 15- to 24-year-old age group, more and more prevention programs are being implemented. One survey shows that the number of schools implementing prevention programs more than doubled between the academic years 1984-1985 to 1986-1987, with programs reaching nearly 200,000 students (Garland, Shaffer, & Whittle, 1989).

Prevention programs have ranged from schoolwide programs designed to increase competence and decrease stress, to phone hotlines designed for crisis intervention. Thus far, the majority of youth suicide prevention programs have been high school-based programs led by teachers or guidance counselors. Most programs last about 4 hours, with goals of raising the awareness of youth about suicide, teaching warning signs, teaching youth to break confidentiality if they suspect a peer is suicidal, and facilitating access to available mental health resources (Garland et al., 1989).

Thus far, few well-controlled suicide prevention studies have been done (see Kalafat, this volume). Although the chapter by Kalafat highlights the potential of the second wave of suicide prevention programs, substantial controversy exists surrounding the success of prevention programs currently in place. Researchers have raised three main concerns about the types of prevention programs currently being implemented. First, "facts" about suicide taught in these programs may not be well validated. Warning signs of suicide, such as giving away possessions and talking about the future in ambiguous terms, have not been empirically validated (Shaffer, Garland, Gould, Fisher, & Trautman, 1989). In addition, although the majority of programs teach that suicide is not related to mental illness but simply a response that anyone might have in the face of overwhelming stress, evidence clearly indicates that suicide is strongly related to psychopathology. Although the rationale of programs may be to decrease the stigma of suicidal ideation so that individuals will seek help, some fear that this view romanticizes suicide, which would not occur if students were taught that a suicide attempt was a sign of severe mental illness (Brent & Perper, 1995). Second, targeting a general student population does not appear to be effective. Of the 172,000 students involved in prevention programs in 1986-1987, according to census data, only 18 would have been expected to commit suicide, leaving the other 1,800 adolescents in the population who committed suicide during these years unassisted (Garland et al., 1989). In addition, the vast majority of adolescents participating in suicide prevention programs already knew the warning signs of suicide, believed that suicidal threats should be taken seriously, believed that mental health professionals were helpful, and knew to break confidentiality if a friend discussed suicidal ideation (Shaffer et al., 1989). Finally, many researchers fear that beyond being ineffective, some suicide prevention programs may actually harm participants. Some evidence suggests that suicide rates increase following the airing of television programs about youth suicide. The amount of publicity given to a local youth suicide is significantly related to the number of copycat suicides following the first suicide (Shaffer et al., 1989). In addition, not only did the views of the most at-risk youth fail to change following a prevention program, many reported feeling more hopeless, less sure that mental health professionals would be of help, and more likely to identify suicide as a possible solution to a problem (Shaffer, Garland, Vieland, Underwood, & Busner, 1991).

One direction for enhancing the efficacy of suicide prevention efforts is to establish a closer link with depression prevention programs. The strong association between depression and suicide clearly suggests that this is an important avenue for future research. As discussed below, both depression and suicide may be best addressed as part of broader preventive interventions that address wide ranges of problems.

Conclusions and Future Directions

We will now consider the progress that has been made in the prevention of depression in young people and outline directions for future research by addressing six key questions for the field. These are key issues to consider in the formulation of goals for *Healthy People 2010* as they pertain to depression in young people.

1. Should we prevent depression in childhood and adolescence?

The evidence is clear that depression represents a significant health and mental health problem for children and adolescents. The prevalence of significant symptoms of depressed mood, symptoms of a syndrome of mixed anxiety/depression, and rates of MDD and DY are all sizeable, particularly among adolescents. Moreover, there is evidence that depressive problems are increasing among children and youth.

In addition to establishing the prevalence of depressive problems, research has shown that there are significant correlates and consequences of depression in young people. These include impairment in academic and interpersonal functioning and disrupted development. The onset of depression in childhood or adolescence also predicts a worse course for the disorder, with an increased likelihood of recurrent episodes during adulthood. The most serious correlate of depression in childhood and adolescence is the dramatic increase in risk for attempted and completed suicide. Although suicide is affected by a number of factors, an episode of major depression increases the risk for a suicide attempt dramatically, and this risk is further magnified when depression is comorbid with disruptive behavior disorders or substance or alcohol abuse. Given the high priority given in *Healthy People 2000* (DHHS, 1991) to reducing the rate of adolescent suicide, further consideration of depression in suicide is essential.

On the basis of the evidence of the prevalence, severity, course, and correlates of depression in childhood and adolescence, it is clear that depression should be a high priority for preventive interventions that are a part of the objectives of *Healthy People 2010*. Early intervention could reduce the risk for associated problems and impairment during childhood and adolescence and reduce the risk for future depression during adulthood as well. From a developmental perspective, late childhood and early adolescence are optimal times for the prevention of depression and, indirectly, the many problems that are associated with depression. Early adolescence appears to be an important time to deter the negative course that is set in motion by the onset of depressive problems at a young age.

2. Can we prevent depression in childhood and adolescence?

Although it is clear that the prevention of depression among children and youth should be a major health priority, the evidence is less clear that we are currently capable of accomplishing this important objective. At best, current intervention efforts can be labeled as promising; at worst, the wide-scale implementation of prevention programs aimed at depression would be premature at the present time.

The promise of current programs is reflected in several features of current research and program development. First, researchers have shown that it is feasible to implement depression prevention programs in schools and in mental health settings. The programs that have been developed have been delivered in an efficient, cost-effective manner that is acceptable to children, adolescents, families, and schools. Second, the initial findings suggest that depressive symptoms can be reduced and that the onset of elevated depressive symptoms and perhaps episodes of MDD and DY can be decreased. Third, there is some evidence that these effects can be maintained at follow-ups as long as 1 to 2 years after the intervention (Clarke et al., 1995; Gillham et al., 1995).

These promising features of depression prevention programs are balanced by several limitations in current research. First, these studies have relied primarily on self-reports of depressed mood or depressive symptoms, rather than indexes of other levels of depressive problems. None of the studies employed the widely used measures that reflect the mixed anxiety/depression syndrome identified by Achenbach (1991b, 1991c) and colleagues. Only one study used standardized interviews to derive *DSM* diagnoses of MDD and DY. Thus, the demonstrated impact of these programs has been primarily limited to only one level of depressive problems, as reported by a single informant. Second, the samples in these studies have been relatively small and limited in their representativeness. Third, although Clarke et al. (1995) and Seligman and his associates (Gillham et al., 1995; Jaycox et al., 1994) reported evidence for follow-up effects at 12 and 24 months, respectively, Kellam et al. (1994) have not yet reported follow-up data on their intervention, and Petersen et al. (in press) reported that initial gains from the intervention were lost at 12 months. Thus, the ability of these programs to truly prevent depression in the long term is unclear. Fourth, none of these studies included measures of other forms of psychopathology that are frequently associated with depression. Given that comorbid problems may play a role in the onset or recurrence of depression, it is essential to include measures of other syndromes and disorders.

3. Should preventive interventions for depression be universal, selective, or indicated in nature?

All three approaches to prevention are represented in these initial intervention studies. Kellam et al. (1994) and Petersen et al. (in press) report on universal interventions administered to all students in public school settings, Seligman and colleagues (Gillham et al., 1995; Jaycox et al., 1994) report on a selective intervention on the basis of cognitive and social risk factors, and Clarke et al. (1995) describe an indicated intervention for adolescents who are already experiencing depressive symptoms. Thus, there is preliminary support for each of these approaches.

A broader perspective on preventive interventions suggests that these types of interventions need to be linked in a hierarchical and sequential fashion (Compas, 1995). That is, these three approaches to prevention are not in competition with one another to determine which is the optimal way to prevent depression or other disorders. They are complementary in the effects that they can have on the incidence and recurrence of a disorder. Universal interventions are important to reduce the incidence in the population as a whole. They will reach the largest proportion of the population and are likely to deter some of the broad risk factors from coming into play. It is unlikely, however, that universal interventions can deliver a sufficient dose nor address risk factors with sufficient specificity to prevent depression in those children and youth who are at high risk. Therefore, universal interventions need to be complemented by selective interventions that are delivered to subgroups within the population who are distinguished on the basis of exposure to personal or contextual risk factors. Because the identification of risk factors is always an imperfect process and no intervention will be completely effective in preventing a problem, selective interventions need to be coordinated with indicated interventions for those children and youth who already evidence significant depressive symptoms.

4. Have the crucial risk factors been addressed in these interventions?

Depression is a heterogeneous problem with multiple sources of risk. Not surprisingly, previous interventions have addressed some, but not all, of the important sources of risk for depression in childhood and adolescence. The most common focus has been on sources of cognitive vulnerability including a negative attributional or explanatory style, dysfunctional or irrational thinking, ineffective strategies for solving social problems, and maladaptive ways of coping with stress. These constitute the major personal or individual sources of vulnerability to depression.

In contrast to the attention given to individual sources of risk, contextual factors have received relatively little attention. Foremost among the contextual sources of risk are family factors, including parental depression, conflict, and maladaptive parenting. None of the interventions described above have directly addressed the role of parental depression and other sources of family stress that are central to the risk for depression in many children and youth. Some promising efforts in this area have been reported by Beardslee and colleagues in their development of a preventive intervention for families of depressed parents (Beardslee et al., 1993; Beardslee, Wright, Rothberg, Salt, & Versage, 1996). Unfortunately, no child outcome data are yet available on this program.

A comprehensive model of depression will need to include both person-centered and contextual risk and protective factors. Previous research has not identified specific risk factors for depression, in part because there may be few risk factors that are indeed specific to this problem. In light of the high rates of co-occurrence and comorbidity associated with depression, a broader perspective on risk and protective factors appears to be warranted.

5. Should preventive interventions specifically target depression, or should they be aimed at multiple problems simultaneously?

One of the defining characteristics of depression in young people is the pattern of comorbidity with other disorders and co-occurrence with other problems. A glaring omission in previous studies has been the evaluation of the impact of interventions on other problems and disorders, including anxiety, disruptive behavior disorders, alcohol and substance abuse, eating disorders, and suicide. This oversight has operated in both directions, that is, interventions designed to prevent a host of other problems have failed to measure their impact on the prevention of depression, just as depression prevention programs have often not measured their effects on other problems.

As more resources are devoted to the prevention of a wide range of problems in children and youth, we run the risk of overburdening institutions such as schools that are asked to deliver these interventions, as well as the ability and willingness of young people themselves to participate in multiple intervention programs. This problem is a direct reflection of delivering interventions to discrete problems or disorders, rather than conceptualizing and implementing programs in a coordinated manner. A perusal of the content of these interventions reveals substantial overlap in their content. For example, interventions designed to prevent aggression and violence (e.g., Elias et al., 1986; Tremblay et al., 1991; Vitaro & Tremblay, 1994), as well as those to prevent substance abuse, contain many elements similar to the depression interventions reviewed above. Common elements include the development of effective social problem-solving skills and adaptive strategies for coping with stress. Depression interventions differ from these other programs somewhat in their emphasis on prevention of self-blame and other negative ways of thinking. An important next step for future research is to evaluate the efficacy of broadly focused preventive interventions for a wider range of problems.

It is possible that integration of preventive interventions can be best achieved at the universal intervention level, whereas more specific interventions will be needed for selective and indicated programs. This will be true, however, only to the extent that unique risk factors are associated with different problems and disorders. As noted above, however, much of the risk research has not delineated specific risk factors for specific disorders. For example, even if we accept that parental depression is the single strongest risk factor for depression in children and adolescents, it is also clear that children of depressed parents are at risk for many problems other than depression. Therefore, interventions based on broad models of risk and protective factors may be required.

6. What are the major methodological hurdles facing researchers in the prevention of depression in young people?

Continued development of preventive interventions for depression depends in part on overcoming methodological problems in this research. Several problems reflect generic issues in prevention research, whereas others are more unique to the problems presented by the characteristics of depression in children and adolescents.

First, larger and more diverse samples need to be included in future depression prevention trials. The relatively small samples in previous studies have limited statistical power for testing intervention effects for the whole sample. Further, the small samples have limited the degree to which follow-up analyses can be conducted on the onset of depressive episodes because these will occur relatively rarely in a specified window of time, even within a high-risk sample. Previous research has included primarily middle-socioeconomic-status Caucasian samples, limiting the generalizability of these findings to more ethnically diverse youth and children and adolescents in poverty.

Better understanding of depressive processes and the development of more sophisticated theoretical models require moving beyond the study of the relationship between depressive symptoms to the analysis of more specific risk factors. Beyond assessing initial depressive symptoms, all the studies described in this chapter hypothesized that specific risk factors, such as family conflict, poor academic achievement, and cognitive processing style, were implicated in causing or maintaining depressive symptoms and geared their intervention to improving weak skills or enhancing needed coping resources. To validate a theory, however, the design of the prevention program must include measurement of depressive symptoms/disorder and of the hypothesized risk and protective factors. There are three steps in analyzing the data. First, the study must demonstrate that a decrease in risk factors or an increase in protective factors is related to the intervention. Second, the study must demonstrate that the changes in risk or protective factors are associated with decreased levels of depression. Third, to demonstrate a preventive effect, the analysis must demonstrate that the prevention group has lower levels of depression than a control group at a long-term follow-up. Several studies have succeeded in doing this well (Gillham et al., 1995; Jaycox et al., 1994).

In most treatment studies, random assignment of individuals to intervention and control groups is used to demonstrate that the intervention, rather than other variables, led to targeted changes. In prevention trials, however, there are several practical constraints to randomization by individual. The majority of prevention programs take place within school classrooms, and it can be difficult and disruptive to randomize children within a classroom to different conditions. In addition, there may be a negative impact on individuals in control groups when they are aware that others are receiving an intervention while they are not. Thus, in prevention trials, groups are often randomized by classroom or school district, rather than by individual, which requires careful assessment of possible between-group differences. Of the four studies presented in this chapter, all either randomized between treatment and control group by individual or paid close attention to equivalence between groups. For example, in the rare cases in which between-group differences were found after careful matching, Petersen et al. (in press) chose to bias the assignment of classrooms to prevention or control conditions against the sought-for effects, thus providing the most stringent test of the prevention program.

Despite gaps in knowledge about the development and course of depressive disorders, considerable information is now available about related risk and protective factors (see above). Although the bulk of knowledge thus far has come from descriptive and epidemiological studies, randomized prevention trials are in many ways ideally suited to test theories about risk and resilience factors. Good prevention studies not only will be based on empirically validated theories but also will be specifically designed to test those theories. Prevention trials can contribute to the understanding of the development and course of depression in two ways. First, using depressive symptoms as risk factors, they can help clarify the relationship between depressive symptoms and depressive disorders. Although this first step will help in deciding when a preventive intervention is called for, it will not suggest the actual shape of the intervention. The second way prevention studies can contribute to basic research is by elucidating the relationship between depressive symptoms and hypothesized causal mechanisms, such as environmental stress, biological predispositions, and cognitive processing styles. Fortunately, it is possible for prevention workers to target both goals within the same study.

Conclusion: Implications for *Healthy Children 2010*

The prevention of depression in young people warrants increased attention on the agenda of prevention researchers and in national health objectives for children and adolescents. The knowledge base of the characteristics, course, and risk factors for depression is now in place. Promising programs have been developed, and initial evaluation data have been reported. There is considerable promise that future research can lead to programs that can make meaningful reductions in depressive symptoms, episodes of MDD, and the many deleterious correlates and consequences of depression in children and youth.

Greater recognition of the scope and significance of depression in young people has a clear place in the development of objectives for *Healthy People 2010*. First, the goal of reducing suicide among youth (Fleming, 1996) will be facilitated by addressing the role of depression as a significant risk factor for suicide. This is particularly true for adolescents who experience other mental health and behavioral problems in combination with depression. Second, the goal of reducing the overall prevalence of mental disorders among children and adolescents (Fleming, 1996) must include the reduction of the prevalence of depression as part of this objective. As noted above, depression should be included as one of the targets of comprehensive preventive interventions. Third, the goals outlined in *Healthy People 2000* include recognition of enhanced quality of life as an essential element of improved health in the broad sense. Reductions in the prevalence of depressive symptoms and disorders will reflect an important step toward improvement in overall quality of life among our nation's children.

References

Achenbach, T. M. (1985). *Assessment and taxonomy of child and adolescent psychopathology.* Beverly Hills, CA: Sage.

Achenbach, T. M. (1991a). *Integrative guide for the 1991 CBCL/4-18, YSR, and TRF Profiles.* Burlington: University of Vermont, Department of Psychiatry.

Achenbach, T. M. (1991b). *Manual for the Child Behavior Checklist and 1991 Profile.* Burlington: University of Vermont, Department of Psychiatry.

Achenbach, T. M. (1991c). *Manual for the Youth Self-Report and 1991 Profile.* Burlington: University of Vermont, Department of Psychiatry.

Achenbach, T. M. (1993). *Empirically based taxonomy.* Burlington: University of Vermont, Department of Psychiatry.

Achenbach, T. M., & Howell, C. T. (1993). Are American children's problems getting worse? A 13-year comparison. *Journal of the American Academy of Child and Adolescent Psychiatry, 32,* 1145-1154.

Achenbach, T. M., Howell, C. T., McConaughy, S. H., & Stanger, C. T. (1995). Six-year predictors of problems in a national sample of children and youth: I. Cross-informant syndromes. *Journal of the American Academy of Child and Adolescent Psychiatry, 34,* 336-347.

Achenbach, T. M., Verhulst, F. C., Baron, G. G., & Akkerhuis, G. W. (1987). Epidemiological comparisons of American and Dutch children: I. Behavioral/emotional problems and competencies reported by parents for ages 4 to 16. *Journal of the American Academy of Child and Adolescent Psychology, 26,* 317-325.

Altmann, E. O., & Gotlib, I. H. (1988). The social behavior of depressed children: An observational study. *Journal of Abnormal Child Psychology, 16,* 29-44.

Ambrose, B., & Rholes, W. S. (1993). Automatic cognitions and symptoms of depression and anxiety in children and adolescents: An examination of the content specificity hypothesis. *Cognitive Therapy and Research, 17,* 289-308.

American Psychiatric Association. (1994). *Diagnostic and statistical manual of mental disorders* (4th ed.). Washington, DC: Author.

Angold, A. (1988). Childhood and adolescent depression: I. Epidemiological and aetiological aspects. *British Journal of Psychiatry, 152,* 601-617.

Angold, A., & Costello, E. J. (1993). Depressive comorbidity in children and adolescents: Empirical, theoretical, and methodological issues. *American Journal of Psychiatry, 150,* 1779-1791.

Angold, A., & Rutter, M. (1992). Effects of age and pubertal status on depression in a large clinical sample. *Development and Psychopathology, 4,* 5-28.

Asarnow, J. R., & Bates, S. (1988). Depression in child psychiatric inpatients: Cognitive and attributional patterns. *Journal of Abnormal Child Psychology, 16,* 601-615.

Aseltine, R. H., Gore, S., & Colton, M. E. (1994). Depression and the social developmental context of adolescence. *Journal of Personality and Social Psychology, 67,* 252-263.

Beardslee, W. R., Salt, P., Perterfield, K., Rothberg, P. C., van de Velde, P., Swatling, S., Hoke, L., Moilanen, D. L., & Wheelock, I. (1993). Comparison of preventive interventions for families with parental affective disorder. *Journal of the American Academy of Child and Adolescent Psychiatry, 32,* 254-263.

Beardslee, W. R., Wright, E., Rothberg, P. C., Salt, P., & Versage, E. (1996). *Response of families to two preventive intervention strategies: Long-term differences in behavior and attitude change.* Manuscript under review.

Brent, D. A., & Perper, J. A., (1995). Research in adolescent suicide: Implications for training, service delivery, and public policy. *Suicide and Life-Threatening Behavior, 25,* 222-230.

Brooks-Gunn, J., Petersen, A. C., & Compas, B. E. (1995). Physiological processes and the development of childhood and adolescent depression. In I. M. Goodyer (Ed.), *The depressed child and adolescent: Developmental and clinical perspectives* (pp. 81-109). New York: Cambridge University Press.

Cantwell, D. P., & Baker, L. (1991). Manifestations of depressive affect in adolescence. *Journal of Youth and Adolescence, 20,* 121-133.

Carlson, G. A. (1994). Adolescent bipolar disorder: Phenomenology and treatment implications. In W. M. Reynolds & H. F. Johnston (Eds.), *Handbook of depression in children and adolescents* (pp. 41-60). New York: Plenum.

Cicchetti, D., Rogosch, F. A., & Toth, S. L. (1994). A developmental psychopathology perspective on depression in children. In W. M. Reynolds & H. F. Johnston (Eds.), *Handbook of depression in children and adolescents* (pp. 97-122). New York: Plenum.

Clarke, G. N., Hawkins, W., Murphy, M., Sheeber, L. B., Lewinsohn, P. M., & Seeley, J.R. (1995). Targeted prevention of unipolar depressive disorder in an at-risk sample of high school adolescents: A randomized trial of a group cognitive intervention. *Journal of the American Academy of Child and Adolescent Psychiatry, 34,* 312-321.

Coie, J. D., Watt, N., West, S. G., Hawkins, D., Asarnow, J., Markman, H., Ramey, S., Shure, M., & Long, B. (1993). The science of prevention: A conceptual framework and some directions for a national research program. *American Psychologist, 48,* 1013-1022.

Cole, D. A. (1991). Change in self-perceived competence as a function of peer and teacher evaluation. *Developmental Psychology, 27,* 682-688.

Cole, D., Martin, J., Powers, B., & Truglio, R. (in press). Modeling causal relations between academic and social competence and depression: A multitrait-multimethod longitudinal study of children. *Journal of Abnormal Psychology.*

Compas, B. E. (1987). Stress and life events during childhood and adolescence. *Clinical Psychology Review, 7,* 275-302.

Compas, B. E. (1995). Promoting successful coping during adolescence. In M. Rutter (Ed.), *Psychosocial disturbances in young people: Challenges for prevention.* New York: Cambridge University Press.

Compas, B. E., Ey, S., & Grant, K. E. (1993). Taxonomy, assessment, and diagnosis of depression during adolescence. *Psychological Bulletin, 114,* 323-344.

Compas, B. E., Grant, K., & Ey, S. (1994). Psychosocial stress and child/adolescent depression: Can we be more specific? In W. M. Reynolds & H. F. Johnston (Eds.), *Handbook of depression in children and adolescents.* New York: Plenum.

Compas, B. E., & Hammen, C. L. (1994). Child and adolescent depression: Covariation and comorbidity in development. In R. J. Haggerty, L. R. Sherrod, N. Garmezy, & M. Rutter (Eds.), *Stress, risk, and resilience in children and adolescents: Processes, mechanisms, and interventions* (pp. 225-267). New York: Cambridge University Press.

Compas, B. E., Oppedisano, G., Connor, J. K., Gerhardt, C. A., Hinden, B., Achenbach, T. M., & Hammen, C. (in press). Gender differences in depressive symptoms in adolescence: Comparison of national samples of clinically-referred and non-referred youth. *Journal of Consulting and Clinical Psychology.*

Compas, B. E., Worsham, N. L., Epping-Jordan, J. E., & Grant, K. E. (1994). When Mom or Dad has cancer: Markers of psychological distress in cancer patients, spouses, and children. *Health Psychology, 13,* 507-515.

Conger, R., Conger, K., Elder, G., Lorenz, F., Simons, R., & Whitbeck, L. (1992). A family process model of economic hardship and adjustment of early adolescent boys. *Child Development, 63,* 526-541.

Cross-National Collaborative Group. (1992). The changing rate of major depression: Cross-national comparisons. *Journal of the American Medical Association, 268,* 3098-3105.

Dodge, K. A., Pettit, G. S., Gregory, S., & Bates, J. E. (1994). Socialization mediators of the relation between socioeconomic status and child conduct problems [Special issue: Children and poverty]. *Child Development, 65,* 649-665.

Downey, G., & Coyne, J. (1990). Children of depressed parents: An integrative review. *Psychological Bulletin, 108,* 50-76.

Elias, M. J., Gara, M., Ubriaco, M., Rothbaum, P. A., Clabby, J. F., & Schuyler, T. (1986). Impact of a preventive social problem solving intervention on children's coping with middle school stressors. *American Journal of Community Psychiatry, 14,* 259-275.

Emslie, G., Rush, A. J., Weinberg, W., Rintelmann, J., & Roffwarg, H. (1994). Sleep EEG features of adolescents with major depression. *Biological Psychiatry, 36,* 573-581.

Fendrich, M., Warner, V., & Weissman, M. M. (1990). Family risk factors, parental depression, and psychopathology in offspring. *Developmental Psychology, 26,* 40-50.

Fleming, J. E., & Offord, D. R. (1990). Epidemiology of childhood depressive disorders: A critical review. *Journal of the American Academy of Child and Adolescent Psychiatry, 29,* 571-580.

Fleming, M. (1996). *Healthy youth 2000: A mid-decade review.* Chicago: American Medical Association, Department of Adolescent Health.

Forehand, R., Wierson, M., Thomas, A. M., Armistead, L., Kempton, T., & Neighbors, B. (1991). The role of family stressors and parent relationships on adolescent functioning. *Journal of the American Academy of Child and Adolescent Psychiatry, 30,* 316-322.

Garber, J., & Hilsman, R. (1992). Cognitions, stress, and depression in children and adolescents. *Child and Adolescent Psychiatric Clinics of North America, 1,* 129-167.

Garland, A., Shaffer, D., & Whittle, B. (1989). A national survey of school-based, adolescent suicide prevention programs. *Journal of the American Academy of Child and Adolescent Psychiatry, 28,* 931-934.

Garrison, C. Z., Jackson, K. L., Marstellar, F., McKeown, R. E., & Addy, C. (1990). A longitudinal study of depressive symptomatology in young adolescents. *Journal of the American Academy of Child and Adolescent Psychiatry, 29,* 581-585.

Ge, X., Conger, R., Lorenz, F., Shanahan, M., & Elder, G. (1995). Mutual influences in parent and adolescent psychological distress. *Developmental Psychology, 31,* 406-419.

Gillham, J. E., Reivich, K. J., Jaycox, L. H., & Seligman, M. E. P. (1995). Prevention of depressive symptoms in school children: A two-year follow-up. *Psychological Science, 6,* 343-351.

Gladstone, T. R. G., & Kaslow, N. J. (1995). Depression and attributions in children and adolescents: A meta-analytic review. *Journal of Abnormal Child Psychology, 23,* 597-606.

Goodman, S. H., Gravitt, G. W., & Kaslow, N. J. (1995). Social problem-solving: A moderator of the relation between negative life stress and depression symptoms among children. *Journal of Abnormal Child Psychology, 23,* 473-485.

Goodyer, I. M., & Altham, P. M. E. (1991). Lifetime exit events and recent social and family adversities in anxious and depressed school-age children and adolescents: I. *Journal of Affective Disorders, 21,* 219-228.

Goodyer, I. M., Wright, C., & Altham, P. (1990). The friendships and recent life events of anxious and depressed school-age children. *British Journal of Psychiatry, 156,* 689-698.

Gore, S., Aseltine, R. H., & Colton, M. E. (1992). Social structure, life stress, and depressive symptoms in a high school aged population. *Journal of Health and Social Behavior, 33,* 97-113.

Gotlib, I. H., & Hammen, C. L. (1992). *Psychological aspects of depression: Toward a cognitive-interpersonal integration.* London: Wiley.

Gotlib, I. H., Lewinsohn, P. M., & Seeley, J. R. (1995). Symptoms versus a diagnosis of depression: Differences in psychosocial functioning. *Journal of Consulting and Clinical Psychology, 63,* 90-100.

Grant, K. E., & Compas, B. E. (1995). Stress and anxious-depressed symptoms among adolescents: Searching for mechanisms of risk. *Journal of Consulting and Clinical Psychology, 63,* 1015-1021.

Hammen, C. (1988). Self-cognitions, stressful events, and the prediction of depression in children of depressed mothers. *Journal of Abnormal Child Psychology, 16,* 347-360.

Hammen, C. (1991). *Depression runs in families: The social context of risk and resilience in children of depressed mothers.* New York: Springer-Verlag.

Hammen, C., Burge, D., & Adrian, C. (1991). Timing of mother and child depression in a longitudinal study of children at risk. *Journal of Consulting and Clinical Psychology, 59,* 341-345.

Hammen, C., Burge, D., Burney, E., & Adrian, C. (1990). Longitudinal study of diagnoses in children of women with unipolar and bipolar affective disorder. *Archives of General Psychiatry, 47,* 1112-1117.

Hammen, C., & Goodman-Brown, T. (1990). Self-schemas and vulnerability to specific life stress in children at risk for depression. *Cognitive Therapy and Research, 14,* 215-227.

Hammen, C., & Rudolph, K. D. (in press). Childhood depression. In E. Mash & R. Barkley (Eds.), *Child psychopathology.* New York: Guilford.

Harrington, R., Fudge, H., Rutter, M., Pickles, A., & Hill, J. (1990). Adult outcomes of childhood and adolescent depression: Psychiatric status. *Archives of General Psychiatry, 47,* 1112-1117.

Hilsman, R., & Garber, J. (1995). A test of the cognitive diathesis-stress model of depression in children: Academic stressors, attributional style, perceived competence, and control. *Journal of Personality and Social Psychology, 69,* 370-380.

Huston, A. C. (Ed.). (1991). *Children in poverty: Child development and public policy.* New York: Cambridge University Press.

Institute of Medicine. (1994). *Reducing risks for mental disorders: Frontiers for preventive intervention research.* Washington, DC: National Academy Press.

Jaycox, L. H., Reivich, K. J., Gillham, J., & Seligman, M. E. P. (1994). Prevention of depressive symptoms in school children. *Behavior Research and Therapy, 32,* 801-816.

Jensen, P. S., Richters, J., Ussery, T., Bloedau, L., & Davis, H. (1991). Child psychopathology and environmental influences: Discrete life events versus ongoing adversity. *Journal of the American Academy of Child and Adolescent Psychiatry, 30,* 303-309.

Jolly, J. B., & Dykman, R. A. (1994). Using self-report data to differentiate anxious and depressive symptoms in adolescents: Cognitive content specificity and global distress. *Cognitive Therapy and Research, 18,* 25-37.

Kandel, D. B., & Davies, M. (1986). Adult sequelae of adolescent depressive symptoms. *Archives of General Psychiatry, 43,* 255-262.

Kaslow, N. J., Brown, R. T., & Mee, L. L. (1994). Cognitive and behavioral correlates of childhood depression: A developmental perspective. In W. M. Reynolds & H. F. Johnston (Eds.), *Handbook of depression in children and adolescents* (pp. 97-122). New York: Plenum.

Kaslow, N. J., & Racusin, G. R. (1990). Childhood depression: Current status and future directions. In A. S. Bellack, M. Hersen, & A. E. Kazdin (Eds.), *International handbook of behavior modification and therapy* (2nd ed., pp. 649-668). New York: Plenum.

Kazdin, A. E. (1990). Evaluation of the Automatic Thoughts Questionnaire: Negative cognitive processes and depression among children. *Psychological Assessment, 2,* 73-79.

Kellam, S. G., Rebok, G. W., Mayer, L. S., Ialongo, N., & Kalodner, C. R. (1994). Depressive symptoms over first grade and their response to a developmental epidemiologically based preventive trail aimed at improving achievement. *Development and Psychopathology, 6,* 473-481.

Kellam, S. G., Werthamer-Larson, L. G., Dolan, L. J., & Brown, C. H. (1991). Developmental epidemiologically based preventive trials: Baseline modeling of early target behaviors and depressive symptoms. *American Journal of Community Psychology, 19,* 563-584.

Keller, M. B., Beardslee, W. R., Dorer, D. J., Lavori, P. W., Samuelson, H., & Klerman, G. R. (1986). Impact of severity and chronicity of parental affective illness on adaptive functioning and psychopathology in children. *Archives of General Psychiatry, 43,* 930-937.

Keller, M. B., Beardslee, W., Lavori, P. W., Wunder, J., Dorer, D. L., & Samuelson, H. (1988). Course of major depression in non-referred adolescents: A retrospective study. *Journal of Affective Disorders, 15,* 235-243.

Kendall, P. C., Stark, K. D., & Adam, T. (1990). Cognitive deficit or cognitive distortion in childhood depression. *Journal of Abnormal Child Psychology, 18,* 255-270.

King, C. A., Naylor, M. W., Segal, H. G., Evans, T., & Shain, B. N. (1993). Global self-worth, specific self-perceptions of competence, and depression in adolescents. *Journal of the American Academy of Child and Adolescent Psychiatry, 32,* 745-752.

Kovacs, M. (1989). Affective disorders in children and adolescents. *American Psychologist, 44,* 209-215.

Kovacs, M., Feinberg, T. L., Crouse-Novak, M. A., Paulauskas, S. L., & Finkelstein, R. (1984). Depressive disorders in childhood: I. A longitudinal prospective study of characteristics and recovery. *Archives of General Psychiatry, 41,* 229-237.

Kovacs, M., & Gatsonis, C. (1994). Secular trends in age of onset of major depressive disorder in a clinical sample of children. *Psychiatric Research, 28,* 319-329.

Leadbeater, B. J., Blatt, S. J., & Quinlan, D. M. (1995). Gender-linked vulnerabilities to depressive symptoms, stress, and problem behaviors in adolescents. *Journal of Research on Adolescence, 5,* 1-29.

Lewinsohn, P. M., Hoberman, H. M., & Rosenbaum, M. (1988). A prospective study of risk factors for unipolar depression. *Journal of Abnormal Psychology, 97,* 251-264.

Lewinsohn, P. M., Rohde, P., & Seeley, J. R. (1995). Adolescent psychopathology: III. The clinical consequences of comorbidity. *Journal of the American Academy of Child and Adolescent Psychiatry, 34,* 510-519.

Lewinsohn, P. M., Rohde, P., & Seeley, J. R. (1996). Adolescent suicidal ideation and attempts: Prevalence, risk factors, and implications. *Clinical Psychology: Science and Practice, 3,* 25-46.

Lewinsohn, P. M., Rohde, P., Seeley, J. R., & Fischer, S. A. (1993). Age-cohort changes in the lifetime occurrence of depression and other mental disorders. *Journal of Abnormal Psychology, 102,* 110-120.

Lewinsohn, P. M., Rohde, P., Seeley, J. R., & Hops, H. (1991). Comorbidity of unipolar depression: I. Major depression with dysthymia. *Journal of Abnormal Psychology, 100,* 205-213.

McCauley, E., Mitchell, J. R., Burke, P., & Moss, S. (1988). Cognitive attributes of depression in children and adolescents. *Journal of Consulting and Clinical Psychology, 56,* 903-908.

McCauley, E., Myers, K., Mitchell, J., Calderon, R., Schloredt, K., & Treder, R. (1993). Depression in young people: Initial presentation and clinical course. *Journal of the American Academy of Child and Adolescent Psychiatry, 32,* 714-722.

McLoyd, V. C. (1990). The impact of economic hardship on Black families and children: Psychological distress, parenting, and socioemotional development. *Child Development, 61,* 311-346.

Nolen-Hoeksema, S., & Girgus, J.S. (1994). The emergence of gender differences in depression during adolescence. *Psychological Bulletin, 115,* 424-443.

Nolen-Hoeksema, S., Girgus, J. S., & Seligman, M. E. P. (1986). Learned helplessness in children: A longitudinal study of depression, achievement, and explanatory style. *Journal of Personality and Social Psychology, 51,* 435-442.

Nolen-Hoeksema, S., Girgus, J. S., & Seligman, M. E. P. (1992). Predictors and consequences of childhood depressive symptoms: A 5-year longitudinal study. *Journal of Abnormal Psychology, 101,* 405-422.

Panak, W. F., & Garber, J. (1992). Role of aggression, rejection, and attributions in the prediction of depression in children. *Development and Psychopathology, 4,* 145-165.

Petersen, A. C., Compas, B. E., & Brooks-Gunn, J. (1992). *Depression in adolescence: Current knowledge, research directions, and implications for programs and policy.* Washington, DC: Carnegie Council on Adolescent Development.

Petersen, A. C., Compas, B. E., Brooks-Gunn, J., Stemmler, M., Ey, S., & Grant, K. E. (1993). Depression in adolescence. *American Psychologist, 48,* 155-168.

Petersen, A. C., Leffert, N., Graham, B., Alwin, J., & Ding, S. (in press). Promoting mental health during the transition into adolescence. In J. Schulenberg, J. L. Muggs, & A. K. Hierrelmann (Eds.), *Health risks and developmental transitions during adolescence.* New York: Cambridge University Press.

Petersen, A. C., Sarigiani, P. A., & Kennedy, R. E. (1991). Adolescent depression: Why more girls? *Journal of Youth and Adolescence, 20,* 247-271.

Puig-Antich, J. (1987). Sleep and neuroendocrine correlates of affective illness in childhood and adolescence: National Invitational Conference: Health futures of adolescents. *Journal of Adolescent Health Care, 8,* 505-529.

Puig-Antich, J., Lukens, E., Davies, M., Goetz, D., Brennan-Quattrock, J., & Todak, G. (1985). Psychosocial functioning in prepubertal major depressive disorders: II. Interpersonal relationships after sustained recovery from affective episodes. *Archives of General Psychiatry, 42,* 511-517.

Quiggle, N. L., Garber, J., Panak, W. F., & Dodge, K. A. (1992). Social information processing in aggressive and depressed children. *Child Development, 63,* 1305-1320.

Robinson, N. S., & Garber, J. (1995). Social support and psychopathology across the life span. In D. Cicchetti & D. Cohen (Eds.), *Developmental psychopathology: Vol. 2. Risk, disorder, and adaptation* (pp. 162-209). New York: John Wiley.

Robinson, N. S., Garber, J., & Hilsman, R. (1995). Cognitions and stress: Direct and moderating effects on depressive versus externalizing symptoms during the junior high school transition. *Journal of Abnormal Psychology, 104,* 453-463.

Rohde, P., Lewinsohn, P. M., & Seeley, J. R. (1991). Comorbidity of unipolar depression: II. Comorbidity with other mental disorders in adolescents and adults. *Journal of Abnormal Psychology, 54,* 653-660.

Rudolph, K. D., Hammen, C., & Burge, D. (1994). Interpersonal functioning and depressive symptoms in childhood: Addressing the issues of specificity and comorbidity. *Journal of Abnormal Child Psychology, 22,* 355-371.

Ryan, N. D., Williamson, D. E., Iyengar, S., Orvaschel, H., Reich, T., Dahl, R. E., & Puig-Antich, J. (1992). A secular increase in child and adolescent onset affective disorder. *Journal of the American Academy of Child and Adolescent Psychiatry, 31,* 600-605.

Shaffer, D., Garland, A., Gould, M., Fisher, P., & Trautman, P. (1989). Preventing teenage suicide: A critical review. In S. Chess & M. E. Hertzig (Eds.), *Annual progress in child psychiatry and child development* (pp. 401-428). New York: Brunner/Mazel.

Shaffer, D., Garland, A., Vieland, V., Underwood, M., & Busner, C. (1991). The impact of curriculum-based suicide prevention programs for teenagers. *Journal of the American Academy of Child and Adolescent Psychiatry, 30,* 588-596.

Stanger, C., Achenbach, T. M., & McConaughy, S. H. (1993). Three-year course of behavioral and emotional problems in a national sample of 4- to 16-year-olds: III. Predictors of signs of disturbance. *Journal of Consulting and Clinical Psychology, 61,* 839-848.

Stanger, C., McConaughy, S. H., & Achenbach, T. M. (1992). Three-year course of behavioral/emotional problems in a national sample of 4- to 16-year-olds: II. Predictors of syndromes. *Journal of the American Academy of Child and Adolescent Psychiatry, 31,* 941-950.

Strober, M., Lampert, C., Schmidt, S., & Morrell, W. (1993). The course of major depressive disorder in adolescents: Recovery and risk of manic switching in a 24-month prospective, naturalistic follow-up of psychotic and nonpsychotic subtypes. *Journal of the American Academy of Child and Adolescent Psychiatry, 32,* 34-42.

Tremblay, R. E., McCord, J., Boileau, H., Charlebois, P., Gagnon, C., Le Blanc, M., & Larivee, S. (1991). Can disruptive boys be helped to become competent? *Psychiatry, 54,* 148-161.

Turner, J. E., & Cole, D. A. (1994). Developmental differences in cognitive diatheses for child depression. *Journal of Abnormal Child Psychology, 22,* 15-32.

U.S. Department of Health and Human Services, Public Health Service. (1991). *Healthy people 2000: National health promotion and disease prevention objectives* (DHHS Publication No. PHS 91-50212). Washington, DC: U.S. Government Printing Office.

Verhulst, F. C., & van der Ende, J. (1992). Six-year developmental course of internalizing and externalizing problem behaviors. *Journal of the American Academy of Child and Adolescent Psychiatry, 31,* 924-931.

Vitaro, F., & Tremblay, R. E. (1994). Impact of a prevention program on aggressive children's friendships and social adjustment. *Journal of Abnormal Child Psychology, 22,* 457-475.

Wagner, B. M., Cole, R. E., & Schwartzman, P. (in press). Comorbidity of symptoms among junior and senior high school suicide attempters. *Suicide and Life-Threatening Behavior.*

Weissman, M. M., Gammon, G. D., John, K., Merikangas, K. R., Warner, V., Prusoff, B. A., & Sholomskas, D. (1987). Children of depressed parents: Increased psychopathology and early onset of major depression. *Archives of General Psychiatry, 44,* 847-853.

Weisz, J. R., Sweeney, L., Proffitt, V., & Carr, T. (1993). Control-related beliefs and self-reported depressive symptoms in late childhood. *Journal of Abnormal Psychology, 102,* 411-418.

Weller, E. B., Weller, R. A., Fristad, M. A., Cantwell, M. L., & Preskorn, S. H. (1986). Dexamethasone suppression test and clinical outcome in prepubertal depressed children. *American Journal of Psychiatry, 143,* 1469-1470.

World Health Organization. (1990). *International classification of diseases and health related problems (ICD-10).* Geneva, Switzerland: Author.

W. T. Grant Foundation Consortium on Depression During Childhood and Adolescence. (1996). *Depression during childhood and adolescence: Bridging the gap between basic research and intervention.* Manuscript under review.

Zahn-Waxler, C., Cummings, E. M., Iannotti, R., & Radke-Yarrow, M. (1984). Young offspring of depressed parents: A population at risk for affective problems. *New Directions for Child Development, 26,* 81-105.

• *CHAPTER 7* •

Prevention of Youth Suicide

JOHN KALAFAT

Suicide consistently ranks as the second or third leading cause of death for adolescents between 15 and 19 years of age. Between 1960 and 1990, the suicide rate for 15- to 19-year-olds more than tripled from 3.6 to 11.3 per 100,000 (Berman & Jobes, 1995). From 1980 to 1992, for persons aged 20 to 24 years, the suicide rate declined 7.2% (from 16.1 to 14.9 per 100,000). It increased, however, among persons aged 15 to 19 by 28.3% (from 8.5 to 10.9) and among persons aged 10 to 14 by 120% (from 0.8 to 1.7). This ominous (and likely underreported) increase in the rates for the younger age group appears to be following the trends for substance abuse. Among persons aged 15 to 19, firearm-related suicides accounted for 81% of the increase in the overall rate from 1980 to 1992 (Centers for Disease Control and Prevention [CDC], 1995a). The incidence of suicide *attempts* among adolescents is considerably higher, with various surveys of adolescents consistently averaging about 10% reported attempts among the respondents. For example, the 1993 National Youth Risk Behavior Surveillance (CDC, 1995b) revealed that 22.9% of females and 15.3% of males reported having made a suicide plan during the previous year. Suicide attempts not only can lead to serious injury but also are associated with significantly higher subsequent completions than among the general adolescent population (Pfeffer et al., 1993). Thus, given the prevalence of all suicide behaviors and the impact of suicide attempts and completions on peers, families, institutions, and communities, suicide has impacts far beyond that implied by base rates of reported completions.

These data have resulted in a variety of national calls for intervention and prevention efforts including *Healthy People 2000* (U.S. Department of Health and Human Services, Public Health Service [DHHS], 1991) objectives 6.6: Reduce suicides of youth ages 15 to 19 to no more than 8.2 per 100,000; and 6.2: Reduce by 15% the incidence of injurious suicide attempts among adolescents aged 14 through 17. *Healthy Communities 2000: Model Standards: Guidelines for Community Attainment of the Year 2000 Health Objectives* (1991) included among its services and protection objectives availability and access to services, public awareness, public information, referral networks, and case finding and surveillance systems. Included among its risk reduction objectives is quality school health education, including a mental health component. The report of the Second World Conference on Injury Control, *Injury Control in the 1990s* (1993), included among its violence (including suicide) reduction recommendations the following: programs to improve the recognition, referral, shelter, and long-term therapeutic interventions for people at high risk for violent injury; programs to address not only the behavior of individuals but also the behavior of community institutions and the community environment; and better dissemination of education materials to people who have influence or access to persons at risk.

Clearly, the institution that has the most influence and access to at-risk youth are schools. Coie et al. (1993) noted that schools offer a logical setting for broad-scale (universal) preventive interventions because 9 out of 10 children in our society are found there. Locally initiated school-based youth suicide prevention and intervention programs have become ubiquitous. The responsibility for such programs is acknowledged by educators (Davis & Sandoval, 1991) and included in education statutes and codes that address the protection of students (Kalafat, 1990). Such programs are also clearly part of a rapidly growing trend for school-based health and mental health initiatives that address what Dryfoos (1994) referred to as the "new morbidities" (p. 2), which include violence-related injuries (Carnegie Council on Adolescent Development, 1988; Christopher, Kurtz, & Howing, 1989).

As these programs have matured, many of them conform to the *Healthy Communities 2000* (1991) and *Injury Control in the 1990s* (1993) recommendations to educate those who have influence and access to youth and have begun to address the institutional and community environment to improve the recognition, referral, and supportive aftercare of suicidal youth (CDC, 1992; Kalafat & Elias, 1995). Although evaluation of these programs remains a critical need (CDC, 1992), results from small-scale evaluations are promising.

This chapter provides an overview of current school-based youth suicide prevention efforts. Rather than review the wide variety of existing broad-based and focused school-based prevention programs, conceptually grounded exemplars for which there are some empirical data have been chosen to illustrate recommended, available youth suicide prevention strategies.

The review will begin with a general prevention framework that informs these programs. The articulation of this framework is important for two reasons. First, these programs share an overarching characteristic of effective interventions in that they are *intentional* (Cowen, 1980). That is, they are based on articulated conceptual frameworks or program logic (Illback, Zins, Maher, & Greenberg, 1990). An understanding of this framework can serve as a guide to those who wish to adapt a cost-efficient youth suicide prevention program to their particular setting and to developments in the field, while preserving its essential elements. Second, general confusion exists about prevention concepts and terminology (Institute of Medicine, 1994), and this lack of understanding of basic prevention concepts and strategies is reflected in criticisms of school-based universal prevention programs that can hamper their dissemination.

Prevention Framework

Silverman and Felner (1995) proposed that a prevention framework should address four questions:

1. What do we mean by the concept *prevention* when applied to suicide?
2. What and where is the focus of suicide intervention (prevention)?
3. What are the goals of suicide prevention programs?
4. Who are the target groups of suicide prevention versus, for example, intervention?

What Is Prevention? The Classic Model

Citing confusion surrounding the public health nomenclature of primary, secondary, and tertiary prevention, the Institute of Medicine (1994) adopted a framework developed by Gordon (1983) that uses a nomenclature that has an intervention focus. This consists of *universal* interventions, which are directed at an entire population; *selective* interventions, which are directed at individuals who are at greater risk for diseases or disorders than the general population; and *indicated* interventions, which are targeted to relatively small groups who are found, by screening programs or other inquiries, to manifest a condition that requires intensive interventions. At least one comprehensive, statewide youth suicide prevention effort has been organized around these concepts (Eggert, Thompson, Randell, & McCauley, 1995).

This new terminology may not clarify programmatic efforts—for example, coping skills classes for students or family support programs can fit into any of the three categories, depending on the target audiences. Others have recommended reformulation of primary, secondary, and tertiary prevention into prevention, early intervention, and treatment, respectively (Felner, Adan, & Silverman, 1992).

On a practical level, a classic prevention framework seems to serve well to organize intervention efforts. This states that the goal of prevention is to reduce the incidence and prevalence of disorders or dysfunctional behaviors in a population by reducing stressors (predisposing or precipitating) associated with the emergence of the disorder and/or enhancing available supports, both internal (e.g., coping skills, knowledge, and attitudes) and external (e.g., individual support networks and supportive contexts or environments; Caplan, 1964).

The Foci of Prevention: Pathways to Suicide

Prevention occurs, by definition, before the disorder or dysfunction is fully manifested, so its focus is on precursors of dysfunction or health. Because of this focus,

> it cannot have as its first order targets of change the disorders it seeks to reduce or other individual level pathologies. Instead, prevention

> will be applied to the enhancement, disruption, or modification, as appropriate, of the unfolding processes (and conditions) that lead to well-being or to serious mental health or social problems . . . with the goals of increasing or decreasing, respectively, the rate or level with which these occur in the target population. (Silverman & Felner, 1995, p. 75)

These potential precursors of dysfunction or health are called, respectively, risk or protective factors (Coie et al., 1993). These are the stressors and supports in Caplan's (1964) framework, and the emphasis in suicide prevention, then, is not so much on suicide behavior per se but on individual and environmental processes that may lead to that state.

Another characteristic of preventive interventions that is contained in the above formulation should be highlighted. The emphasis on addressing a priori unfolding processes that lead to the emergence of suicidal behavior requires that some attempt be made to explicate the developmental trajectories or evolutionary history of youth suicide (Felner et al., 1992). As one moves along that trajectory, the conditions targeted become progressively more severe and specific to the dysfunctional outcome, which, in this case, is, again, suicidal behavior.

Thus, to mount a youth suicide prevention program within the framework that has been described so far, one must seek to identify risk and protective factors (stressors and supports) in the adolescent population that can be reduced or enhanced, respectively, such that the trajectory toward suicidal behavior will be attenuated or interrupted. As the trajectory moves closer to suicidal behavior, these factors will move from broad-based risk/protective factors (e.g., social problem solving) to those more specific to the emerging crisis of the suicidal state (e.g., helpful responses to troubled or suicidal youth).

Efforts to identify specific risk factors associated with suicide have been unsuccessful to date. Felner et al. (1992) describe "an almost bewildering array of conditions that have been cited as contributing to suicidal risk" (p. 428). Risk factors that have been identified have been described as sensitive but not specific, in that they produce significantly high false positive rates (Garland & Zigler, 1993). Coie et al. (1993) noted that specific forms of dysfunction are typically associated with many risk factors and that diverse disorders share fundamental risk factors in common. As Felner et al. point out, risk factors considered for suicide have high levels of associations with a broad array of other disorders, which are themselves often employed as predictors of youth suicide. Moreover, youth epidemiological studies have yielded a clear picture of the comorbidity of a variety of disorders, and suicide is no exception; comorbidity with substance abuse, depression, and social and behavioral problems (conduct disorders) have been demonstrated (Rutter, 1989). One of the bases for the comorbidity of such phenomena as suicide, substance abuse, and conduct disorders may be that they share similar underlying functions. At the least, they may represent ineffective responses to stressful situations. Finally, Coie et al. noted that the salience of risk factors may fluctuate developmentally, such that indexes of risk at one age do not necessarily identify risk at all ages. This prompted them to indicate that "as a general rule, prevention is best made from proximal risk factors" (p. 1014).

Given that "it would be difficult to find some life experience, adaptive demand, or psychological difficulty that has not been shown to relate to suicide in one way or another" (Felner et al., 1992, p. 428), one can understand why it is difficult to develop a youth suicide prevention program that targeted the reduction of relevant stressors or risk factors. Research on risk factors continues and appears to dominate federal funding priorities (e.g., National Institute of Mental Health, 1994). Although current risk factors that have been posited as associated with suicide risk do not yet constitute reliable predictors, they can serve as markers of troubled youth who require early intervention in any case.

In the meantime, applied suicide prevention efforts must identify potentially effective strategies. Both broad-based and focused school-based prevention programs have tended to emphasize the strategy of enhancing internal and external resources. In contrast to the somewhat confusing array of risk factors, there is evidence that protective factors, such as strong social support and well-developed coping skills, may reduce the likelihood of a range of disorders or dysfunctions, even in the presence of a variety of conditions of risk or vulnerability (Felner, DuBois, & Adan, 1991; Weissberg, Caplan, & Harwood, 1991). Coie et al. (1993) stated that "enhancing protective factors may be the strategy of choice in cases in which risk factors are difficult to identify in advance . . . or to eliminate altogether" (p. 1014). This seems to echo a conclusion proposed by Caplan (1964), as part of his classic prevention model: "In the absence of a knowledge of the causes of mental disorders, primary prevention must be directed toward improving nonspecific helping resources in the community" (p. 30). This strategy may be particularly important for the prevention of youth suicide because there is troubling evidence that a number of variables that have been associated with youth suicide are associated with reductions in support levels.

Bell-Dolan, Foster, and Christopher (1995) found significantly higher levels of anxiety and depression in rejected and withdrawn girls compared with neglected and popular girls. These authors reviewed studies indicating the unpopularity of anxious and depressed youth. These studies were correlational, however, and thus provided no evidence whether rejection caused anxiety and depression or vice versa. In a longitudinal study, Hirsch and DuBois (1992) found anxiety and depression prospectively associated with low levels of peer support during transition to seventh grade, at midyear, and again at the end of seventh grade. Two other studies suggest that depressed youth may elicit negative social responses. Connolly, Geller, Morton, and Kutcher (1992) found that depressed adolescents were rated less favorably by peers than nondepressed adolescents after a brief interaction. Mullins et al. (1995) found that depressed fourth- to sixth-grade children elicited negative social responses from teachers. Joiner (1994; Joiner, Alfano, & Metalsky, 1992) also found that depressive symptomatology led to negative reactions in others.

Dubow, Kausch, Blum, Reed, and Bush (1989) found that junior high and high school students who experienced the most severe suicidal ideation in the past year also experienced more negative life events, lower levels of family support, and less school involvement than nonideators. Garrison, Addy, Jackson, McKeown, and Waller (1991) found that undesirable life events and self-report measures of low family adaptability (rigidity) and cohesion (disengagement) were significant predictors of suicidal ideation in a longitudinal study. Kienhorst, DeWilde, Diekstra, and Wolters (1995) found that suicide attempters reported family and peer problems occurring prior to their attempt and identified isolation as the main reason for the 6 months prior to their attempt being worse than before. These and other studies provide evidence for a relationship between low family and peer support and suicidal risk in adolescents (Hawton, O'Grady, Osborn, & Cole, 1982; Topol & Resnikoff, 1982).

Also, interpersonal conflict and losses are among the most commonly reported precipitants for completed and attempted suicide in adolescents (Brent, Perper, Moritz, Baugher, Balach, & Schweers, 1993; Shaffer & Gould, 1987).

Finally, Clark and Fawcett (1992) described a phenomenon among suicidal individuals that they termed *help negation.* They contended that this negation is due to the hopelessness and pessimism characteristic of the constricted cognitive/affective state of a suicidal crisis, but there is some evidence that this hopelessness and pessimism may be more generally characteristic of these individuals outside the crisis state (Rudd, Joiner, & Rajab, 1995).

In regard to external supports, these studies portray a trajectory toward suicidal behavior composed of the experience of stressful (often interpersonal) life events, a (at least perceived) lack of support from family and friends, perhaps the exhibition of behavior and affect that may attenuate supportive responses, a lack of integration into the school environment, and a general pattern of increasing isolation (Trout, 1980). To the extent that this pattern of withdrawal is interrupted at all, troubled and suicidal youth tend to turn to peers for support.

Research has indicated that many suicidal youth confide their concerns more often to peers than adults (Brent, Perper, Kolko, & Goldstein, 1988; Clark, 1993; Dubow et al., 1989; Kalafat & Elias, 1992; Spirito, Overholser, Ashworth, Morgan, & Benedict-Drew, 1988). These studies indicate that 40% to 60% of female adolescents and 25% to 40% of male adolescents report personally knowing a teen who had attempted suicide. This phenomenon has emphasized the importance of peers in the school-based prevention of youth suicidal behavior and prompted the authors of one psychological autopsy study to comment that "the role of friends and peers in the early recognition of suicidal behavior and prevention of suicide cannot be overemphasized" (Shafii et al., 1984, p. 293).

Some adolescents, however, particularly some male adolescents, do not respond in an empathic and helpful way to potentially or overtly suicidal peers (Norton, Durlak, & Richards, 1989; Overholser, Hemstreet, Spirito, & Vyse, 1989; Wellman & Wellman, 1986). As few as 25% of these peer confidants may tell an adult about their suicidal peer (Kalafat & Elias, 1992; Kalafat, Elias, & Gara, 1993). The concerns raised by these findings are reinforced by the general literature on adolescent help seeking. These and other studies consistently find a trend toward peers as primary sources of support for troubled adolescents (Harman, Armsworth, & Henderson, 1989; Wintre, Hicks, McVey, & Fox, 1988). Youth who are disturbed (including those who are depressed, suicidal, and substance abusers) favor peers over adults more than do nondisturbed youth (Naginy & Swisher, 1990; Offer, Howard, Schonert, & Ostrov, 1991; Wills & Vaughan, 1989). Of critical importance to school-based interventions is that school personnel are among the last choices for talking about personal concerns (Hutchinson & Reagan, 1987; Meagher & Clark, 1982; Wells & Ritter, 1979). On the basis of these studies, *it is reasonable to consider reluctance to seek adult help as a risk factor that increases the probability of negative or injurious outcomes for a variety of disturbed youth.* Again, because many of the problem behaviors displayed by troubled youth tend to occur together, a program that promotes help seeking may affect more than one behavior and thus generate a greater return on the school's investment.

Conversely, *contact with helpful adults may be considered a protective factor.* One of the protective factors for resilient youth (i.e., youth who do well despite stressful environments) is involvement with a significant adult figure (Garmezy, 1983). For young adolescents, studies suggest that family support is a major influence on self-esteem and self-efficacy and consistently show stress-buffering effects (Greenberg, Siegel, & Leitch, 1983; Larson, 1983; Wills, 1985). Also, the findings concerning the prominence of peer groups in teens' lives prompted Cauce and Srebnik (1989) to suggest that peer networks affect youth behavior both in the support they provide and the values they promote. These values may serve to support or undermine the goals of prevention programs. Certainly, the value placed on keeping confidences and not confiding in adults represents a teen value that must be addressed in prevention programs aimed at enhancing the efficacy of peers in the early detection of troubled and suicidal adolescents. Cauce and

Srebnik called for better ways to channel students' energies into activities that promote mutual help. The Carnegie Council on Adolescent Development listed among its Recommendations for Fully Healthy Adolescents, "Willingness and ability to use the available information and services, especially when provided by family, youth organizations, educators, mentors, and constructive role models" (Hechinger, 1992, p. 9).

There is also evidence that the *provision* of help by youth may be beneficial to them. Adolescents' prosocial values have been directly related to multiple indexes of their social competence and inversely related to several serious adolescent problem behaviors (Allen, Aber, & Leadbeater, 1990; Allen, Weissberg, & Hawkins, 1989). Also, empirical studies of children participating in helping interactions indicate that these interactions may shape children's prosocial behavior and reduce problematic behavior (Allen, Philliber, & Hoggson, 1990; Staub, 1979). Such prosocial competencies may carry over to a variety of current and future challenging situations faced by youth, thus further amplifying the effects of programs that emphasize mutual support (Silverman & Felner, 1995).

The Goals of Suicide Prevention Programs

The findings that troubled youth frequently turn to peers for support and that encounters between suicidal youth and peers are fairly common point to a clear need to prepare youth to respond to these encounters in prosocial, effective, and helpful ways. This entails convincing adolescents to break confidences and tell adults. There is now an increasing consensus among those who provide school-based youth suicide prevention programs that one important objective of these programs is to increase the probability that troubled or suicidal youth and their peer confidants will turn to adults before their concerns become overwhelming and/or injurious (CDC, 1992; Kalafat & Ryerson, 1993).

In addition to focusing on peers, these programs also seek to enhance the ability of adults in schools and families to identify and respond to troubled (i.e., before suicidal ideation occurs) and suicidal (i.e., ideation and behavior) youth. The overall goal of such programs within the present prevention framework is to enhance the responsiveness and supportiveness of key elements in the environments of youth to interrupt the pathway toward suicidal behavior.

Given the low base rates of many disorders and that nonspecific predisposing and precipitating conditions may be responsible for the expression of many disorders, Coie et al. (1993) suggested that an emphasis on identifying risk and protective factors unique to specific disorders is less likely to be productive than an attempt to discover those that are common to many disorders. They further contended that most generic risk and protective factors lend themselves to preventive interventions consonant with broad community mental health approaches and that "prevention theory can specify universal interventions to be administered to unselected populations if they are known to have potential benefits and no adverse effects for participants" (p. 1017). Help seeking on one's own or one's peer's behalf appears to be a generic protective factor that can be addressed through population-focused or universal prevention programs.

The Target Groups

By now, it is apparent that prevention programs are by definition population focused. All adolescents should be targeted in programs that emphasize the prosocial values and behaviors of mutual support. In regard to the timing of interventions, transitional periods such as the entry into middle school from elementary school or into high school from middle or elementary school may be most appropriate (Eccles et al., 1993; Felner & Adan, 1988; Hirsch & DuBois, 1992). Ninth graders appear to be a particularly appropriate target for intervention because peer conformity for antisocial behavior may peek at this age (Berndt, 1979). Also, at least one study of a community sample found that suicidal ideation peaked in 9th grade, following transition to high school (Dubow et al., 1989). In another study, 9th graders were more likely to ignore suicidal peers than 11th graders (Kalafat & Elias, 1992). They are also less likely to be familiar with any adults in the school. Finally, they are members of the age cohort for which the increase in suicide rate between 1980 and 1992 was greatest among youth. Comprehensive programs have included booster sessions for later grades—for example, how to find help on college campuses and in the community (Kalafat & Underwood, 1989).

Features of Comprehensive School-Based Prevention Programs

Comprehensive programs are multilevel, multicomponent interventions that include the following components, usually implemented in this order:

1. *Administrative consultation* ensures that policies and procedures for responding to at-risk students, attempts, and completions are in place and ensures that community linkages exist for close coordination of referrals to, and return of students from, community gatekeepers.
2. *School gatekeeper training* is provided for all faculty and staff (including such staff as bus drivers and cafeteria workers) on the identification of, initial response to, and effective referral of students who are troubled and at risk. This sometimes includes the establishment of in-school crisis response teams made up of faculty, staff, and administrators.
3. *Parent training* covers similar material as the school gatekeeper training, as well as means restriction strategies.
4. *Community gatekeeper training* incorporates policies and procedures for effective response and coordination with schools and families. This sometimes includes training in the treatment of depressed and suicidal adolescents. Community crisis teams and media campaigns have also been implemented.
5. *Student classes* usually consist of four to five class periods included in the health curriculum. Classes include a variety of media and involve students in discussions and role plays to prepare them to recognize and respond to troubled peers and to destigmatize seeking adult help.
6. *Postvention interventions* are provided by external consultants to schools and communities in which a suicide completion or serious attempt has occurred. These interventions consist of standard steps designed to process faculty, student, and community reactions to the event; facilitate grief work; and prevent imitative acts among identified vulnerable peers.

School officials may be hesitant to commit what appears to be a significant amount of time and resources to a phenomenon that is less visible to them than other problems, such as interpersonal violence. These programs, however, were developed in school settings and have evolved cost-efficient implementation procedures. Crisis response teams, community linkages, and outreach to parents are already part of effective schools' repertoires for addressing a variety of problems. Well-developed sets of policies and procedures can be easily adapted to particular schools. The educator and parent training can be completed in 1 to 2 hours each, with brief annual updates. Again, the mutual help message of the student lessons is relevant to a variety of issues faced by students and, as will be described later in this chapter, can be combined with general problem-solving lessons that have a broad application to student issues.

The student lessons of established programs were developed in collaboration with educators and thus share additional features that facilitate their efficient adaptation to school settings. They contain developmentally appropriate, detailed lesson plans that eschew mental health jargon and comply with the educational and protective mission of schools. These lessons include the instructional sequence that is necessary for teaching skills: demonstration, practice, feedback, and practice (Gagne, 1985). They have also been successfully adapted to multicultural settings (Ryerson, 1990). Finally, they are designed to be taught by regular classroom teachers. This promotes ownership of the program and enhances school-based supports in the form of adults who are informed and willing to discuss sensitive issues. These lessons have been packaged for turnkey implementation (Kalafat & Underwood, 1989), or, to ensure fidelity, teachers selected by the school can be provided additional initial training.

Some schools also include peer support or helper programs. Descriptions of examples of each of these components are included in a comprehensive overview by the CDC (1992). These programs, then, share many features that have been posited as characteristic of effective school-based prevention programs (Weissberg & Elias, 1993).

Evaluation of School-Based Prevention Programs

School-based youth suicide programs that have addressed help seeking to various degrees have been in existence since 1980. They have undergone several iterations since the initial grassroots responses to school requests for assistance. First-generation school programs were characterized by attempts to address a variety of topics such as depression, stress, suicide dynamics and etiology, warning signs, and help seeking. They lacked focus, and evaluation results were mixed. Either program effects on student knowledge and attitudes toward suicidal peers and intervening on their behalf were not found (Shaffer, Garland, Vieland, Underwood, & Busner, 1991), or knowledge gains were found for both genders while positive attitude changes were found for only female students (Overholser et al., 1989; Spirito et al., 1988).

Drawing on the experiences of initial programmatic efforts, many second-generation programs were more focused on preparing students to respond to encounters with at-risk peers and to seek adult help. The evaluations of these programs, although few in number, have been encouraging. Ciffone (1993) assessed the impact of health classes aimed at increasing understanding of the nature of suicide and increasing the number of students who endorse the option of taking suicidal threats seriously and seeking help on behalf of a potentially suicidal peer. He found that exposure to the program resulted in shifts in responses from undesirable to desirable in all six items addressing help seeking for oneself or a troubled peer that were significantly greater than in comparison groups.

A colleague and I (Kalafat & Elias, 1994) evaluated a published curriculum (Kalafat & Underwood, 1989) using a Solomon four-groups design and found that students who participated in the four suicide response health classes, as compared with controls, showed significant gains in relevant knowledge about suicide and significantly more positive attitudes toward help seeking and intervening with potentially suicidal peers. No gender or pretesting effects were found. Student reactions to the curriculum were positive and emphasized the use of the classes for helping them with friends' problems, as was the intent of the program.

These studies employed self-report questionnaires, and another study (Kalafat & Gagliano, 1996) employed simulations to assess the responses of trained and untrained students, as has been successfully done with simulations in the counseling (Berven, 1985) and medical education fields (Hubbard, 1978). Assessed were student responses in simulations of both suicidal and troubled (not explicitly suicidal) peers to evaluate a curriculum that aimed at destigmatizing mental health services and help seeking in general and that also included practice in responding to suicidal peers. Two vignettes were employed (from the Kalafat et al., 1993 study): (a) low ambiguity—peer says, "Sometimes I think I might as well kill myself," and (b) high ambiguity—peer writes essay titled "(Final) Family Decisions." Participants, compared with controls, showed significant increases in the "tell an adult" responses to the vignettes. Although more class participants wrote "tell an adult" responses to both vignettes at the posttest, the actual percentages of responses in this category at posttest (unambiguous: 40.4% treatment, 1.8% control; ambiguous: 28.8% treatment, 0% control) indicate the need for further work in this area.

These studies provide encouraging initial data concerning proximal outcomes for student curricula. As noted previously, however, a critical need remains for large-scale studies of comprehensive programs. The question also persists whether these knowledge and attitude changes translate into performance in actual situations. To date, a number of programs have reported increased referrals (self and other) following program implementation, but no controlled studies have systematically tracked such referral patterns (CDC, 1992).

Efforts to assess distal outcomes of school-based youth suicide prevention programs—reductions in the incidence of suicide attempts and completions—are fraught with difficulties. First, the goal of most programs is the early identification and referral of at-risk youth, but, as will be discussed later in this chapter, the results of treatment of at-risk persons, and adolescents in general, are not impressive. Second, no reliable morbidity (attempts) data are available (Moscicki, 1995). Third, as Weissberg et al. (1991) pointed out, prevention programs must first assess the extent of implementation fidelity and institutionalization to demonstrate sustained impact. Finally, because of the low incidence of suicide completions, a program not only must be faithfully implemented but also must be widely disseminated and institutionalized for years to be able to demonstrate any epidemiological impact.

Data are available for one comprehensive school-based program that has fulfilled these criteria. The Adolescent Suicide Awareness Program (ASAP; Ryerson, 1990) is essentially the same type of program previously discussed (evaluated by Kalafat & Elias, 1994) and is the program on which the simulation intervention (Kalafat & Gagliano, 1996) was modeled.

A hallmark of ASAP has been a set of specific implementation and dissemination procedures. To ensure greater program fidelity and to ensure the school community linkages that are an essential component of ASAP, the preferred implementation strategy is to train a core of consultants from a mental health or crisis agency. Those consultants, in turn, disseminate ASAP to schools in their service area. ASAP consultants employ a train, demonstration, feedback method in which they (a) provide the consultants with an 8-hour ASAP workshop, (b) implement ASAP in a school while being observed by the consultants, and (c) observe the consultants implementing ASAP. In turn, ASAP is implemented in schools by training a core of school personnel, demonstrating the educational program components to them in their schools, and observing their provision of the educational components (gatekeeper, parent, and student training).

In the county in which ASAP originated, a populous Northeastern county containing a multiethnic middle-class and blue-collar population, ASAP was implemented in 40 of 52 public and private high schools from 1982 to 1987. A 10-year follow-up survey (Ryerson, 1993), to which 31 of 46 public secondary schools in the target county responded, revealed that 30 of the 31 respondents still provided the student curriculum. In general, student classes were reduced in length from the original program, probably because of the need to address additional morbidities such as interpersonal violence and AIDS. Only 5 schools reported continuing faculty training, 3 reported continuing parent training, and 27 reported having in-school crisis teams (a recommended means of providing accessible response to troubled students).

In addition, 11 county schools that had participated in the first round of ASAP implementation (1983 to 1984) were interviewed using a survey questionnaire based on the literature on the institutionalization of innovations (see Fairweather, Tornatzky, Fergus, & Avellar, 1982). Of particular interest was the *fidelity adaptation* issue regarding the degree to which programs can be adapted to local contexts without compromising the essential components of the program (Blakey et al., 1987). Results indicated that 9 of the 11 schools continued to provide ASAP 10 years after the original implementation (Ryerson, 1993). Every school had updated materials (e.g., statistics and videos), deleted some materials (e.g., section on adolescent development), and added content (e.g., problem solving, other self-destructive behavior). Five had converted a pullout workshop into classes in the health curriculum. Only one reported change raised concern about program integrity: One school converted the workshop into three classes, which was half the original dosage.

In schools that had retained the program for years, a number of elements that are critical for the institutionalization of innovative programs were present. These included (a) the ability to adapt the program to the school structure and to new findings; (b) a specific individual who retained responsibility for the program; (c) administrative support; and (d) a supportive organizational context in the form of policies, community linkages, and clear connection to the school's mission.

To assess the possible epidemiological impact of a carefully implemented, widely disseminated systemic program, the suicide rates for the county and state were compared (Table 7.1). Although these results cannot be causally linked to the ASAP dissemination, they do provide encouraging data from a county saturated by a prevention program and also provide further evidence against the persistent myth that talking about suicide with adolescents will prompt suicidal behavior.

In addition to evaluations of the student portion of school programs, evaluations of school gatekeeper training have yielded gains in knowledge of suicide warning signs and community resources and attitudes toward intervening with and referring at-risk youth (Reisman & Scharfman, 1991; Shaffer, Garland, & Whittle, 1988). Evaluations of community gatekeeper training programs

Table 7.1 Suicide Rates for 15 to 24 Age Group for Bergen County (NJ) and the State of New Jersey

	New Jersey	*Bergen County*
Preimplementation 1978 to 1982	8.72	7.26
Implementation 1983 to 1987	8.66	7.53 (6.98)*
Postimplementation 1988 to 1992 (continuing operation)	7.90	4.38

NOTE: Separate rates for ages 15 to 19 and ages 20 to 24 are not available for state or county.
* This figure excludes a cluster of four suicides of adolescents who had dropped out of a school that did not have a program.

have shown significant increases in suicide intervention knowledge and skills (Tanney, 1989; Tierney, 1988). Several school-based programs, although not controlled studies, report after program implementation increased self- and other referrals and, in particular, increased calls to local hotlines (CDC, 1992). Hotlines are particularly accessible to adolescents because they are anonymous "low cost" help-seeking options that require no transportation, payment, or parental knowledge. There is some evidence for a preventive effect of suicide prevention centers (which are mainly hotlines) in the form of a negative correlation between the number of centers in states and the suicide rates (Lester, 1993).

Issues in School-based Prevention

The universal youth suicide prevention approach that has been described is not without controversy. Two issues deserve at least brief overviews: means restriction and student curricula. A third issue involves the availability of competent, accessible adults and has significant programmatic implications for school-based prevention efforts.

Means restriction is a recommended part of the parents component. Means restriction refers to prevention efforts that reduce access to common means of committing suicide. For adolescents, the most common means of committing suicide is firearms. In 1988, among males aged 15 to 24, 64% of all suicides were committed with guns; for females, this rate was 45% (CDC, 1992). As was previously noted, firearms account for 81% of the increase in adolescent suicides between 1980 and 1992.

For most adolescents, suicide appears to be an impulsive act carried out in response to a particular precipitant (Rosenberg & Mercy, 1991; Shaffer, Garland, Gould, Fisher, & Trautman, 1988). Research has indicated that the risk of suicide doubles if a firearm is in the house, even if it is locked up (Brent et al., 1991; Brent, Perper, Moritz, Baugher, Schweers, & Roth, 1993). A number of studies have shown a positive association between strict handgun control laws and low firearm-related suicide rates (Lester, 1996; Loftin, McDowall, Wiersema, & Cottey, 1991). Evidence for switching to other means is mixed for the total population and has not been studied for adolescents, although results of studies on restricting access to lethal means other than firearms show a strong preventive effect (Lester, 1996). Thus, one goal of *Healthy People 2000* (DHHS, 1991) was a 20% reduction in the proportion of people who possess weapons that are inappropriately stored and therefore dangerously available. The CDC (1992) has also identified restriction of access to firearms as a major strategy for the prevention of youth suicide.

According to experts, including the National Rifle Association and the Sporting Arms and Ammunition Manufacturers Institute, the safe handling of firearms requires that guns be stored unloaded in a locked area separate from ammunition (Zimring & Hawkins, 1983). The major reason U.S. gun owners give for ownership, however, is protection, and thus the majority keep guns loaded and unlocked (Weil & Hemenway, 1992).

Specific strategies for reducing the availability of guns, including firearm disposal and safe storage, are available (e.g., Handgun Epidemic Lowering Plan, 1996), but this remains a contentious issue in this country. For example, in July 1996, the House of Representatives slashed $2.6 million from the National Center for Injury Prevention and Control, a branch of the CDC that had planned to use the funds for research on firearm-related injuries. Republican lawmakers accused the injury center of promoting research that advocates gun control (Walker, 1996). Given that means restriction appears to be one of the most effective youth suicide prevention strategies, efforts will continue in this area. For example, the American Association of Suicidology has received a grant to develop effective means restrictions strategies (Berman, 1996).

A second issue that has plagued prevention efforts in this area is the persistent myth that discussions with students about suicide will somehow prompt suicidal behavior among them. This myth stems in part from a specious analogy between discussions with students in an effort to promote mutual support and help seeking and imitation by vulnerable adolescents following media depiction of suicidal acts (CDC, 1994) and imitative suicidal behavior following suicides of peers of vulnerable youth (Brent et al., 1992). Carefully designed programs eschew any media depiction of suicidal behavior. As with discussion of any sensitive material that touches students' current lives, experienced teachers know the need, and well-designed programs include reminders for the provision of opportunities to process or follow up individual students' reactions. Therefore, these classroom discussions of responses to suicide are no more equivalent to media depictions or actual suicide completions (which are followed by suspension of classroom lessons and institution of postvention procedures) than are discussions of drugs and interpersonal violence equivalent to media depiction or modeling of these phenomena. This argument also incorrectly assumes that such classroom discussions represent the students' initial exposure to the topic or phenomenon, which is no more true for suicide than for sex education.

A second source for this myth is an often-cited article by Shaffer et al. (1990). This study reported the responses to first-generation school programs of self-reported suicide attempters, as compared with self-reported nonattempter program participants. The numbers of attempters available for these comparisons were small (35 for some analyses, 17 for other analyses) because some schools did not employ all the questions (many of the differences were for males, which involved sample sizes of 10 and 4 for the two sets of analyses). Although the overall responses of these students to the programs were generally positive, a greater percentage of the attempters, compared with nonattempters, reported negative reactions on some items. A variety of methodological concerns and plausible rival hypotheses (as opposed to harmful effects on participants) as to the meaning of these responses were noted by the authors themselves in another report (Shaffer, Garland, & Whittle, 1988) and by other researchers (Clark, 1990; Kalafat, 1991). Although Shaffer et al. (1990) noted that "even if the program did upset a minority of the attempters, perhaps arousing thoughts and feelings of their own situation, that would not necessarily be dangerous" (p. 3155), they continued to express concerns. The study was followed by a spate of strident headlines such as "stirs depression" and "killing our kids," as well as by references to harmful or iatrogenic effects by otherwise responsible researchers. The facts are best summarized by the following quotes: "There is no evidence of increased suicidal ideation or behavior among program participants" (CDC, 1992, p. 66). "Furthermore, numerous research and intervention efforts have been completed without any reports of harm" (Potter, Powell, & Kachur, 1995, p. 87). Again, this is exemplified by the results of the ASAP dissemination.

The third issue arises in relation to prevention strategies that involve referring at-risk and suicidal adolescents to treatment or urging troubled youth and their peer confidantes to turn to adults in the school. The former strategy may appear tenuous because of the lack of evidence for the efficacy of treatment of individuals who have made prior suicide attempts (CDC, 1992; Muehrer, 1990). As Felner et al. (1992) pointed out, however, this should not be surprising, given how late in the developmental stage of their problems suicide attempters are. Programs that focus on earlier identification and referral and that lower barriers to help seeking may bring troubled youth to treatment at a more amenable stage of their problems. The early detection goal of school-based programs is to identify and assist troubled youth prior to, or at the latest, at, the ideation stage that precedes overt behavior. Still, this area is troubling because adolescents are well known for their resistance to treatment and for high dropout rates (Sommers-Flanagan & Sommers-Flanagan, 1995) and because of the probably not-unrelated lack of preparation of many providers for working with suicidal clients (Bongar & Harmatz, 1991). The shift to school-based services provided by individuals more familiar with and to students may enhance the psychological and cultural accessibility of assistance for troubled adolescents (Dryfoos, 1994).

Given the current strong resistance of students toward using adults in their schools as helpers, however, providing training to students and school gatekeepers on the early identification and referral of troubled adolescents and attempting to convince them of the importance of breaking confidences in special situations is only half the battle (Kalafat & Elias, 1995). There has been a call for ecological or transactional programs (Felner & Felner, 1989) that address the nature of the environment confronted by individuals. For the most part, this is a call for attending to generalization issues that have long been a concern of organizational trainers. Strategies for ensuring that knowledge and skills learned in the classroom are applied or translate into performance outside the classroom include arranging positive contingencies for such performance and removing barriers to the performance. For school-based programs that emphasize help seeking, this means that such training must be complemented by efforts to provide supportive and culturally, psychologically, and temporally accessible adults to students in their schools and to address organizational issues that serve as barriers to help seeking in schools.

Toward this end, focus groups of 9th- and 11th-grade students have been conducted to identify barriers to their seeking help from adults in their schools (Ross & Kalafat, 1996). In addition to particular characteristics of adults in whom they would and would not confide, these students identified systemic or school organizational characteristics that appear to attenuate seeking help from adults in the school. They indicated that a central characteristic of adults in whom they would confide was that they and the adult had gotten to know each other fairly well. They then pointed out that the way schools are organized, which is characterized by multiple periods occurring in rapid succession and teachers' inability to track students within a class year or across years, precludes teachers and other school personnel from forming relationships with students that encourage sharing of concerns. This is particularly true for 9th graders, who are dealing with a major transition from elementary or middle schools and do not know anyone in the school well. Guidance counselors, in particular, were characterized as overworked and under time pressures that precluded their giving the message that they would be willing to sit and listen to students. Moreover, there did not appear to be facilities for such private conversations in many of the schools.

A second major barrier to talking to adults in schools were the dual roles occupied by teachers and counselors. That is, both teachers and counselors carried out disciplinary and evaluative functions that made students cautious about revealing personal problems to them.

Finally, students noted that confidentiality was rarely honored. Part of this appears to be a "teachers' lounge" phenomenon, and part a genuine confusion as to what interactions with adolescents at which ages may be kept confidential. This issue appears to be widespread, as confirmed by informal discussions with school personnel and consultants from a number of states, as well as in a project that involved the enhanced coordination between schools and a regional mental health system for the safe return of students to schools after hospitalization for suicidal ideation or behavior (Kalafat & Mackey, 1994). This effort prompted the development of well-received workshops on confidentiality for school personnel.

These concerns about depersonalizing school organizational environments have been noted in the literature. A report on the education of young adolescents (Carnegie Council on Adolescent Development, 1988) noted that keeping students and teachers together in teams in which they can develop a sense of belonging and interconnectedness reduces the degree of flux that students must confront and provides for increased support that may reduce the development of psychosocial difficulties. A review of prevention programs aimed at the interrelated behaviors of low achievement, dropout, delinquency, and substance abuse reveals that this call has been answered by the development of programs aimed at creating a sense of community (Purkey & Smith, 1983). Specifically, these programs involve a variety of strategies for engaging youth in the operations of their schools and thus promoting bonding with the school (Hawkins & Weis, 1985). Strategies have included providing students opportunities for increased decision making about rules, skills to make such contributions, and praise and recognition for their contributions (Natriello, Pallas, McDill, McPartland, & Royster, 1988). Also, schools have been reorganized to provide students with enhanced interactions with teachers (Felner & Adan, 1988), and large schools have been organized as schools-within-schools that reduced "overstaffing" and limited niches that had led to alienation and limited participation and had attenuated a sense of responsibility by students (Linney & Seidman, 1989). These organizational changes have been shown to enhance achievement and reduce a variety of forms of deviancy. As with specific suicide prevention curricula, most of these programs feature strong peer involvement in buddy/tutoring programs to increase involvement and reduce alienation (Cowen, Hightower, Pedro-Carroll, & Work, 1989; Jason & Rhodes, 1989).

These strategies for involvement and bonding seem particularly suited to the suicidal process that is characterized by social isolation, alienation, withdrawal, and low social supports. They have been included in at least one school-based indicated suicide intervention program that has sought to increase at-risk adolescents' sense of support from teachers and peers and their involvement in school activities (Eggert, Thompson, Herting, & Nicholas, 1994).

In sum, the search for general protective factors has led to the development and implementation of school-based youth suicide prevention programs that teach students help-seeking and help-providing knowledge, attitudes, and skills. Given the prevalence of encounters between actively or potentially suicidal youth and their peers, these programs provide a problem-centered (i.e., relevant to issues that students are currently dealing with) starting point for teaching students an important component of a prosocial behavioral repertoire.

These programs are taking the first steps toward ecological programming by exploring school organizational barriers to helpful contacts between students and adults in the school and are complemented by efforts to increase student involvement in the schools. Such efforts to enhance the supportiveness of the school environment can also be complemented by addressing the other major support system for youth through the growing movement to enhance family support, functioning, and involvement with schools (Booth & Dunn, 1996).

The focus of school-based youth suicide prevention programs is at a point in the trajectory toward suicidal behavior that is quite proximal to the emergence of such undesirable outcomes. Although this proximal emphasis may be necessary, given the lack of established long-range predictors or prevention strategies (Coie et al., 1993), it is recognized that this is not a sufficient universal prevention strategy. Many factors, such as the co-occurrence of a variety of dysfunctional behaviors and their shared risk and protective elements, as well as the limited capacity of schools to absorb and implement a variety of categorical programs, point to the need for programs that address more generic protective factors that may operate earlier in the etiology of the problems of youth.

Problem-Solving Competency: A General Protective Factor

Successful strategies from prevention programs aimed at related adolescent deviant behaviors can be combined with current promising school-based suicide prevention efforts (Kalafat & Elias, 1995). The goal of enhancing supports in the educational and family contexts provides a bridge to other prevention efforts that enhance protective factors. One set of prevention programs particularly relevant to suicide includes those that promote social problem-solving/decision-making competencies.

The acquisition of competencies, particularly social problem-solving competencies, has shown considerable promise as a protective factor for a variety of the unavoidable stressors and challenges with which many adolescents must contend (Durlak, 1983; Elias et al., 1993; Kornberg & Caplan, 1980). Space limitations prevent a comprehensive review of these programs, which can be obtained from a number of sources (e.g., Elias et al., 1993; Weissberg, Caplan, & Sivo, 1989). For present purposes, the next sections will provide an overview of their conceptual basis, their particular relevance to suicide, and some of the evidence for their impact on dysfunctional behaviors, including suicide.

Essentially, competency consists of the knowledge and abilities to respond to environmental demands and the related self-appraisal that one has the ability to meet such demands (Masterpasqua, 1989). Symptoms or psychological disorders appear when individuals sense that the competencies with which they engage their environment are stretched beyond their limit (Zigler & Glick, 1986). According to Masterpasqua, the individual's implicit self-statement becomes "I just don't have what it takes and there's nothing I can do about it" (p. 1367). A core component of competency is the ability to recognize possibilities and generate alternatives (Tyler, 1978). Elias, Gara, Schuyler, Branden-Muller, and Sayette (1991) posited that "conceptually, children's ability or inability to cope with decision making situations, particularly when under stress, is viewed as a primary link in a sequence of interpersonal behavior that may eventuate in positive social functioning or in . . . psychopathology" (p. 409). A number of studies indicate that childhood patterns of deficits in adaptational competencies predict the emergence of maladjustments in adulthood (Kohlberg, Ricks, & Snarey, 1984).

This conceptualization is clearly related to the processes of hopelessness and cognitive constriction (inability to see or generate alternatives) that mediate suicide (Beck, Steer, Beck, & Newman, 1993; Schneidman, 1989). Note the similarity in the quote from

Masterpasqua (1989) and Schneidman's (1989) "There is nothing I can do (except commit suicide), and there is no one who can help me (with the pain that I am suffering)" (p. 18). In regard to their relevance to social or interpersonal problem-solving interventions, such cognitive states appear to have interpersonal implications. As reviewed earlier, there is evidence that depression may undermine supportive responses from others, and a recent study demonstrated that hopelessness mediated both loneliness and suicidality (Joiner & Rudd, 1996).

A number of studies have found greater cognitive problem-solving deficits in suicidal adolescents, compared with psychiatric and normal controls, including generation of fewer alternatives, less accurate appraisals, repetitive use of ineffective solutions, avoidant responses, and emotional responses to problematic situations (Asarnow, Carlson, & Guthrie, 1987; McLeavey, Daly, Murray, O'Riordan, & Taylor, 1987; Orbach, Bar-Joseph, & Dror, 1990; Rotheram-Borus & Trautman, 1990; Sadowski & Kelly, 1993). It follows, then, that developing social problem-solving competencies in youth may provide them with personal resources that would permit them to effectively cope with challenging situations and thus not feel so helpless and hopeless that suicide becomes a considered alternative.

Adolescent suicide attempts are most often precipitated by common stressful events such as interpersonal conflict, rejection and humiliation, and getting into trouble (Dubow et al., 1989; Shaffer & Gould, 1987; Spirito, Overholser, & Stark, 1989). Thus, programs that teach adolescents how to cope or problem solve in response to stressful events may be an important component of prevention efforts. There is evidence that social problem-solving training prepares individuals to respond more effectively to stressors and attenuates ineffective responses, including suicide.

Elias et al. (1986) and Elias et al. (1991) provided extended social problem-solving curricula to grade school students. In follow-up assessments in middle and high school, they found that participants, compared with controls, responded more effectively to stressors, were less likely to engage in vandalism or aggression, and were less likely to use alcohol or tobacco. Subsequent analyses found social problem-solving skills to be a consistent mediator of students' responses to stressors.

Dubow, Schmidt, McBride, Edwards, and Merk (1993) assessed the impact of a 13-session problem-solving curriculum and found program participants, compared with controls, able to generate a greater number of effective solutions and to express greater self-efficacy in response to vignettes of specific stressful situations such as divorce, moving, and self-care. Some effects were stronger at a 5-month follow-up assessment.

Weissberg and Elias (1993) noted that children have limited capacities to transfer and generalize skills, attitudes, and knowledge for dealing with stressors from one domain to another. Thus, Caplan et al. (1992) and Felner et al. (1992) recommended a combination of general skills training with domain-specific instructions as a means of preventing particular psychosocial problems. Caplan noted the successful application of social competence training to depression, impulsivity, and aggression as supportive of this approach and described a project that combined a structured problem-solving program with specific sessions on substance abuse into a 20-session curriculum. Inner-city and suburban 6th- and 7th-grade students were randomly assigned to the curriculum or a control group. Curriculum participants showed significant increases in quantity and effectiveness of coping skills and teacher (not blind to condition) ratings of social adjustment and interpersonal effectiveness (conflict resolution, impulse control, and popularity). Self-reports of substance use showed generally positive outcomes; controls showed increases in intentions to use beer and hard liquor and excessive alcohol use, whereas participants did not. Both groups showed increases in intentions to use cigarettes, marijuana, and wine; no differences were found in reported changes in frequency of substance use.

Orbach and Bar-Joseph (1993) evaluated a combined universal prevention program that included a session on suicide. Seven 2-hour meetings were devoted to a wide range of topics: depression and happiness, family issues, feelings of helplessness, coping with failure, coping with stress, problem solving, and coping with suicidal urges. The sessions emphasized sharing, universalizing of experiences, problem-solving alternatives, and self- and peer help approaches. Students were randomly assigned to experimental and control classes in six high schools and completed questionnaires on suicidal tendencies, hopelessness, ego identity, and coping ability before and after the program. Significant positive changes were found for the class participants compared with controls in reduction of suicidal feelings, increased ego identity cohesion, and ability to cope with problems.

In an indicated intervention, McLeavey, Daly, Ludgate, and Murray (1994) randomly assigned self-poisoning patients (average age = 24) to either a 5-hour interpersonal problem-solving skills training group or individual crisis-oriented problem reduction sessions that did not include specific skills training. A number of problem-solving measures were included in the assessment battery that was administered prior to the interventions and at 3-week and 6-month follow-ups. Participants were followed for 1 year to assess for repeated self-poisoning acts. Interpersonal problem-solving skills and the ability to cope with everyday problematic situations significantly improved for the experimental group but not for the control group. At 1-year follow-up, the self-poisoning act was repeated by 10.5% of the experimental participants and 25% of the control participants.

Overall, these studies provide evidence that teaching individuals problem-solving skills may help them cope with a variety of stressors, may attenuate dysfunctional behaviors such as substance use (which often co-occurs with suicide), and may provide a viable alternative to suicidal feelings and behaviors. It is possible that such problem-solving competencies may serve as protective factors that along with other supports, may attenuate the risk of developing suicidal behaviors.

As is the case with evaluations of school-based suicide prevention programs, these represent a set of generally well-designed, controlled evaluations of specific programs that with the possible exception of the 2-year program implemented by Elias et al. (1991), were relatively brief interventions. None of them represented the institutionalized multiyear, ecological, or systemic programming recommended by Weissberg and Elias (1993). A number of these investigators reported nested effects by classes or schools, thus reemphasizing the need for careful implementation procedures.

On the positive side, the evaluations of school-based suicide prevention and problem-solving/competence programs lend empirical support to a prevention strategy that has a solid conceptual basis. The enhancement of problem-solving competencies, sense of self-efficacy, and prosocial help-seeking/help-providing behaviors, combined with organizational changes in schools and the families and communities with which they and their students interact, could provide a powerful counterbalance to the stressors and personal vulnerabilities with which youth must contend.

Conclusion

Weissberg and Elias (1993) reviewed a number of national calls for comprehensive kindergarten through 12th grade school health programming that would provide students and families with exposure to a range of cognitive, affective, and skill development approaches that contribute to overall competence with respect to physical, mental-emotional, and social health. They recommended that such programming synthesize the strengths of many currently available prevention programs into a larger coordinated effort called Comprehensive Social Competence and Health Education (C-SCAHE). They noted gaps in program scope, intensity, and duration between this ideal and the current program models that have been implemented and evaluated in schools to date; and called for a sustained, collaborative 20-year effort to establish, evaluate, and disseminate K-12 C-SCAHE programming.

That 20-year figure is well advised, given the difficulty involved in establishing even limited, demonstrably effective innovations in schools and the daunting moving target created by the expanding incidence of new morbidities among youth. In the shorter run, common conceptual bases and individual controlled studies suggest the promise of combining generic problem-solving training with focused, domain-specific training in such areas as suicide prevention into ecological prevention programs.

The *Healthy People 2000: Midcourse Review and 1995 Revisions* (DHHS, 1995) reported that for youth aged 15 to 24, the reduction of mortality was the only life stage goal not met in 1990. This report indicated that "real progress is needed in curbing both interpersonal violence and self-inflicted violence to achieve the year 2000 target" (p. 11). The lack of progress for self-inflicted injury is not surprising because suicide receives far less media, political, and fiscal attention than does homicide, although it is a more prevalent manner of death. It appears that many federal and school officials have erroneously concluded that the youth suicide problem has been solved despite the absence of a commitment to support large-scale evaluations of promising applied prevention programs. Goals and concerns have not translated into funding for the development or evaluation of comprehensive prevention programs (Berman & Jobes, 1995; Potter, 1994). The reduction in emphasis on school-based programs was reflected in a 1994 national Gallup survey of adolescents in which respondents were significantly less likely than in a 1991 survey to report that their school and community were doing anything regarding adolescent suicide (Zimmerman, 1994).

This retreat from concern about youth suicide is particularly unfortunate at this time, not only because of the continued prevalence of youth suicidal behaviors but also because of the convergence of compelling conceptual and empirical support for effective school-based prevention programming. It is past time to commit sufficient resources to establish and evaluate such prevention programs in grade levels that precede major school transitions, with boosters in subsequent grades. Evaluation should include careful assessment of implementation fidelity as well as a multilevel outcome evaluation that assesses (a) participant acceptance of the program; (b) acquisition of knowledge, skills, and, attitudes; (c) necessary organizational changes; (d) the application or performance of learning; and (e) distal impacts associated with such organizational changes and performance (Kirkpatrick, 1975). By enhancing adolescents' coping competencies and prosocial repertoire, and the supportiveness of their community contexts, such programs may not only reduce the incidence of self-destructive behaviors but also contribute to the development of healthy people and healthy communities.

References

Allen, J. P., Aber, J. L., & Leadbeater, B. J. (1990). Adolescent problem behaviors: The influence of attachment and autonomy. *Psychiatric Clinics of North America, 13,* 455-467.

Allen, J. P., Philliber, S., & Hoggson, N. (1990). School-based prevention of teen-age pregnancy and school dropout: Process evaluation of the national replication of the Teen Outreach program. *American Journal of Community Psychology, 18,* 505-524.

Allen, J. P., Weissberg, R. P., & Hawkins, J. (1989). The relation between values and social competence in early adolescence. *Developmental Psychology, 25,* 458-464.
Asarnow, J. R., Carlson, G. A., & Guthrie, D. (1987). Coping strategies, self perceptions, hopelessness, and perceived family environments in depressed and suicidal children. *Journal of Consulting and Clinical Psychology, 55,* 361-366.
Beck, A. T., Steer, R. A., Beck, J. S., & Newman, C. F. (1993). Hopelessness, depression, suicidal ideation, and clinical diagnosis of depression. *Suicide and Life-Threatening Behavior, 23,* 139-145.
Bell-Dolan, D., Foster, S. L., & Christopher, J. M. (1995). Girls' peer relations and internalizing problems: Are socially neglected, rejected, and withdrawn girls at risk? *Journal of Child Clinical Psychology, 24,* 463-473.
Berman, A. L. (Chair). (1996, April). *The prevention of youth suicide by firearms.* Panel presentation at the annual conference of the American Association of Suicidology, St. Louis, MO.
Berman, A. L., & Jobes, D. A. (1995). Suicide prevention in adolescents (age 12-18). *Suicide and Life-Threatening Behavior, 25,* 143-154.
Berndt, T. J. (1979). Developmental changes in conformity to peers and parents. *Developmental Psychology, 15,* 608-616.
Berven, N. L. (1985). Reliability and validity of standardized case management simulations. *Journal of Counseling Psychology, 32,* 397-409.
Blakey, C. H., Mayer, J. P., Gottshalk, R. G., Schmitt, N., Davidson, W. S., Roitman, D. B., & Emshoff, J. G. (1987). The fidelity-adaptation debate: Implications for the implementation of public sector social programs. *American Journal of Community Psychology, 15,* 253-268.
Bongar, B., & Harmatz, M. (1991). Clinical psychology graduate education in the study of suicide: Availability, resources, and importance. *Suicide and Life-Threatening Behavior, 21,* 231-244.
Booth, A., & Dunn, J. F. (1966). *Family-school links: How do they affect educational outcomes?* Mahwah, NJ: Lawrence Erlbaum.
Brent, D. A., Perper, J., & Allman, C., Moritz, G. M., Wartella, M. E., & Zelenak, J. P. (1991). The presence and accessibility of firearms in the homes of adolescent suicides. *Journal of the American Medical Association, 266,* 2989-2995.
Brent, D. A., Perper, J., Kolko, D. J., & Goldstein, C. E. (1988). Risk factors for adolescent suicide: A comparison of adolescent suicide victims with suicidal inpatients. *Archives of General Psychiatry, 45,* 581-588.
Brent, D. A., Perper, J., Moritz, G., Allman, C., Friend, A., Schweers, J., Roth, C., Balach, L., & Harrington, K. (1992). Psychiatric effects of exposure to suicide among friends and acquaintances of adolescent suicide victims. *Journal of the American Academy of Child and Adolescent Psychiatry, 31,* 629-640.
Brent, D. A., Perper, J., Moritz, G., Baugher, C. R., Balach, L., & Schweers, J. (1993). Stressful life events and adolescent suicide. *Suicide and Life-Threatening Behavior, 23,* 179-187.
Brent, D. A., Perper, J., Moritz, G., Baugher, C. R., Schweers, J., & Roth, C. (1993). Firearms and adolescent suicide: A community case-control study. *American Journal of Diseases of Children, 147,* 1066-1071.
Caplan, G. (1964). *Principles of preventative psychiatry.* New York: Basic Books.
Caplan, W., Weissberg, R. P., Grober, J. S., Sivo, P. J., Grady, K., & Jacoby, C. (1992). Social competence promotion with inner-city and suburban young adolescents:

Effects on social adjustment and alcohol use. *Journal of Consulting and Clinical Psychology, 60,* 56-63.

Carnegie Council on Adolescent Development. (1988). *Review of school-based health services.* New York: Carnegie Foundation.

Cauce, A. M., & Srebnik, D. S. (1989). Peer networks and social support: A focus for preventive efforts with youths. In L. A. Bond & B. E. Compas (Eds.), *Primary prevention and promotion in the schools* (pp. 235-254). Newbury Park, CA: Sage.

Centers for Disease Control and Prevention. (1992). *Youth suicide prevention programs: A resource guide.* Atlanta, GA: Author.

Centers for Disease Control and Prevention. (1994). Suicide contagion and the reporting of suicide: Recommendations from a national workshop. *Morbidity and Mortality Weekly Report, 43*(RR-6), 13-18.

Centers for Disease Control and Prevention. (1995a). Suicide among children, adolescents, and young adults. *Morbidity and Mortality Weekly Report, 44*(15), 289-291.

Centers for Disease Control and Prevention. (1995b). Youth risk behavior surveillance: United States, 1993. *Morbidity and Mortality Weekly Report, 44*(SS-1).

Christopher, G. M., Kurtz, P. D., & Howing, P. T. (1989). The status of mental health services for youth in the school and community. *Children and Youth Services Review, 11,* 159-174.

Ciffone, J. (1993). Suicide prevention: A classroom presentation to adolescents. *Social Work, 38,* 196-203.

Clark, D. C. (1990, December). School-based suicide prevention. *Suicide Research Digest, 4,* 1-3.

Clark, D. C. (1993). Suicidal behavior in childhood and adolescence: Recent studies and clinical implications. *Psychiatric Annals, 23,* 271-283.

Clark, D. C., & Fawcett, B. (1992). Review of empirical risk factors for evaluation of the suicidal patient. In B. Bongar (Ed.), *Suicide: Guidelines for assessment, management, and treatment* (pp. 16-48). New York: Oxford University Press.

Coie, J. D., Watt, N. F., West, S. G., Hawkins, J. D., Asarnow, J. R., Markham, J. J., Raney, S. L., Shure, M. B., & Lang, B. (1993). The science of prevention: A conceptual framework and some directions for a national research program. *American Psychologist, 48,* 1013-1022.

Connolly, J., Geller, S., Morton, P., & Kutcher, S. (1992). Peer response to social interactions with depressed adolescents. *Journal of Clinical Child Psychology, 21,* 365-370.

Cowen, E. L. (1980). The wooing of primary prevention. *American Journal of Community Psychology, 8,* 258-284.

Cowen, E. L., Hightower, A. D., Pedro-Carroll, J. A., & Work, W. C. (1989). School-based models for primary prevention programming with children. *Prevention in Human Services, 7,* 133-160.

Davis, J. M., & Sandoval, J. (1991). *Suicidal youth: School-based intervention and prevention.* San Francisco: Jossey-Bass.

Dryfoos, J. G. (1994). *Full-service schools: A revolution in health and social services for children, youth, and families.* San Francisco: Jossey-Bass.

Dubow, E. F., Kausch, D. F., Blum, M. C., Reed, J., & Bush, E. (1989). Correlates of suicidal ideation and attempts in a community sample of junior high and high school students. *Journal of Clinical Child Psychology, 18,* 158-166.

Dubow, E. F., Schmidt, D., McBride, J., Edwards, S., & Merk, F. L. (1993). Teaching children to cope with stressful experiences: Initial implementation and evaluation of a primary prevention program. *Journal of Consulting and Clinical Psychology, 22,* 428-440.

Durlak, J. A. (1983). Social problem-solving as a primary prevention strategy. In R. D. Felner, L. A. Jason, J. N. Moritsuge, & S. S. Farber (Eds.), *Preventive psychology: Theory, research, and practice* (pp. 31-48). New York: Pergamon.

Eccles, J. S., Midgley, C., Wigfield, A., Buchanan, C. M., Reuman, D., Flanagan, C., & MacIver, D. (1993). Development during adolescence: The impact of stage-environment fit on young adolescents' experience in schools and families. *American Psychologist, 48,* 90-101.

Eggert, L. L., Thompson, E. A., Herting, J. R., & Nicholas, L. J. (1994). A prevention research program: Reconnecting at-risk youth. *Issues in Mental Health Nursing, 15,* 107-135.

Eggert, L. L., Thompson, E. A., Randell, B. P., & McCauley, E. (1995). *Youth suicide prevention plan for Washington State.* Olympia: Washington State Department of Health.

Elias, M. J., Gara, M. A., Schuyler, T. F., Branden-Muller, L. R., & Sayette, M. A. (1991). The promotion of social competence: Longitudinal study of a preventive school-based program. *American Journal of Orthopsychiatry, 61,* 409-417.

Elias, M. J., Gara, M. A., Ubriaco, M., Rothbaum, P. A., Clabby, J. F., & Schuyler, T. (1986). Impact of a social problem solving intervention on children's coping with middle-school stressors. *American Journal of Community Psychology, 14,* 259-275.

Elias, M. J., Weissberg, R. P., Hawkins, J. D., Perry, C. L., Zins, J. E., Dodge, K. A., Kendall, P. C., Rotheram-Borus, M. J., Jason, L. A., & Wilson-Brewer, R. (1993). The school-based promotion of social competence: Theory, research, and practice. In R. J. Haggerty, N. Garmezy, M. Rutter, & L. Sherrod (Eds.), *Stress, risk, and resilience in children and adolescents: Processes, mechanisms, and interventions.* New York: Cambridge University Press.

Fairweather, G. W., Tornatzky, L. G., Fergus, E., & Avellar, J. (1982). *Innovation and social process.* New York: Pergamon.

Felner, R. D., & Adan, A. M. (1988). The school transitional project: An ecological intervention and evaluation. In R. H. Price, E. L. Cowen, R. P. Lorion, & J. Ramos-McKay (Eds.), *14 ounces of prevention* (pp. 111-122). Washington, DC: American Psychological Association.

Felner, R. D., Adan, A. M., & Silverman, M. M. (1992). Risk assessment and prevention of youth suicide in schools and educational contexts. In R. W. Maris, A. L. Berman, J. T. Maltsberger, & R. I. Yufit (Eds.), *Assessment and prediction of suicide* (pp. 420-447). New York: Guilford.

Felner, R. D., DuBois, D. L., & Adan, A. M. (1991). Community-based intervention and prevention: Conceptual underpinnings and progress toward a science of community intervention and evaluation. In C. E. Walker (Ed.), *Clinical psychology: Historical and research foundations* (pp. 459-510). New York: Plenum.

Felner, R. D., & Felner, T. W. (1989). Primary prevention programs in the educational context: A transactional-ecological framework and analysis. In L. A. Bond & B. E. Compas (Eds.), *Primary prevention and promotion in the schools* (pp. 13-49). Newbury Park, CA: Sage.

Gagne, R. M. (1985). *The conditions of learning.* New York: Holt, Rinehart & Winston.

Garland, A. F., & Zigler, E. (1993). Adolescent suicide prevention: Current research and social policy implications. *American Psychologist, 48,* 169-182.

Garmezy, N. (1983). Stresses of childhood. In N. Garmezy & M. Rutter (Eds.), *Stress, coping and development in children.* New York: McGraw-Hill.

Garrison, C. Z., Addy, C. L., Jackson, K. L., McKeown, R. E., & Waller, J. L. (1991). A longitudinal study of suicidal ideation in young adolescents. *Journal of the American Academy of Child and Adolescent Psychiatry, 30,* 597-603.

Gordon, R. (1983). An operational classification of disease prevention. *Public Health Reports, 96,* 107-109.

Greenberg, M. T., Siegel, J. M., & Leitch, C. J. (1983). The nature and importance of attachment relationships to parents and peers during adolescence. *Journal of Youth and Adolescence, 12,* 373-386.

Handgun Epidemic Lowering Plan (HELP) Network. (1996). *The HELP handgun disposal handbook: A prescription for safety.* Chicago: Author.

Harman, M. J., Armsworth, M. W., & Henderson, D. L. (1989, Fall). Rural Texas: To whom do children with problems turn? *TACD Journal,* 107-113.

Hawkins, J., & Weis, J. (1985). The sociodevelopmental model: An integrated approach to delinquency prevention. *Journal of Primary Prevention, 6,* 73-97.

Hawton, K., O'Grady, J., Osborn, M., & Cole, D. (1982). Adolescents who take overdoses: Their characteristics, problems, and contacts with helping agencies. *British Journal of Psychiatry, 140,* 118-123.

Healthy communities 2000: Model standards: Guidelines for community attainment of the year 2000 health objectives. (1991). Washington, DC: American Public Health Association.

Hechinger, F. M. (1992). *Fateful choices: Healthy youth for the 21st century.* New York: Hill & Wang.

Hirsch, B. J., & DuBois, D. L. (1992). The relation of peer social support and psychological symptomatology during the transition to junior high school: A two-year longitudinal analysis. *American Journal of Community Psychology, 20,* 333-348.

Hubbard, J. P. (1978). *Measuring medical education: The tests and experience of the National Board of Medical Examiners* (2nd ed.). Philadelphia: Lea & Febiger.

Hutchinson, R. L., & Reagan, C. A. (1987). Problems for which seniors would seek help from guidance counselors. Washington, DC: Educational Resources Information Center.

Illback, R. J., Zins, J. E., Maher, C. A., & Greenberg, R. (1990). An overview of principles and procedures of program planning and evaluation. In T. B. Gutkin & C. R. Reynolds (Eds.), *The handbook of school psychology* (pp. 799-820). New York: John Wiley.

Injury control in the 1990s: A national plan for action. (1993). Atlanta, GA: Centers for Disease Control and Prevention.

Institute of Medicine. (1994). *Reducing risk for mental disorder: Frontiers for preventive intervention research.* Washington, DC: National Academy Press.

Jason, L., & Rhodes, J. (1989). Children helping children: Implications for prevention. *Journal of Primary Prevention, 9,* 203-212.

Joiner, T. E., Jr. (1994). Contagious depression: Existence, specificity to depressed symptoms, and the role of reassurance-seeking. *Journal of Personality and Social Psychology, 67,* 287-296.

Joiner, T. E., Jr., Alfano, M. S., & Metalsky, G. I. (1992). When depression breeds contempt: Reassurance-seeking, self-esteem, and rejection of depressed college students by their roommates. *Journal of Abnormal Psychology, 101,* 165-173.

Joiner, T. E., Jr., & Rudd, M. D. (1996). Disentangling the interrelations between hopelessness, loneliness, and suicidal ideation. *Suicide and Life-Threatening Behavior, 26,* 19-26.

Kalafat, J. (1990). Suicide intervention in the schools. In A. R. Roberts (Ed.), *Contemporary perspectives on crisis intervention and prevention* (pp. 447-474). Englewood Cliffs, NJ: Prentice Hall.

Kalafat, J. (1991, April). *Avoiding premature closure: Early data on the evaluation of school programs.* Panel presentation at the annual conference of the American Association of Suicidology, Boston.

Kalafat, J., & Elias, M. (1992). Adolescents' experience with and response to suicidal peers. *Suicide and Life-Threatening Behavior, 22,* 315-321.

Kalafat, J., & Elias, M. (1994). An evaluation of adolescent suicide intervention classes. *Suicide and Life-Threatening Behavior, 24,* 224-233.

Kalafat, J., & Elias, M. (1995). Suicide prevention in an education context. *Suicide and Life-Threatening Behavior, 25,* 123-133.

Kalafat, J., Elias, M., & Gara, M. A. (1993). The relationship of bystander intervention variables to adolescents' responses to suicidal peers. *Journal of Primary Prevention, 13,* 231-244.

Kalafat, J., & Gagliano, C. (1996). The use of simulations to assess the impact of an adolescent suicide response curriculum. *Suicide and Life-Threatening Behavior, 26,* 359-364.

Kalafat, J., & Mackey, K. (1994, April). *The school return of youths hospitalized for suicidal behavior.* Paper presented at the annual conference of the American Association of Suicidology, New York.

Kalafat, J., & Ryerson, D. (1993, April). *Current practices in school based suicide programs.* Workshop presented at the annual conference of the American Association of Suicidology, San Francisco.

Kalafat, J., & Underwood, M. (1989). *Lifelines: A school based adolescent suicide response program.* Dubuque, IA: Kendall/Hunt.

Kienhorst, I. C. W. M., DeWilde, E. J., Diekstra, R. F. W., & Wolters, W. H. G. (1995). Adolescents' image of their suicide attempt. *Journal of the American Academy of Child and Adolescent Psychiatry, 34,* 623-628.

Kirkpatrick, D. (1975). *Evaluating training programs.* Madison, WI: American Society for Training and Development.

Kohlberg, L., Ricks, D., & Snarey, J. (1984). Childhood development as a predictor of adaptation in adulthood. *Genetic Psychology Monographs, 110,* 91-172.

Kornberg, M. S., & Caplan, G. (1980). Risk factors and preventive interventions in child psychotherapy: A review. *Journal of Primary Prevention, 1,* 71-133.

Larson, R. W. (1983). Adolescents' daily experience with family and friends: Contrasting opportunity systems. *Journal of Marriage and Family, 45,* 739-750.

Lester, D. (1993). The effectiveness of suicide prevention centers. *Suicide and Life-Threatening Behavior, 23,* 263-267.

Lester, D. (1996, April). *Controlling crime facilitators: Evidence from research on homicide and suicide.* Paper presented at the annual conference of the American Association of Suicidology, St. Louis, MO.

Linney, J. A., & Seidman, E. (1989). The future of schooling. *American Psychologist, 44,* 336-340.

Loftin, C., McDowall, D., Wiersema, B., & Cottey, T. J. (1991). Effects of restrictive licensing of handguns on homicide and suicide in the District of Columbia. *New England Journal of Medicine, 325,* 1615-1620.

Masterpasqua, F. (1989). A competence paradigm for psychological practice. *American Psychologist, 44,* 1366-1371.

McLeavey, B. C., Daly, R. J., Ludgate, J. W., & Murray, C. M. (1994). Interpersonal problem-solving skills training in the treatment of self-poisoning patients. *Suicide and Life-Threatening Behavior, 24,* 382-394.

McLeavey, B. C., Daly, R. J., Murray, C. M., O'Riordan, J., & Taylor, M. (1987). Interpersonal problem solving deficits in self-poisoning patients. *Suicide and Life-Threatening Behavior, 17,* 33-49.

Meagher, N., & Clark, J. (1982, March). Fewer adolescents discuss problems with school staff. *Phi Delta Kappan,* 494-497.

Moscicki, E. K. (1995). Epidemiology of suicidal behaviors. *Suicide and Life-Threatening Behavior, 25,* 22-35.

Muehrer, P. (1990). *Conceptual research models for preventing mental disorders* (DHHS Publication No. ADM 90-1713). Rockville, MD: National Institute of Mental Health.

Mullins, L. L., Chard, S. R., Hartman, V. L., Bowbly, D., Rich, L., & Burke, C. (1995). Relation between depressive symptomatology in school children and social response of teachers. *Journal of Clinical Child Psychology, 24,* 474-482.

Naginy, J. L., & Swisher, J. D. (1990). To whom would adolescents turn with drug problems? Implications for school professionals. *High School Journal, 73,* 80-85.

National Institute of Mental Health. (1994). *NIMH suicide research program.* Rockville, MD: Author.

Natriello, G., Pallas, A., McDill, E., McPartland, J., & Royster, D. (1988). *An examination of the assumptions and evidence of alternative drop-out prevention programs in high school* (Rep. No. 365). Baltimore: Johns Hopkins University, Center for Research on Elementary and Middle Schools. (ERIC Documentation Reproduction No. ED-299374)

Norton, E. M., Durlak, J. A., & Richards, M. H. (1989). Peer knowledge of and reactions to adolescent suicide. *Journal of Youth and Adolescence, 18,* 427-437.

Offer, D., Howard, K. J., Schonert, K. A., & Ostrov, E. (1991). To whom do adolescents turn for help? Differences between disturbed and nondisturbed adolescents. *Journal of the American Academy of Child and Adolescent Psychiatry, 30,* 623-630.

Orbach, I., & Bar-Joseph, H. (1993). The impact of a suicide prevention program for adolescents on suicidal tendencies, hopelessness, ego identity, and coping. *Suicide and Life-Threatening Behavior, 23,* 120-129.

Orbach, I., Bar-Joseph, H., & Dror, N. (1990). Styles of problem solving in suicidal individuals. *Suicide and Life-Threatening Behavior, 20,* 56-64.

Overholser, J. C., Hemstreet, A. H., Spirito, A., & Vyse, S. (1989). Suicide awareness programs in the schools: Effects of gender and personal experience. *Journal of the American Academy of Child and Adolescent Psychiatry, 28,* 925-930.

Pfeffer, C. R., Klerman, G. L., Hurt, S. W., Kakuma, T., Peskin, J. R., & Siefker, C. A. (1993). Suicidal children grow up: Rates and psychological risk factors for suicide attempts during follow-up. *Journal of the American Academy of Child and Adolescent Psychiatry, 32,* 106-113.

Potter, L. (1994, April). *Reducing the toll: Means to an end.* Paper presented at the annual conference of the American Association of Suicidology, New York.

Potter, L., Powell, K. E., & Kachur, S. P. (1995). Suicide prevention from a mental health perspective. *Suicide and Life-Threatening Behavior, 25,* 82-91.

Purkey, S. C., & Smith, M. S. (1983). Effective schools: A review. *Elementary School Journal, 83,* 427-453.

Reisman, B. A., & Scharfman, M. A. (1991). *Teenage suicide prevention workshops for guidance counselors* [Trainer's manual and resource materials]. Douglastown, NY: Pride of Judea Medical Center.

Rosenberg, M. L., & Mercy, J. A. (1991). Introduction. In M. L. Rosenberg & M. A. Fenely (Eds.), *Violence in America: A public health approach.* New York: Oxford University Press.

Ross, C., & Kalafat, J. (1996). *Barriers to seeking help from adults in schools.* Manuscript in preparation.

Rotheram-Borus, M. J., & Trautman, P. D. (1990). Cognitive style and pleasant activities among female adolescent suicide attempters. *Journal of Consulting and Clinical Psychology, 58,* 554-561.

Rudd, M. D., Joiner, T. E., & Rajab, M. H. (1995). Help negation after acute suicidal crisis. *Journal of Consulting and Clinical Psychology, 63,* 499-503.

Rutter, M. (1989). Isle of Wright revisited: Twenty-five years of child psychiatric epidemiology. *Journal of the American Academy of Child and Adolescent Psychiatry, 28,* 633-653.

Ryerson, D. (1990). Suicide awareness education in schools: The development of a core program and subsequent modifications for special populations or institutions. *Death Studies, 14,* 371-390.

Ryerson, D. (1993, April). *A ten-year follow-up of a multi-site school program.* Paper presented at the annual conference of the American Association of Suicidology, San Francisco.

Sadowski, C., & Kelly, M. L. (1993). Social problem solving in suicidal adolescents. *Journal of Consulting and Clinical Psychology, 61,* 121-127.

Schneidman, E. S. (1989). Overview: A multidimensional approach to suicide. In D. Jacobs & H. N. Brown (Eds.), *Suicide: Understanding and responding* (pp. 1-30). Madison, CT: International Universities Press.

Shaffer, D., Garland, A., Gould, M., Fisher, P., & Trautman, P. (1988). Preventing teenage suicide: A critical review. *Journal of the American Academy of Child and Adolescent Psychiatry, 27,* 675-687.

Shaffer, D., Garland, A., Vieland, V., Underwood, M., & Busner, C. (1991). The impact of curriculum-based suicide prevention programs for teenagers. *Journal of the American Academy of Child and Adolescent Psychiatry, 30,* 588-596.

Shaffer, D., Garland, A., & Whittle, B. (1988). *An evaluation of youth suicide prevention programs: New Jersey adolescent suicide prevention project: Final project report.* Trenton: New Jersey Division of Mental Health and Hospitals.

Shaffer, D., & Gould, M. S. (1987). *Progress report: Study of completed and attempted suicides in adolescents* (Contract No. RO1-MH-38198). Bethesda, MD: National Institute of Mental Health.

Shaffer, D., Vieland, V., Garland, A., Rojas, M., Underwood, M., & Busner, C. (1990). Adolescent suicide attempters: Response to suicide prevention programs. *Journal of the American Medical Association, 264,* 3151-3155.

Shafii, M., Whittinghill, J. R., Dolen, D. C., Pearson, V. D., Derrick, A., & Carrington, S. (1984). Psychological reconstruction of completed suicide in childhood and adolescence. In H. S. Sudak, A. B. Ford, & N. B. Rushforth (Eds.), *Suicide in the young* (pp. 271-294). Boston: Wright-PSG.

Silverman, M. M., & Felner, R. D. (1995). The place of suicide prevention in the spectrum of prevention: Definitions of critical terms and constructs. *Suicide and Life-Threatening Behavior, 25,* 70-81.

Sommers-Flanagan, J., & Sommers-Flanagan, R. (1995). Psychotherapy techniques with treatment-resistant adolescents. *Psychotherapy, 32,* 131-140.

Spirito, A., Overholser, J., Ashworth, S., Morgan, J., & Benedict-Drew, C. (1988). Evaluation of a suicide awareness curriculum for high school students. *Journal of the American Academy of Child and Adolescent Psychiatry, 27,* 705-711.

Spirito, A., Overholser, J., & Stark, L. J. (1989). Common problems and coping strategies: II. Findings with adolescent suicide attempters. *Journal of Abnormal Child Psychology, 17,* 213-221.

Staub, E. (1979). *Positive social behavior and morality: Vol. 2. Socialization and development.* New York: Academic Press.

Tanney, B. L. (1989). Preventing suicide by improving the competencies of care-givers. In *Report of the Secretary's Task Force on Youth Suicide: Vol. 3. Preventions and interventions in youth suicide* (DHHS Publication No. ADM 89-1623, pp. 213-223). Washington, DC: U.S. Government Printing Office.

Tierney, R. J. (1988). *Comprehensive evaluation for suicide intervention training.* Unpublished doctoral dissertation, University of Calgary, Alberta, Canada.

Topol, P., & Resnikoff, M. (1982). Perceived peer and family relationships, hopelessness, and locus of control as factors in adolescent suicide attempts. *Suicide and Life-Threatening Behavior, 12,* 141-150.

Trout, D. L. (1980). The role of social isolation in suicide. *Suicide and Life-Threatening Behavior, 10,* 10-23.

Tyler, L. E. (1978). *Individuality.* San Francisco: Jossey-Bass.

U.S. Department of Health and Human Services, Public Health Service. (1991). *Healthy people 2000: National health promotion and disease prevention objectives* (DHHS Publication No. PHS 91-50212). Washington, DC: U.S. Government Printing Office.

U.S. Department of Health and Human Services, Public Health Service. (1995). *Healthy people 2000: Midcourse review and 1995 revisions.* Washington, DC: U.S. Government Printing Office.

Walker, P. V. (1996, August 2). Scientists decry lawmakers' decision to slash support for firearms research. *Chronicle of Higher Education, 42*(47), 19-21.

Weil, D. S., & Hemenway, D. (1992). Loaded guns in the home: Analysis of a national random survey of gun owners. *Journal of the American Medical Association, 267,* 3033-3077.
Weissberg, R. P., Caplan, M., & Harwood, R. L. (1991). Promoting competent young people in competence-enhancing environments: A systems-based perspective on primary prevention. *Journal of Consulting and Clinical Psychology, 59,* 830-841.
Weissberg, R. P., Caplan, M., & Sivo, P. J. (1989). A new conceptual framework for establishing school-based social competence promotion programs. In L. A. Bond & B. E. Compas (Eds.), *Primary prevention and promotion in the schools* (pp. 255-296). Newbury Park, CA: Sage.
Weissberg, R. P., & Elias, M. J. (1993). Enhancing young people's social competence and health behavior: An important challenge for educators, scientists, policymakers, and funders. *Applied & Preventive Psychology, 2,* 179-190.
Wellman, M. M., & Wellman, R. J. (1986). Sex differences in peer responsiveness to suicide ideation. *Suicide and Life-Threatening Behavior, 3,* 360-378.
Wells, C. E., & Ritter, K. (1979). Paperwork, pressure, and discouragement: Student attitudes toward guidance services and implications for the profession. *Personnel and Guidance Journal, 58,* 170-175.
Wills, T. A. (1985). Supportive functions of interpersonal relationships. In S. Cohen & S. L. Syme (Eds.), *Social support and health* (pp. 61-82). Orlando, FL: Academic Press.
Wills, T. A., & Vaughan, R. (1989). Social support and substance use in early adolescence. *Journal of Behavioral Medicine, 12,* 321-339.
Winter, M. G., Hicks, R., McVey, G., & Fox, J. (1988). Age and sex differences in choice of consultation for various types of problems. *Child Development, 59,* 1046-1055.
Zigler, E., & Glick, M. (1986). *A developmental approach to adult psychopathology.* New York: John Wiley.
Zimmerman, J. K. (1994, Fall). Gallup survey of adolescent suicidality. *Newslink, 20,* 6-7.
Zimring, F. E., & Hawkins, J. (1983). *The citizen's guide to gun control.* New York: Macmillan.

• *CHAPTER 8* •

Promoting Healthy Dietary Behaviors

CHERYL L. PERRY
MARY STORY
LESLIE A. LYTLE

The purpose of this chapter is to review the research to date on promoting healthy dietary behaviors in youth. Healthy dietary behaviors involve the adoption and maintenance of eating patterns that include a variety of foods (U.S. Department of Agriculture [USDA], 1992) and sufficient nutrients (U.S. Department of Health and Human Services [DHHS], 1988) and yet are not excessive in calories, fat, sodium, or sugar (USDA, 1995). Therefore, this chapter is concerned with the dietary behaviors of all children and adolescents, not just young people who exhibit problems such as obesity or eating disorders. This focus was selected because of the critical role of diet in the prevention of chronic diseases and the high prevalence of less-than-optimal eating behaviors across the population.

The importance of changing dietary behaviors to promote the health of children and adolescents is reflected in *Healthy People 2000: National Health Promotion and Disease Prevention Objectives* (DHHS, 1991a). Of the 21 nutrition objectives for the year 2000, eight pertain to children and adolescents and are shown in Table 8.1. Concern for the dietary behaviors of all youth has clearly

Table 8.1 *Healthy People 2000:* Nutrition Objectives for Children and Adolescents

- Reduce overweight to a prevalence of no more than 15% among adolescents aged 12 through 19.
- Reduce growth retardation among low-income children aged 5 and younger to less than 10%.
- Reduce dietary fat intake to an average of 30% of calories or less and average saturated fat intake to less than 10% of calories among people aged 2 and older.
- Increase to at least 50% the proportion of overweight people aged 12 and older who have adopted sound dietary practices combined with regular physical activity to attain an appropriate body weight.
- Increase calcium intake so that at least 50% of youth aged 12 through 24 consume three or more servings daily of foods rich in calcium.
- Reduce iron deficiency to less than 3% among children aged 1 through 4 and women of childbearing age.
- Increase to at least 90% the proportion of school lunch and breakfast services and child care food services with menus that are consistent with the nutrition principles in the *Dietary Guidelines for Americans.*
- Increase to at least 75% the proportion of the nation's schools that provide nutrition education from preschool through 12th grade, preferably as part of quality school health education.

SOURCE: U.S. Department of Health and Human Services, Public Health Service (1991a).

become a national priority and remains so even after reviewing progress since 1990 (DHHS, 1995b).

The first section of this chapter presents a case for the importance of addressing healthy dietary behaviors with children and adolescents, on the basis of the impact of these behaviors on short- and long-term health. The second section presents a review of nutrition education programs that have attempted to change these behaviors, a model for health promotion that is specific to young people's dietary behaviors, and a list of future research needs in this area. This review, then, not only provides evidence for the importance of the *Healthy People 2000* objectives but also provides direction on how they might best be achieved.

The Importance of Healthy Dietary Behaviors in Youth

Impact on Short-Term and Long-Term Health

Diet is critical to health, affecting both short-term and long-term health. During childhood and adolescence, good nutrition and dietary behaviors are important to achieve full growth potential, to promote health and well-being, and to reduce risk of chronic diseases in adulthood.

Children require sufficient energy, protein, and other nutrients for growth as well as maintenance of body functions. Growth continues at a steady rate during childhood but accelerates dramatically during adolescence, creating significant increases in calories and nutrient intake needs to support the rapid growth rate and increase in lean body mass and body size (Story, 1992). During puberty, adolescents achieve the final 15% to 20% of linear height, gain 50% of their adult body weight, and accumulate up to 40% of skeletal mass (Gong & Heald, 1994). Inadequate intake of protein, energy, or certain vitamins and minerals will be reflected in slow growth rates, delayed sexual maturation, inadequate mineralization of bones, and low body reserves of micronutrients (Story, 1992; DHHS, 1988).

In addition to the impact on growth and development, children's diets are important to ensure overall health and well-being. Dietary practices affect young people's risk for a number of immediate health problems, including iron deficiency, obesity, eating disorders, undernutrition, and dental caries (Story, 1992; DHHS, 1988). Inadequate nutrition also lowers resistance to infectious diseases and may adversely affect the ability to function at peak mental and physical ability (DHHS, 1988). Recent research provides evidence that undernutrition during any period of childhood can have detrimental effects on the cognitive development of children, affecting concentration, learning, and academic achievement (Center on Hunger, Poverty, and Nutrition Policy, 1995). Undernutrition may occur among low-income children experiencing hunger and among food-restricting dieters. Short-term studies looking at the relationship between omitting breakfast and cognitive performance have reported that inadequate nutrition compromises learning (Pollitt, 1995; Simeon & Grantham-McGregor, 1989). For example, Pollitt found that well-nourished children ages 9 to 11 who skipped breakfast had higher rates of inaccurate responses to problem solving. Furthermore, low-income elementary school students who participated in the School Breakfast Program showed greater improvements in standardized test scores and had reduced rates of tardiness and absences compared with children who qualified for the program but did not participate (Meyers, Sampson, Weitzman, Rogers, & Kayne, 1989).

There is also concern about long-term health because certain dietary patterns, developed in childhood and carried into adulthood, may in combination with other behavioral, genetic, or environmental factors result in an increased risk for chronic diseases, such as heart disease, osteoporosis, and some types of cancer later in life. Some of the physiological processes that lead to diet-related chronic diseases have their onset during childhood. For example, a variety of studies have indicated that the process of atherosclerosis begins in childhood (Moller, Taubert, Allen, Clark, & Lauer, 1994; DHHS, 1991b). Fatty streaks have been found in children as young as 3 and have occurred in a progressively greater proportion of children with increasing age. Intimal plaques have been found in adolescents (Moller et al., 1994).

Four of the ten leading causes of death in adults are diet-related chronic diseases: coronary heart disease, certain cancers, strokes, and diabetes (DHHS, 1988). Poor diet and sedentary activity patterns together account for at least 300,000 adult deaths each year in the United States and are second only to tobacco use as the major behavioral contributors to death (McGinnis & Foege, 1993). Like tobacco use, eating behaviors are modifiable risk factors that begin early in life. These behaviors of are particular concern because they appear to track, that is, behavior patterns learned in childhood are predictive of behaviors and risk factors later in life (discussed in more detail below). Childhood and adolescence, then, offer opportunities to influence the establishment of healthful lifelong eating patterns. Preventing or slowing chronic disease processes in childhood and adolescence could extend the years of healthy life for many Americans (DHHS, 1991b).

Tracking and Covariation of Risk Factors and Eating Behaviors

Studies have shown that physiologic risk factors for cardiovascular disease (elevated cholesterol levels and obesity) and behavioral risk factors (diets high in total fat and saturated fat and low physical activity levels) are widely prevalent among children and adolescents (Moller et al., 1994; Perry, Kelder, & Klepp, 1994b; DHHS, 1988, 1991b). There is also evidence that behavioral risk factors for cardiovascular disease and obesity track from childhood to adulthood. Kelder, Perry, Klepp, and Lytle (1994) examined the tracking of food choices and physical activity during a 6-year period for students beginning in the 6th grade and continuing through 12th grade. A clear pattern of tracking was observed; in the 6th grade, those in the highest quintile for healthy food choices or hours of exercise a week largely remained in that quintile, and the lowest remained low. This suggests that the development of healthy dietary patterns during childhood may be particularly important in the prevention of diet-related chronic diseases later in life.

Several studies have related childhood cholesterol levels to later young adult levels. Of the six major studies tracking cardiovascular disease physiological risk factors in childhood—the Muscatine Study (Lauer, Lee, & Clarke, 1988), the Bogalusa Heart Study (Freedman, Shear, Srinivasan, Webber, & Berenson, 1985), the Cincinnati Study (Laskarezewski et al., 1979), the Cittadella Study (Pagman et al., 1982), the Beaver County Study (Orchard, Donahue, Kuller, Hodge, & Drash, 1983) and the Cardiovascular Risk in Young Finns Study (Porkka, Viikari, & Akerblom, 1991)—all indicated that total cholesterol and low- and high-density lipoprotein cholesterol measurements in childhood and adolescence were predictive of adult values. This has implications for dietary behaviors in youth because dietary fat intake is associated with cholesterol measurements, and primary prevention of elevated cholesterol levels may require lower-fat dietary patterns among young people.

Tracking of weight and body mass index from childhood into the adult years is also evident, with many overweight children becoming overweight adults. Clarke and Lauer (1993) found that from 48% to 75% of children in the upper quintile of body mass index ranked again in the upper quintiles as adults. The risk of overweight children becoming overweight adults increases with age. Serdula and colleagues (1993) reviewed 16 studies on the relationship between obesity in childhood and in adulthood and found that although 26% to 41% of obese preschool children became obese as adults, 42% to 62% of obese school-age children were obese as adults. Stunkard and Burt (1967) reported that the odds against obese 13-year-olds becoming normal-weight adults were 4:1; if they had not reduced their weight by the end of adolescence, the odds increased to 28:1.

In addition, eating behaviors do not occur in isolation from other health behaviors among children and adolescents. During the past decade, a number of studies have looked at the interrelationship (also referred to as covariation or clustering) between health behaviors among adolescents. Some of these have examined unhealthy eating behaviors, dieting, or unsafe weight loss methods and their association to other health behaviors (French, Story, Downes, Resnick, & Blum, 1995; Lytle, Kelder, Perry, & Klepp, 1995; Lytle & Roski, in press; Neumark-Sztainer, Story, & French, 1996). Lytle and Roski recently reviewed nine studies on the covariance or clustering of health behaviors in adolescents that included a measure of eating behavior. Of the nine studies, seven showed modest associations between unhealthy eating and other health-compromising behaviors. In general, the highest correlations were observed between lack of exercise and poor diet. Lytle et al. (1995) examined the relationships between a food choice score, an activity score, and smoking prevalence in a cohort of students as they moved from 6th to 12th grade. After the 8th grade, students who reported making fewer healthy food choices also had lower physical activity patterns and were more likely to smoke cigarettes.

The results from these studies on physiologic risk factors, obesity, and dietary behaviors indicate a consistent pattern of tracking from childhood and adolescence into adulthood. In addition, poor eating patterns are correlated with other health-compromising behaviors that are of concern. These data suggest that eating behaviors consolidate prior to and during adolescence and place some individuals at risk for chronic diseases in adulthood. Clearly, programs aimed at establishing healthy dietary practices, the prevention of obesity, and the primary prevention of other chronic diseases should be implemented in childhood and adolescence. In particular, school health programs need to promote the development of a healthy lifestyle across multiple, related behaviors.

Current Dietary Intakes, Eating Patterns, and Nutrition Concerns of Youth

As the 20th century draws to a close, it is of interest to review the dietary behaviors of youth in the United States. What are U.S. children eating? Are the problems of unhealthy diet outlined above evident among youth in the United States or primarily among small subgroups?

The nutritional problems of children and adolescents have changed drastically during the past century. With the exception of iron deficiency, overt nutrient deficiencies are not public health problems today as they commonly were earlier in this century and as recently as the 1940s (DHHS, 1988). As problems of nutrient deficiency diseases and undernutrition have diminished, they have been replaced by public health problems of dietary excesses and imbalances.

National surveys show that most children do not consume a diet that meets the USDA's (1995) *Dietary Guidelines for Americans* (Kennedy & Goldberg, 1995; McDowel et al., 1994). Dietary excesses of total fat, saturated fat, and sodium are common among youth and are found in all income groups, racial/ethnic groups, and both sexes (McDowel et al., 1994). Although the level of total fat and saturated fat in the diets of all Americans has been declining since the early 1980s, current average intakes for children and adolescents (33% to 34% of calories from fat and 12% of calories from saturated fat) still exceed the recommendations of 30% of calories from fat and less than 10% of calories from saturated fat. In the Third National Health and Nutrition Examination Survey (NHANES III) data, school-age children and adolescents were more likely than other age groups to exceed the recommendations for fat and saturated fat (Lewis, Crane, Moore, & Hubbard, 1994). In the 1989-1991 USDA Continuing Survey of Food Intake by Individuals (CSFII), more than 90% of teenage boys exceeded the recommendations for total fat, saturated fat, and sodium (2,400 mg sodium/day; Kennedy & Goldberg, 1995). Dietary cholesterol has declined steadily across all age groups, in part because of a decline in egg consumption during the past 20 years. Now, almost 90% of children meet the dietary recommendation for cholesterol (300 mg cholesterol/day).

Dietary fiber is also low in the diets of many children and adolescents. Compared with current dietary intakes, the new fiber recommendations (age of child plus 5 grams per day for youth ages 2-18) would require a 25% to 50% increase in fiber consumption for preadolescents and a 70% to 100% increase for many adolescents (Williams, 1995). One reason for the low fiber intake is the low consumption of fruits and vegetables. Of the five major food groups, children are most likely to have an inappropriate number of servings from the fruit and vegetable group (Kennedy & Goldberg, 1995). In the national Youth Risk Behavior Surveillance Survey, 60% of adolescents reported eating no vegetables, and 40% ate no fruit on the day preceding the survey (Kann et al., 1995).

Nationally representative surveys have shown that the average intake of protein and many vitamins and minerals meets or exceeds the recommended dietary allowances (Alaimo et al., 1994; Kennedy & Goldberg, 1995). Exceptions include vitamins B_6, folate, A, and E and the minerals zinc, calcium, and iron (for adolescent girls). Given the importance of calcium and bone health in the potential prevention of osteoporosis, it is of concern that calcium intake of adolescent girls starts to decline at puberty, the time of maximal requirements. Females 12 to 19 years consume an average of only 68% of the recommended dietary allowance for calcium, making it unlikely that many will reach their full genetic potential for bone mass development (Kennedy & Goldberg, 1995).

Other nutrition-related concerns include overweight, unsafe weight-loss methods, eating disorders, low physical activity levels, and hypercholesterolemia among children and adolescents. Overweight is a major public health problem in the United States and has increased significantly in the past 30 years among children and adults. The NHANES III data indicated that 22% of children and adolescents (ages 6-18) were overweight, on the basis of a body mass index greater than the 85th percentile (Troiana, Flegal, Kuczmarski, Campbell, & Johnson, 1995). The prevalence of eating disorders ranges from 1% to 5% among adolescent girls and is associated with serious morbidities (DHHS, 1988). Although difficult to measure and document, hunger and insufficient food resources are of concern among youth in low-income families.

In addition to changes in dietary intakes, dramatic changes have also occurred in children's and adolescents' eating patterns during the past two decades. Today, youth are eating more frequently throughout the day, obtaining a greater proportion of their energy and nutrient intake from snacks, and eating more meals away from home (Kennedy & Goldberg, 1995). According to the National Adolescent Student Health Survey, almost 90% of adolescents ate at least one snack the previous day, with one fourth eating four or more snacks. Almost two thirds of these snacks were categorized as high-fat or high-sugar foods (chips, soda, candy, ice cream, and cake; American School Health Association, 1988).

In addition, almost half of the family food expenditures (46%) are for food and beverages served outside the home, with 34% of the total food dollar spent on fast foods. Fast-food restaurants capture 83% of restaurant visits by young people under 18 years of age (DHHS, 1991a). Away-from-home eating is associated with higher calorie, fat, and saturated fat intake than at-home eating (Troiana et al., 1995). Foods most often ordered for children under age 6 at restaurants include soft drinks, hamburgers, cheeseburgers, french fries, pizza, and ice cream—foods that tend to be high in saturated fatty acids, total fat, cholesterol, and calories. These same foods plus fried chicken are among the items 6- to 17-year-olds are most likely to order (DHHS, 1991a). A shift toward eating more meals out has also contributed to decreased milk intake because milk is consumed most often at home. Only 7% of adolescents order milk in a fast-food restaurant (National Dairy Council, 1995).

Recommendations for Healthy Eating

The most recent *Dietary Guidelines for Americans* (USDA, 1995) developed by the USDA and DHHS provide a framework for healthful diets for all healthy Americans 2 years of age and older and include the following seven recommendations:

1. Eat a variety of foods.
2. Balance the food you eat with physical activity—maintain or improve your weight.

3. Choose a diet with plenty of grain products, vegetables, and fruits.
4. Choose a diet low in fat, saturated fat, and cholesterol.
5. Choose a diet moderate in sugars.
6. Choose a diet moderate in salt and sodium.
7. If you drink alcoholic beverages, do so in moderation (intended for adults only). (pp. 1-43)

These guidelines focus on the overall modifications that are needed to reduce the risk of diet-related chronic diseases. *The Food Guide Pyramid* (USDA, 1992), designed to help Americans choose foods consistent with the *Dietary Guidelines for Americans,* provides recommendations for daily servings of food (see Figure 8.1).

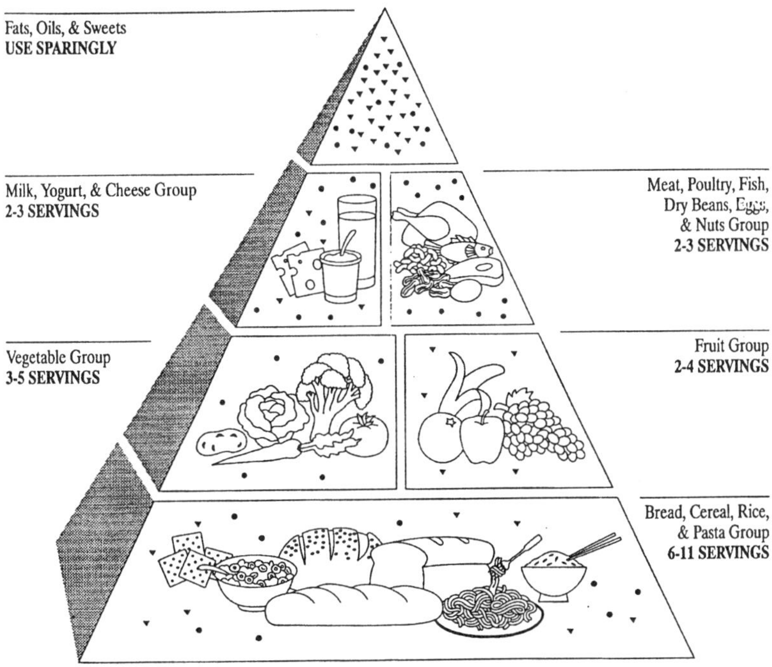

Figure 8.1. Food Guide Pyramid: A Guide to Daily Food Choices
SOURCE: U.S. Department of Agriculture (1992).

The number of servings in each food group is expressed as a range and depends on several factors including growth status, age, gender, body size, and activity level. The lower number of servings in each food group is the minimum needed, whereas adolescents who are physically active require the larger number of servings from each group. The pyramid encourages the three basic principles of a healthful diet—variety, balance, and moderation—and is based on the concept of proportionality, that is, eating more foods from the groups at the base of the pyramid. This is best visualized by imagining a dinner plate divided into four sections: Three sections are filled with vegetables, fruits, and grains, and the fourth with a lower-fat choice from the meat/bean group. A glass of milk is added to complete the five major food groups.

Promoting Healthy Eating Behaviors Among Children and Adolescents

Given the immediate and potential health risks from poor dietary behaviors, nutrition education clearly needs as its primary goal to affect the eating behaviors of children and adolescents. Likewise, positive dietary behaviors need to be sustained, given the evidence of tracking of health behaviors in adolescence (Kelder et al., 1994), and to become part of a healthy lifestyle, given the evidence for the covariation of health behaviors among adolescents (Lytle, Kelder, Perry, & Klepp, 1995; Lytle & Roski, in press). The major outcomes of intervention should be the attainment of behavior patterns consistent with the *Dietary Guidelines* (USDA, 1995). Therefore, population-based and communitywide efforts that encourage healthful dietary behaviors among all children and adolescents are seen as optimal, with communities of color and those of lower socioeconomic status at greatest need and therefore of highest priority (Cook & Martin, 1995; Ervin & Reed, 1993; Kennedy & Goldberg, 1995; DHHS, 1988, 1995a).

The most traditional way to influence children's eating behaviors has been through nutrition education. A survey of 1,000 schools across the country showed that 99% of public schools offered nutrition education somewhere within the curriculum (U.S. Department of Education, 1996). For kindergarten through eighth grade, half or more of all schools had district or state requirements for nutrition education. Nutrition education has been evolving during the last several decades not only to include didactic, knowledge-based nutrition information but also to include, and ideally emphasize, interventions that target the personal, socioenvironmental, and behavioral factors that influence the adoption and maintenance of eating behaviors in youth.

To date, nutrition education has used an information dissemination model emphasizing cognitive information based on nutrition science. Functions of the nutrients, food sources of nutrients, and diet and disease connections (often focusing on rarely occurring deficiency diseases such as scurvy or pellagra) have predominated the content. This knowledge-based model is often referred to as the Knowledge, Attitude, Behavior (KAB) model, which assumes that increasing cognitive knowledge about nutrition will result in positive attitudes toward choosing a healthful diet, which will eventually result in the behavior of choosing a healthful diet (Contento et al., 1995; Lytle-Trenkner & Kelder, 1991). Research findings indicate that the KAB model is effective in increasing students' knowledge of nutrition facts but unsuccessful in influencing students to choose healthful diets.

Since the mid-1980s, nutrition education has been infused with influences from the behavioral sciences. The application of behavior change theory and behaviorally based approaches to nutrition education have been tested and evaluated. Behaviorally based programs target behavior change directly through the provision of increased opportunities to try healthful foods, environmental support for healthful eating behaviors, and a variety of behavior change strategies to model, reinforce, and provide incentives for making healthful choices. Nutrition education programs that focus on behavior change, rather than knowledge acquisition, have had some solid successes in improving the diets and food choices of children.

Several comprehensive reviews of nutrition education with young people have recently been undertaken, providing insights to help guide future directions. Lytle-Trenkner and colleagues conducted reviews of school-based nutrition education programs and school food service interventions from the 1980s (Lytle, Kelder, & Snyder, 1993; Lytle-Trenkner & Kelder, 1991). Contento, Manning, and Shannon (1992) published a review with conclusions that were consistent with most of those made by Lytle-Trenkner and Kelder. In 1995, Lytle and Achterberg published conclusions based on a review of 43 articles including in-school and out-of-school nutrition programs. Contento et al. (1995) expanded that review to include programs for preschool children. Articles were included in the above reviews if they were published since 1980 and were based in the United States. Because the last review has only recently been published, this section will provide a summary of these extensive reviews (Contento et al., 1995; Contento et al., 1992; Lytle & Achterberg, 1995; Lytle et al., 1993; Lytle-Trenkner & Kelder, 1991). The reader is encouraged to read these reviews for greater detail on specific studies.

Preschool Studies

Nutrition programs for preschool children most typically occur because of federally administered programs, such as the Special Supplemental Program for the Women, Infants, and Children (WIC) program and Head Start, and state or local day care settings and preschool programs. State and local programs often rely on materials and information provided by the Nutrition Education and Training (NET) program. WIC programs, administered by USDA, provide food supplements, health services, and nutrition education to pregnant and postpartum women, infants, and young children. The WIC program has been shown to be effective in reducing health risks of pregnant women, infants, and young children through the provision of foods and other health services (Armotrading, Probart, & Jackson, 1992; Batten, Hirshman, & Thomas, 1990; Kennedy & Gershoff, 1982; Kotelchuck, Schwarz, Anderka, & Finison, 1984; Metcoff et al., 1985). The unique benefits of the nutrition education component of WIC have not been studied in isolation from the other WIC services.

Likewise, the Head Start program, administered by USDA, also has been shown to have a positive effect on the nutritional status of preschool children through reimbursed meals and supplements provided to children of low-income families qualifying for the program. Some evaluations have been conducted to ascertain the effectiveness of the nutrition education component of Head Start and were included in the following literature review. The reader is referred to Byrd-Bredbenner, Marecic, and Bernstein (1993) for a more in-depth discussion of the Head Start program. NET was established by Congress in 1977 to teach children, prekindergarten through 12th grade, the value of a nutritionally balanced diet through positive lunchroom experiences and through classroom curricular activities. The literature reviews referred to in the following section includes some nutrition programs that were funded by NET.

A review of the literature by Contento et al. (1995) shows that although many nutrition education programs and activities have been developed for preschool children (most under the auspices of WIC, Head Start, or the NET program), few have undergone a rigorous evaluation assessing their effectiveness. Contento and colleagues identified 23 published studies of nutrition education programs for preschool children and divided the discussion of the studies into those using a knowledge-based approach and those using a behaviorally based approach. They conclude that the KAB model was effective in increasing nutrition-related knowledge but had minimal impact on attitudes and behaviors. A behaviorally focused approach, targeting specific eating behaviors (such as choosing fruits and vegetables and choosing low-fat milk rather than whole milk), has been shown to increase food preferences. Studies with young children indicate that increased exposure to healthful foods (Birch, McPhee, Shoba, Pirok, & Steinberg, 1987; Sullivan & Birch, 1990), positive role models who taste and enjoy healthful foods (Birch, 1980), and the tone of the social interaction surrounding eating experiences (Birch, Zimmerman, & Hind, 1980) have been positive influences for healthful eating practices for young children. Using foods as incentives or rewards, however, does not result in an increase in the preferred behavior (Birch, Marlin, & Rotter, 1984). In addition, Contento et al. (1995) found that involving families with interactive home-based programs and providing hands-on food and activity-based lessons were more likely to result in positive behavior change, stressing the importance of developmentally appropriate learning activities and materials.

To summarize, nutrition programs for young children should concentrate on increasing children's exposure to healthful food through increased opportunity to taste, smell, touch, and prepare foods. Family involvement and support for the development of positive attitudes toward eating, providing opportunities to try new foods, and providing easy access to healthful food choices are important in influencing eating behaviors for this age group.

Community-Based Programs

A limited number of studies target preschool or school-age children in settings other than school, preschool, or day care. Nader et al. (1989), Baranowski et al. (1990), and Wagner, Winett, and Walbert-Rankin (1992) developed programs for families with a goal of positively influencing children's nutrition-related behaviors and attitudes. In the Nader et al. and Baranowski et al. programs, parents and their children were invited to attend nutrition education programs in a community setting. Both studies focused on cardiovascular disease risk reduction (i.e., consumption of low-fat and low-sodium diets) and involved evening sessions. The Nader et al. study showed significant changes in behavioral and physiologic outcomes in the children. Baranowski et al. reported favorable effects for the consumption of high-fat and high-sodium foods but mixed results on other behavioral and psychosocial measures. Low participation rates and attrition were problems in both community-based studies.

Wagner et al. (1992) studied the effectiveness of a grocery store-based program using an interactive computer intervention to educate families and to guide food-purchasing decisions targeting recommendations made by the National Cancer Institute. Results indicate that the intervention had some positive effects for influencing healthful snack preference and entrée choice and for increased knowledge of children.

Although research has been published regarding nutrition education in after-school settings (Connor et al., 1986) and during summer camp experiences (Anliker, Drake, Pacholski, & Litle, 1993) for school-age children, the programs and outcome measures were knowledge based and did not report on behavioral change. After-school programs have a disadvantage in that children prefer less structured activities after school, and intact groups of children may not be available for sequential instruction. Lytle and Achterberg (1995) suggested that if nutrition programming is to be used in after-school settings, activities should include individual learning modules; nutrition activities using computer-interactive programs may be ideal.

School-Based Studies

The majority of studies examining the effectiveness of nutrition education programs on children's eating behaviors and nutrition-related health outcomes have occurred in schools. Schools are a logical place to intervene on children's nutrition practices because the vast majority of children attend school and spend 6 to 8 hours of each weekday in school. Schools provide opportunities for practicing healthful eating behaviors because more than half of students eat one meal in school, and as many as 10% of students eat two meals in school (Dwyer, 1995). In addition, schools are staffed with professionals trained in teaching children.

School-based nutrition education programs may take several forms. Nutrition education programs may (a) stand alone as isolated nutrition education units taught at the classroom level with no tie-in to other school nutrition programs (nutrition curricula); (b) include some family-based activities to link classroom content with family; (c) consist of lessons integrated into other subject areas (i.e., using nutrition-related examples in math or social science class); (d) include planned linkages between what is taught in the classroom and nutrition education activities in the school cafeteria (i.e., school cafeteria promotions for fresh fruits and vegetables occurring simultaneously with a classroom unit on increasing fruit and vegetable consumption; or (e) be part of an overall comprehensive school health program that links nutrition with other health curricula and health services in the school and includes nutrition concerns in developing a school policy to promote a healthful school environment.

The content of school-based nutrition education programs also includes a myriad of options. In 1995, the U.S. Department of Education (1996) conducted a survey of 1,000 principals in the United States to determine what topics were covered in nutrition education in their schools. Topics indicated by 90% or more of the schools participating in the survey included relationships between diet and health, finding and choosing healthy foods, nutrients and their food sources, the dietary guidelines and goals, and reading food labels. Data obtained in this survey indicate that the KAB approach to nutrition education is still quite prevalent. This emphasis on relationships between diet, health, nutrients, and food sources suggests that abstract nutrition science, rather than behavioral skills, is being taught. Even curricula covering the dietary guidelines may emphasize knowledge acquisition, rather than behavior change, if the lesson focuses on what the dietary guidelines are rather than how to use them to guide food choices.

Literature reviews of nutrition programs have shown that nutrition education in schools can be effective in improving aspects of children's eating behaviors and, in some cases, can positively affect physiological outcomes such as serum cholesterol (Contento et al., 1995; Contento et al., 1992; Lytle & Achterberg, 1995; Lytle-Trenkner & Kelder, 1991). In their review of United States-based research, Lytle and Achterberg identified six elements of school nutrition programs that are critical for creating eating behavior change:

1. Programs should be behaviorally based and theory driven.
2. Family involvement should be incorporated into programs for younger children.
3. Programs for middle to senior high school students should include self-assessment of eating patterns.
4. Behavior change programs should include intervening in the school environment.
5. Behavior change programs should include intervening in the larger community.
6. Programs should include intensive instruction or intervention time.

These six elements suggest that nutrition education programs need to be guided by behavioral theories, include components that link an intensive classroom curriculum to changes in school food service, and include opportunities for healthy eating at home and in the community. Contento et al. (1995) echo those same elements as essential in effective nutrition programs.

The Centers for Disease Control and Prevention (CDC, 1996) recently published "Guidelines for School Health Programs to Promote Healthy Eating," providing a template for the development of comprehensive school nutrition programs to be used by school districts, nutrition educators, and health professionals working with school-based nutrition programs. Seven recommendations have been made (Table 8.2) that incorporate what has been learned about effective nutrition programs. These recommendations rein-

Table 8.2 Recommendations for School Health Programs Promoting Healthy Eating

1. Adopt a coordinated school nutrition policy that promotes healthy eating through classroom lessons and a supportive school environment.
2. Implement nutrition education from preschool through secondary school as part of a sequential, comprehensive school health education curriculum designed to help students adopt healthy eating behaviors.
3. Provide nutrition education through developmentally appropriate, culturally relevant, fun, participatory activities that involve social learning strategies.
4. Coordinate school food service with other components of the comprehensive school health program to reinforce messages on healthy eating.
5. Provide staff involved in nutrition education with adequate preservice and ongoing in-service training that focuses on teaching strategies for behavioral change.
6. Involve family members and the community in supporting and reinforcing nutrition education.
7. Regularly evaluate the effectiveness of the school health program in promoting healthy eating, and change the program as appropriate to increase its effectiveness.

SOURCE: Centers for Disease Control and Prevention (1996).

force the need for (a) environmental support that includes a school policy encouraging healthful options in the school, reinforcement and modeling of healthy food-related behaviors, and school and district commitment to provide adequate training and time for nutrition programming; (b) a behaviorally based nutrition curriculum that is part of a comprehensive school health program and is of adequate duration to impact behavior; and (c) the recognition of the importance of school, family, and community linkages and partnering.

To date, a comprehensive school nutrition program reflecting all the recommendations made and spanning children's entire school career has not been evaluated for effectiveness, with results published in the peer review literature. The CDC recommendations have been based on effective programs that have incorporated pieces of a comprehensive nutrition program. The Class of 1989 study and the Child and Adolescent Trial for Cardiovascular Health (CATCH) included many of the elements identified as essential for an effective nutrition education program and thereby serve as examples of what can be accomplished in schools to change eating behaviors of youth.

The Class of 1989 Study

The Class of 1989 study was part of the Minnesota Heart Health Program (MHHP; Blackburn et al., 1984), focusing on adolescent cardiovascular risk reduction through school and communitywide programs (Perry, Klepp, & Sillers, 1989). Two of the six MHHP communities participated in an evaluation of adolescent school-based programs, in combination with communitywide programs, to affect eating, physical activity, and smoking behaviors in a cohort of youth as they progressed from 6th through 12th grade. The Class of 1989 study used behaviorally based curricula and social learning theory to guide intervention strategies (Perry & Jessor, 1985). Nutrition-related lessons were linked to other health content areas, particularly smoking prevention and physical activity. These linkages allowed skills and knowledge related to practicing healthy lifestyles to be reinforced and emphasized across content areas. In addition, students in Class of 1989 schools were exposed to communitywide messages that affected social and cultural norms about heart healthful behaviors and environmental changes through restaurant and grocery store programs. Likewise, the students' parents and teachers were receiving the same communitywide messages as well as communitywide screening for cardiovascular risk factors and adult-centered risk factor education programs on smoking cessation, physical activity, and healthy eating patterns and interventions.

The school-based nutrition interventions occurred in 6th grade, through a one-session program designed to promote packing and eating a healthful school lunch (the Lunch Bag program) and in the 10th grade through a 10-session curriculum (Slice of Life). Slice of Life used self-assessment, modeling, experiential activities, goal setting, and peer leadership to influence healthful eating and physical activity. Physical activity interventions were linked with the nutrition-related activities in the classroom curriculum (Kelder, Perry, & Klepp, 1993; Perry et al., 1987).

As part of the evaluation, more than 1,000 students in the reference and intervention communities completed surveys for 7 consecutive school years, from their 6th through 12th grades

(1983-1989). Results from the Class of 1989 study indicate that those students exposed to the community and school-based intervention, emphasizing behaviorally based messages with school and community linkages, reported healthier food choices as compared with students in the reference community in all but a few years of the 7-year study (Kelder, Perry, Lytle, & Klepp, 1995). Likewise, students in the intervention group reported less frequently adding salt to foods as compared with students in the reference community. In addition, students in the intervention community had lower smoking rates and more positive physical activity measures compared with same-age students in the reference community (Kelder et al., 1993; Perry, Kelder, Murray, & Klepp, 1992). The outcomes from the Class of 1989 study are important because they show that behavioral health education in schools that is implemented during multiple school years and with complementary community programs can positively affect cardiovascular-related health behaviors of adolescents in the community (Perry, Kelder, & Klepp, 1994a). Generalizability of the Class of 1989 study is limited because the population was primarily Caucasian and from the north-central United States.

The Child and Adolescent Trial for Cardiovascular Health

CATCH was the largest multicenter field trial ever funded by the National Heart, Lung, and Blood Institute to evaluate school and family interventions to reduce cardiovascular risk factors in elementary school children (Luepker et al., 1996; Perry, Parcel, et al., 1992; Perry et al., 1990). More than 5,100 children from four states and 96 schools, including Caucasian, African American, and Hispanic children, participated in CATCH from their 3rd- through 5th-grade school years. The intervention was based on social learning theory with a strong behavioral emphasis. The intervention included a school environment component, 3 years of sequential, classroom-based curricula, and family involvement. The school environmental interventions included (a) modification of the school food service to reduce fat and sodium in foods offered through the school breakfast and lunch programs, (b) modification of physical activity classes to increase students' level of moderate to vigorous physical activity during gym class, and (c) promotion of school policy to eliminate tobacco use on the school premises.

The classroom curricula included 12 to 16 sessions in third through fifth grade. Behaviors targeted in the curricula included choosing lower-fat and lower-sodium foods, choosing to engage in regular physical activity, and making the decision not to start smoking. A link was made to families through take-home activity packets completed by parent and child that complemented and expanded the classroom-based lessons. In addition, families were invited to attend a family fun night at the end of the CATCH unit in the third and fourth grades. These family fun nights included games, activities, healthful snacks, and an aerobic dance routine performed by the students.

CATCH was evaluated through a large battery of physiological, behavioral, and psychosocial measures assessing change at both the school and individual level (Luepker et al., 1996) from baseline (fall 1991), when the students were in the third grade, to follow-up (spring 1994), when the students were in the fifth grade. After three school years, intervention schools as compared with control schools had significantly reduced the fat and saturated fat content of school meals (Osganian et al., 1996) and had increased the level of moderate to vigorous physical activity and vigorous physical activity during physical education class (Luepker et al., 1996). In addition, at the student level, students in the intervention schools were consuming diets lower in total fat and saturated fat without compromising energy intake or other vitamin or mineral intake (Luepker et al., 1996; Lytle et al., 1996). The majority of the scales assessing psychosocial constructs, including knowledge, food choice, and perceived social norms, showed significant gains in the intervention group as compared with the control group (Edmundson et al., 1996). Assessment of physiological measures related to cardiovascular disease (e.g., total blood cholesterol, systolic and diastolic blood pressure, and body mass index) did not show intervention effects (Luepker et al., 1996; Webber et al., 1996).

The CATCH trial was important in showing that school-based programs involving school food service, classroom curriculum, family programs, and physical education are feasible to implement in most U.S. schools. In addition, the trial showed that the school environment could be modified without undue financial or resource hardship, that children could modify their health-related behaviors and psychosocial factors, and that the interventions tested were generalizable across four different regional areas and across children from varied ethnic backgrounds. The elements lacking in CATCH were links to the broader community and integration within a comprehensive school health program spanning the children's school years.

Long-Term Outcomes

Studies looking at the long-term effects of youth-centered nutrition programs and interventions are rare. Little is known regarding how youth exposed to any type of nutrition program use information and acquired skills to make food choices during their adult lives. Studies considering the long-term effects, even during students' school years, indicate that the effects of successful interventions tend to dissipate through time. One-shot nutrition education units, even if they are behaviorally based and experiential, are not sufficient for a lifetime of eating-related decisions, skills, and healthful habits. Certainly, implementation of the CDC (1996) guidelines, stressing a comprehensive school health program, including a lifestyle-related message across all health content areas presented throughout children's schooling and providing an environment that models and reinforces healthful life choices, would maximize the potential for outcomes of nutrition programs.

A Conceptual Model for Child and Adolescent Eating Behavior

A conceptual model or theory is useful in understanding the mutable and immutable variables that influence eating behaviors, affect change, and lead to the solidification of healthful lifestyle habits. One of the important criteria for effective nutrition programming is the use of a behavioral model as a guide. The majority of nutrition education programs that have been successful in achieving behavior change or health outcomes have used social learning theory as the guiding conceptual model (Bandura, 1977, 1986; Baranowski, Perry, & Parcel, 1996).

Social learning theory has identified environmental, personal, and behavioral factors that are predictive of a given behavior (Bandura, 1977) and have the potential for behavior change (Baranowski et al., 1997). To use social learning theory, the specific factors that significantly influence eating behaviors among youth need to be identified. Those factors that are also amenable to intervention serve as the primary targets for intervention (Baranowski et al., 1997; Perry, Lytle, & Kelder, 1994). Environmental factors are those aspects of the environment that support, permit, encourage, or discourage engagement in a particular behavior. They include food availability, parenting style and practices, family and peer influences, influential role models, cultural and social norms, social support, and specific opportunities. Personal factors are personality dispositions, cognitions, and affective factors that increase or decrease the likelihood of an individual engaging in a given behavior, such as personal attitudes and beliefs, self-efficacy and control, knowledge, functional meanings of food, and perceived body image. Behavioral factors affect behavior directly and include a person's behavior repertoire, behavioral intentions, reinforcements, skills, and coping responses. To successfully change eating patterns to improve nutritional health of youth, interventions should be aimed at modification of factors at each of the three levels.

An overall model for improving eating behavior of youth is shown in Figure 8.2. The goal of promoting healthy eating behavior is to achieve both short- and long-term health objectives. These health outcomes are, in part, dependent on the adoption of specific dietary behaviors, and their maintenance throughout life, that are suggested by the *Dietary Guidelines* (USDA, 1995). Changes in these dietary behaviors should be the outcomes sought and measured in nutrition education efforts. To make changes in these behaviors, specific psychosocial factors, as discussed above, need to be targeted. These are environmental, personal, and behavioral factors that have been suggested by social learning theory (Baranowski et al., 1997) and, to some extent, by research on the etiology of eating behavior (Perry et al., 1994b), although considerably more research is needed on the latter. How these psychosocial factors manifest must be evaluated for the specific intervention group prior to program development. For example, potent role models for elementary age children clearly include parents; by junior high and high school, peers rival parents in importance. Likewise, access to recommended foods may be difficult for children of low-income families and needs to be considered in program development. Finally, the type of intervention and its components

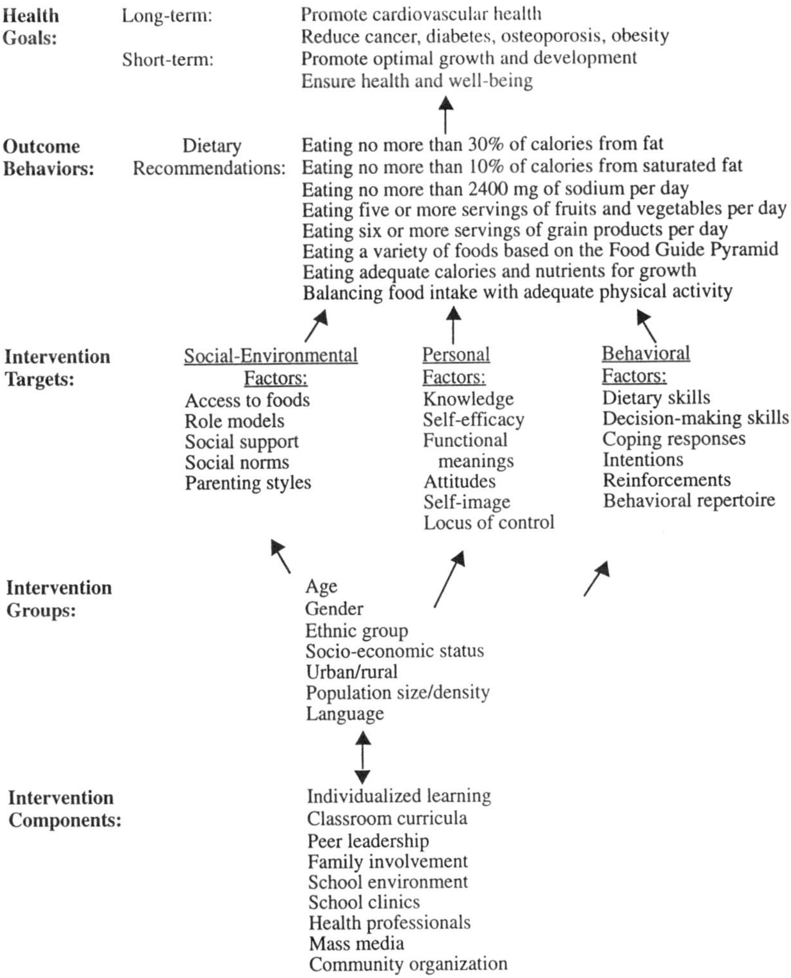

Figure 8.2. Promoting Healthy Dietary Behaviors Among Children and Adolescents: A Conceptual Model

can be addressed on the basis of what is most appropriate for the specific intervention group, what is feasible economically and politically, and what will be most influential in changing the targeted psychosocial factors. From the outcomes of intervention programs to date, it appears that multicomponent, multiyear programs are necessary for demonstrable change. Using this model, programs to change eating behaviors among young people can be constructed, using appropriate end points, targeting key factors, and considering the special needs and opportunities of the intervention group.

Future Directions

If the linkages between psychosocial factors, which are the targets of intervention, and eating behaviors are examined, several gaps in knowledge and research are noteworthy. The following research directions, based on our conceptual model, examine these linkages and may provide new directions to improve programs to change eating behaviors among youth.

Social and environmental factors greatly affect food and eating-related behaviors. Much of the advancement in nutrition education programs during the past two decades has been in acknowledging the importance of the environment in influencing food choices and then intervening in this area. More needs to be done, however. The teaching of media literacy, which has been used in drug abuse prevention efforts (Perry & Kelder, 1992), could be applied to nutrition education. Research shows that children are a targeted market segment for food manufacturers and food distributors. Kotz and Story (1994) analyzed television advertisements aired on Saturday morning (prime-time viewing for young children) and found that more than half the advertisements were for foods that would fit into the food guide pyramid under fats, oils, and sweets. None of the advertisements were for fruits and vegetables. The important role of children as consumers is also evident in the increase in direct advertising in schools in recent years. A study by Consumers Union Education Services (1995) found that advertising for soft drinks, fast-food restaurants, candy, and chips is ubiquitous in the school environment. Children cannot even escape television advertisements in schools. *Channel 1,* a daily news program broadcast to millions of students in grades 6 through 12, includes two minutes of paid commercials of each 12-minute segment. These advertisements are for products that include candy bars, snack chips, and soda pop (Story & Neumark-Sztainer, 1996). Nutrition education needs to spend more time educating children and adolescents on how they are influenced by the media so that they can resist advertising pressure by using the effective strategies from substance abuse prevention programs.

Another lesson to be learned from the smoking prevention and substance abuse prevention literature is to expand the use of peer leaders and peer educators in nutrition education to create positive peer influences (Komro, Perry, Veblen-Mortenson, & Williams, 1994; Perry et al., 1996). Only a limited amount of published work reports nutrition education programs that have used peer educators (Anliker et al., 1993; Perry et al., 1987). Given the importance of peers in the decisions of adolescents, more evaluated work on the use of peers as positive role models and advocates for healthy eating behaviors is needed.

Parenting style is another social-environmental influence that needs further study. Jackson, Bee-Gates, and Henriksen (1994) considered how parenting style affected initiation of smoking. Authoritative parenting has been defined as parenting skills that facilitate children's development of personal, social, and academic competencies by balancing responsiveness and control. Non-authoritative parenting was defined as excessively controlling and providing little support for children's individuation or development of autonomy. Authoritative parenting was associated with lower rates of smoking initiation, intention to smoke, and experimentation with smoking.

The association between parenting style and eating behaviors is supported by the work of Satter (1996), which suggested that excessive parental control over what and how much is consumed by their children worked against children's ability to learn to respond to natural physiological cues of hunger and satiety, placing children at risk for obesity and eating disorders. Little is known about how to positively affect parenting style to improve children's abilities and opportunities to choose healthful foods and regulate their intake in nonclinical settings.

To be able to better influence personal factors, more work needs to be done on how children learn the functional meanings of foods. Functional meanings of foods are the reasons people give for eating particular foods or for particular dietary patterns (Perry & Jessor, 1985). For example, young people may eat to stay healthy but also to have fun with friends or deal with boredom. Certainly, if parents reward children with sweets for good behavior or a good report card, children learn that sweet foods are highly valued foods and a way to reward oneself. Likewise, if children see parents or other adult family members use food to cope with boredom, stress, or frustration, they will surely learn that eating is a way to deal with life's problems (Lytle & Achterberg, 1995). We cannot expect children to learn healthy eating and coping strategies entirely from textbooks or formal lessons; children will learn functional meanings of foods by how significant others in their physical and social environment use foods. Interventions addressing the functional meanings of foods for individuals in the junior and senior high school levels might include self-assessment of eating behaviors, highlighting not just what is consumed but cues to eating and outcome expectancies of eating.

Functional meanings of foods are also taught within the school setting when pizza coupons are used as incentives for reading and when candy bars are passed out to those completing assignments on time. Until school policy begins to address the use of food in schools for incentives and reinforcements, schools will continue to send children a mixed message that says, "Do what I say but not what I do." The functional meaning of foods in the school environment must be addressed by adopting school policies surrounding the availability and use of foods in the school environment (Story & Neumark-Sztainer, 1996).

Another personal factor that has been inadequately studied is how adolescents' need to "individuate" may influence their eating behaviors. As adolescents set out to find out who they are and try on new identities, eating behavior might be affected. There is some evidence (Donovan, Jessor, & Costa, 1993; Lytle & Roski, in press) that healthful eating behaviors are related to other healthful behaviors in youth, whereas risk-taking behaviors are related to making less healthful food choices and to eating disorders (Neumark-Sztainer, 1996). This need for individuation may explain the large number of adolescents who become vegetarian (Johnston & Haddad, 1996). The notion that individuation might affect multiple adolescent behaviors suggests that programs to promote healthy eating behaviors cannot be implemented in isolation of other social behaviors or without regard for the processes of development that are inherent to adolescence.

Finally, at the level of behavioral factors, more work needs to be done in providing students with relevant, hands-on skills for meal planning and food preparation. With the quickening pace of U.S. society and the increasing prevalence of dual-career families, children often do not learn how to plan and prepare healthful meals. Rather, they learn how to order pizza or stop for takeout! Moreover, adolescents are increasingly responsible for preparing their own meals and snacks (Crockett & Sims, 1995). Both in school and in the family setting, children need opportunities to learn how to plan and prepare quick but healthful meals. If food classes are offered in schools, the emphasis should not be on food science applications (i.e., how to bake bread or the proper temperature for frying) but rather on simple and quick meal planning and preparation. It will be a challenge to find time in schools and in homes to teach children how to choose and prepare healthful diets. Yet it is a challenge we, as a nation, must tackle for the short- and long-term health of our children.

Healthy People 2010

In *Healthy People 2000,* eight nutrition objectives were written for children and adolescents (DHHS, 1991a; Table 8.1). The *Midcourse Review and 1995 Revisions* (DHHS, 1995b) reported notable progress in reducing growth retardation among children of low-income families and some progress in lowering fat consumption. Still, the overwhelming majority of Americans, including youth, eat a higher-fat diet and insufficient fruits and vegetables. Moreover, the prevalence of overweight has increased markedly among all age groups. For adolescents aged 12 to 19, there was a 40% increase in the prevalence of overweight in one decade. Clearly, despite explicit nutrition objectives, the introduction of the food guide pyramid, new food labels, and revised dietary guidelines, the year 2000 nutrition objectives will not, for the most part, be realized.

Although the *Healthy People 2000* document provides clear behavioral objectives, only a portion of those objectives address the question "how?" How do we, as a nation, change the dietary behaviors of children and adolescents? Without recourse to etiologic research on how eating behaviors develop and consolidate, a clearly articulated conceptual model, and successful behavioral intervention methods, it will be difficult to create a coordinated national plan that can influence eating behaviors, particularly normative behaviors such as those contributing to a high-fat diet, insufficient fruit and vegetable intake, and overweight. Therefore, it is recommended that in *Healthy People 2010,* greater attention be paid to the conditions, environments, and policies that can support and sustain healthier choices among young people. The answer to the question, "how," thereby, should be evident in the objectives themselves.

First, nutrition education programs that have been successful in research trials need to be widely disseminated. As noted in the chapter, several school-based programs for children have demonstrated significant behavioral changes. Likewise, school food service interventions have been able to make changes in the content of foods that are served at school, and those changes were associated with healthier dietary behaviors among the students (Luepker et al., 1996). Yet monies to systematically implement these programs in schools are limited. Getting what "works" broader and sustained national support should therefore be a priority.

Second, the focus of nutrition education needs to broaden. Eating behaviors do not occur in isolation of other social behaviors of young people. In particular, poorer eating behaviors and less physical activity co-occur. Nutrition objectives need to be considered within the context of the promotion of a healthy lifestyle for youth. For example, engaging in both daily physical activity and healthy eating behaviors are necessary to reverse the trend of increasing overweight and obesity among America's young people. This implies that more time should be devoted within schools to both these behaviors and more opportunities created outside school for healthier convenience foods, snacks, and recreational activities.

Finally, the norms, opportunities, and role models for healthy eating behavior in the larger social environment should be conscientiously addressed. It is clear that when behavioral education in classrooms is complemented by school food service changes, parental involvement, and communitywide change, healthier eating behaviors among young people are more likely to be sustained. Moreover, the media messages, available convenience foods, restaurant offerings, and even grocery store promotions and environments should be considered as necessary targets in developing healthier dietary behaviors with youth. By turning attention in *Healthy People 2010* from individual behavior to the social environment that supports behavior, the objectives for the next century would be consistent with the research to date on what factors most powerfully influence young people's behavior as well as what is effective in changing their eating behaviors. This larger concern is also consistent with the ambitious aims and intent of a national strategy for significantly improving the health of all Americans. It is not too soon to begin to talk about "how" if we want to make a difference in the health of our nation's children.

References

Alaimo, K., McDowel, M. A., Briefel, R. R., Bischof, A. M., Laughman, C. R., Loria, C. M., & Johnson, C. L. (1994). *Dietary intakes of vitamins, minerals and fiber of persons ages 2 months and over in the United States: Third national health and nutrition examination survey, phase I, 1988-91.* Hyattsville, MD: National Center for Health Statistics.

American School Health Association, Association for the Advancement of Health Education, Society for Public Health Education. (1988). *A report on the health of America's youth.* Oakland, CA: Third Party.

Anliker J. A., Drake L. T., Pacholski J., & Litle, W. (1993). Impacts of a multi-layered nutrition education program: Teenagers teaching children. *Journal of Nutrition Education, 25,* 140-143.

Armotrading, D. C., Probart C. K., & Jackson, R. T. (1992). Impact of WIC utilization rate on breastfeeding among international students at a large university. *Journal of the American Dietetic Association, 92,* 352-353.

Bandura, A. (1977). *Social learning theory.* Englewood, NJ: Prentice Hall.

Bandura, A. (1986). *Social foundations of thought and action.* Englewood Cliffs, NJ: Prentice Hall.

Baranowski, T., Henske, J., Simons-Morton, B., Palmer, J., Tiernan, K., Hooks, P. C., & Dunn, J. K. (1990). Dietary change for cardiovascular disease prevention among Black-American families. *Health Education Research, 5,* 433-443.

Baranowski, T., Perry, C. L., & Parcel, G. S. (in press). How individuals, environments, and health behavior interact: Social cognitive theory. In K. Glanz, F. M. Lewis, & B. Rimer (Eds.), *Health education and health behavior* (pp. 153-178). San Francisco: Jossey-Bass.

Batten, S., Hirshman, J., & Thomas, D. (1990). Impact of the special supplemental food program on infants. *Journal of Pediatrics, 117,* S101-S109.

Birch, L. L. (1980). Effect of peer models' food choices and eating behaviors on preschoolers' food preferences. *Child Development, 51,* 489-496.

Birch, L. L., Marlin, D. W., Rotter, J. (1984). Eating as the "means" activity in a contingency: Effects on young children's food preference. *Child Development, 55,* 431-439.

Birch, L. L., McPhee, L., Shoba, B. C., Pirok, E., & Steinberg, L. (1987). What kind of exposure reduces children's food neophobia? *Appetite: Journal of Intake Research, 9,* 171-178.

Birch, L. L., Zimmerman, S. I., & Hind, H. (1980). The influence of social-affective context on the formation of children's food preference. *Child Development, 51,* 856-861.

Blackburn, H., Luepker, R. V., Kline, F. G., Bracht, N., Carlaw, R., Jacobs, D., Mittelmark, M., Stauffer, L., & Taylor, H. L. (1984). The Minnesota Heart Health Program: A research and demonstration project in cardiovascular disease prevention. In J. D. Matarazzo, S. M. Weiss, J. A. Herd, N. E. Miller, & S. M. Weiss (Eds.), *Behavioral health: A handbook for health enhancement and disease prevention* (pp. 1171-1178). Silver Springs, MD: John Wiley.

Byrd-Bredbenner, C., Marecic, M. L., & Bernstein, J. (1993). Development of a nutrition education curriculum for Head Start children. *Journal of Nutrition Education, 25,* 134-139.

Center on Hunger, Poverty, and Nutrition Policy. (1995). *Statement on the link between nutrition and cognitive development in children.* Medford, MA: Tufts University School of Nutrition.

Centers for Disease Control and Prevention. (1996). Guidelines for school health programs to promote healthy eating. *Morbidity and Mortality Weekly Report, 45,* 1-41.

Clarke, W. R., & Lauer, R. M. (1993). Does childhood obesity track into adulthood? *Critical Reviews in Food Science and Nutrition, 33,* 423-430.

Connor, M. K., Smith, L. G., Fryer, A., Erickson, S., Fryer, S., & Drake, J. (1986). Future fit: A cardiovascular health education and fitness project in an after-school setting. *Journal of School Health, 56,* 329-333.

Consumers Union Education Services. (1995). *Captive kids: Commercial pressures on kids at school.* Yonkers, NY: Consumers Union of the United States.

Contento, I., Balch, G. I., Bronner, Y. L., Lytle, L. A., Maloney, S. K., Olson, C. M., & Swadener, S. S. (1995). The effectiveness of nutrition education and implications for nutrition education policy, programs, and research: A review of research. *Journal of Nutrition Education, 36,* 277-420.

Contento, I. R., Manning, A. D., & Shannon, B. (1992). Research perspective on school-aged nutrition education. *Journal of Nutrition Education, 24,* 247-260.

Cook, J. T., & Martin, L. S. (1995). *Differences in nutrient adequacy among poor and non-poor children.* Medford, MA: Tufts University School of Nutrition.

Crockett, S. J., & Sims, L. S. (1995). Environmental influences on children's eating. *Journal of Nutrition Education, 27,* 235-249.

Donovan, J. E., Jessor, R., & Costa, F. M. (1993). Structure of health-enhancing behavior in adolescence: A latent-variable approach. *Journal of Health and Social Behavior, 34,* 346-362.

Dwyer, J. (1995). The school nutrition dietary assessment study. *American Journal of Clinical Nutrition, 61,* 173S-177S.

Edmundson, E., Parcel, G. S., Feldman, H. A., Elder, J., Perry, D. L., Johnson, C. C., Williston, B. J., Stone, E., Yang, M., Lytle, L., & Webber, L. (1996). The effects of the Child and Adolescent Trial for Cardiovascular Health upon psychosocial determinants of diet and physical activity behavior. *Preventive Medicine, 25,* 442-454.

Ervin, B., & Reed, D. (Eds.). (1993). *Nutrition monitoring in the U.S.: Chartbook 1. Selected findings from the national nutrition monitoring and related research program.* Hyattsville, MD: Public Health Service.

Freedman, D. S., Shear, C. L., Srinivasan, S. R., Webber, L. S., & Berenson, G. S. (1985). Tracking of serum lipids and lipoproteins in children over an 8-year period: The Bogalusa Heart Study. *Preventive Medicine, 14,* 203-216.

French, S. A., Story, M., Downes, B., Resnick, M. D., & Blum, R. W. (1995). Frequent dieting among adolescents: Psychosocial and health behavior correlates. *American Journal of Public Health, 85,* 695-701.

Gong, E. J., & Heald, F. P. (1994). Diet, nutrition and adolescence. In M. E. Shils, J. A. Olson, & M. Shike (Eds.), *Modern nutrition in health and disease* (pp. 759-769). Philadelphia: Lea & Febiger.

Jackson, C., Bee-Gates, D. J., & Henriksen, L. (1994). Authoritative parenting, child competencies, and initiation of cigarette smoking. *Health Education Quarterly, 21,* 103-116.

Johnston, P. K., & Haddad, E. H. (1996). Vegetarian and other dietary practices. In V. I. Rickert (Ed.), *Adolescent nutrition: Assessment and management* (pp. 57-88). New York: Chapman & Hill.

Kann, L., Warren, C. W., Harris, W. A., Collins, J. L., Douglas, K. A., Collins, M. E., Williams, B. I., Ross, J. G., & Kolbe, L. J. (1995). Youth risk behavior surveillance: United States, 1993. *Morbidity and Mortality Weekly Report, 44,* 1-55.

Kelder, S. H., Perry, C. L., & Klepp, K.-I. (1993). Community-wide exercise health promotion: Outcomes from the Minnesota Heart Health Program and class of 1989 study. *Journal of School Health, 63,* 218-223.

Kelder, S. H., Perry, C. L., Klepp, K.-I., & Lytle, L. A. (1994). Longitudinal tracking of adolescent smoking, physical activity, and food choice behaviors. *American Journal of Public Health, 84,* 1121-1126.

Kelder, S. H., Perry, C. L., Lytle, L. A., & Klepp, K.-I. (1995). Community-wide nutrition education: Long-term outcomes of the Minnesota Heart Health Program. *Health Education Research, 10,* 119-131.

Kennedy, E. T., & Gershoff, S. (1982). Effect of WIC supplemental feeding on hemoglobin and hematocrit of prenatal patients. *Journal of the American Dietetic Association, 80,* 227-230.

Kennedy, E., & Goldberg, J. (1995). What are American children eating? Implications for public policy, 1995. *Nutrition Reviews, 53,* 111-126.

Komro, K. A., Perry, C. L., Veblen-Mortenson, S., & Williams, C. L. (1994). Peer participation in Project Northland: A community-wide alcohol use prevention project. *Journal of School Health, 64,* 318-322.

Kotelchuck, M., Schwarz, J. B., Anderka, M. T., & Finison, K. S. (1984). WIC participation and pregnancy outcomes: Massachusetts statewide evaluation project. *American Journal of Public Health, 74,* 1086-1092.

Kotz, K., & Story, M. (1994). Food advertisements during children's Saturday morning television programming: Are they consistent with dietary recommendations? *Journal of the American Dietetic Association, 94,* 1296-1300.

Laskarezewski, P., Morrison, J. A., Groot, I., Kelly, K. A., Mellies, M. J., Khoury, P., & Glueck, C. J. (1979). Lipid and lipoprotein tracking in 108 children over a four year period. *Pediatrics, 64,* 584-591.

Lauer, R. M., Lee, J, & Clarke, W. R. (1988). Factors affecting the relationship between childhood and adult cholesterol levels: The Muscatine study. *Pediatrics, 82,* 309-318.

Lewis, C. J., Crane, N. T., Moore, B. J., & Hubbard, V. S. (1994). Healthy people 2000: Report in the 1994 nutrition progress review. *Nutrition Today, 29,* 6-15.

Luepker, R. V., Perry, C. L., McKinlay, S. M., Nader, P. R., Parcel, G. S., Stone, E. J., Webber, L. S., Elder, J. P., Feldman, H. A., Johnson, C. C., Kelder, S. H., & Wu, M. (for the CATCH Collaborative Group). (1996). Outcomes of a field trial to improve children's dietary patters and physical activity. *Journal of the American Medical Association, 275,* 768-776.

Lytle, L. A., & Achterberg, C. (1995). Changing the diet of America's children: What works and why? *Journal of Nutrition Education, 27,* 250-260.

Lytle, L. A., Kelder, S. H., Perry, C. L., & Klepp, K.-I. (1995). Covariance of adolescent health behaviors: The class of 1989 study. *Health Education Research, 10,* 133-146.

Lytle, L. A., Kelder, S. H., & Snyder, M. P. (1993). A review of school food service research. *School Food Service Research Review, 17,* 7-14.

Lytle, L. A., & Roski, J. (in press). Unhealthy eating and other risk taking behavior: Are they related? *Annals of the New York Academy of Sciences.*

Lytle, L. A., Stone, E. J., Nichaman, M. S., Perry, C. L., Montgomery, D. H., Nicklas, T. A., Zive, M. M., Mitchell, P., Dwyer, J. T., Ebzery, M. K., Evans, M. A., & Galati, T. P. (1996). Changes in nutrient intakes of elementary school children following a school-based intervention: Results from the CATCH study. *Preventive Medicine.*

Lytle-Trenkner, L. A., & Kelder, S. H. (1991). *Nutrition education and school food service intervention as components of comprehensive school health education: Final report to the American Cancer Society's advisory committee on technology transfer of behavioral research.* Atlanta, GA: American Cancer Society.

McDowel, M. A., Briefel, R. R., Alaimo, K., Bischof, A. M., Caughman, C. R., Carroll, M. D., Loria, C. M., & Johnson, C. L. (1994). *Energy and macronutrient intakes of persons ages 2 months and over in the United States: Third national health and nutrition examination survey, phase I, 1988-91.* Hyattsville, MD: National Center for Health Statistics.

McGinnis, J. M., & Foege, W. H. (1993). Actual causes of death in the United States. *Journal of the American Medical Association, 270,* 2207-2212.

Metcoff, J., Costiloe, P., Crosby, W. M., Dutta, S., Sandstead, H. H., Milne, D., Bodwell, C. E., & Majors, S. H. (1985). Effect of food supplementation (WIC) during pregnancy on birth weight. *American Journal of Clinical Nutrition, 41,* 933-947.

Meyers, A. F., Sampson, A. E., Weitzman, M., Rogers, B. I., & Kayne, H. (1989). School breakfast program and school performance. *American Journal of Diseases and Children, 143,* 1234-1238.

Moller, J. H., Taubert, K. A., Allen, H. D., Clark, E. B., & Lauer, R. (1994). Cardiovascular health and disease in children: Current status. *Circulation, 89,* 923-930.

Nader, P. R., Sallis, J. F., Patterson, T. I., Abramson, I. S., Rupp, J. W., Senn, K. L., Atkins, C. J., Roppe, B. E., Morris, J. A., Wallace, J. D., & Vega, W. A. (1989).

A family approach to cardiovascular risk reduction: Results from the San Diego family health project. *Health Education Quarterly, 16,* 229-244.

National Dairy Council. (1995). *Meeting calcium requirements with food.* Rosemont, IL: Author.

Neumark-Sztainer, D. (1996). School-based programs for preventing eating disturbances. *Journal of School Health, 66,* 64-71.

Neumark-Sztainer, D., Story, M., & French, S. (1996). Covariates of unhealthy weight loss behaviors and other high risk behaviors. *Archives of Pediatric and Adolescent Medicine, 150,* 304-308.

Orchard, T. J., Donahue, R. P., Kuller, L. H., Hodge, P. N., & Drash, A. L. (1983). Cholesterol screening in childhood: Does it predict adult hypercholesterolemia? The Beaver County experience. *Journal of Pediatrics, 103,* 687-691.

Osganian, V., Feldman, H., Wu, M., Luepker, R., McKenzie, T., Zive, M., Webber, L., & Parcel, G. (1996). Tracking of physiological variables in the CATCH study. *Preventive Medicine.*

Pagman, A., Ambrosio, G. D., Vincenzi, M., Mormino, P., Maiolino, P., Gerin, L., Barbieri, E., Cappelletti, F., & Dal Palu, C. (1982). Precursors of atherosclerosis in children: The Cittadella study. Follow-up and tracking of total serum cholesterol, triglycerides, and blood glucose. *Preventive Medicine, 11,* 381-390.

Perry, C. L., & Jessor, R. (1985). The concept of health promotion and the prevention of adolescent drug abuse. *Health Education Quarterly, 12,* 169-184.

Perry, C. L., & Kelder, S. H. (1992). Models for effective prevention. *Journal of Adolescent Health, 13,* 355-363.

Perry, C. L., Kelder, S. H., & Klepp, K.-I. (1994a). Communitywide cardiovascular disease prevention with young people: Long-term outcomes of the class of 1989 study. *European Journal of Public Health, 4,* 188-194.

Perry, C. L., Kelder, S. H., & Klepp, K.-I. (1994b). The rationale behind early prevention of cardiovascular disease in young people. *European Journal of Public Health, 4,* 156-162.

Perry, C. L., Kelder, S. H., Murray, D. M., & Klepp, K.-I. (1992). Community-wide smoking prevention: Long-term outcomes of the Minnesota Heart Health Program and the class of 1989 study. *American Journal of Public Health, 82,* 1210-1216.

Perry, C. L., Klepp, K.-I., Halper, A., Dudovitz, B., Golden, D., Griffin, G., & Smyth, M. (1987). Promoting healthy eating and physical activity patterns among adolescents: A pilot study of "Slice of Life." *Health Education Research, 2,* 93-103.

Perry, C. L., Klepp, K.-I., & Sillers, C. (1989). Community-wide strategies for cardiovascular health: The Minnesota Heart Health Program youth program. *Health Education Research, 4,* 87-101.

Perry, C. L., Lytle, L. A., & Kelder, S. H. (1994). Teaching healthful eating habits. In L. J. Filer, R. M. Lauer, & R. V. Luepker (Eds.), *Prevention of atherosclerosis and hypertension beginning in youth* (pp. 256-263). Philadelphia: Lea & Febiger.

Perry, C. L., Parcel, G. S., Stone, E. J., Nader, P. N., McKinlay, S. M., Luepker, R. V., & Webber, L. S. (1992). The Child and Adolescent Trial for Cardiovascular Health (CATCH): Overview of the intervention program and evaluation methods. *Cardiovascular Risk Factors, 2,* 36-44.

Perry, C. L., Stone, E. J., Parcel, G. S., Ellison, R. C., Nader, P., Webber, L. S., & Luepker, R. V. (1990). School-based cardiovascular health promotion: The Child and Adolescent Trial for Cardiovascular Health (CATCH). *Journal of School Health, 60,* 406-413.

Perry, C. L., Williams, C. L., Veblen-Mortenson, S., Toomey, T., Komro, K. A., Anstine, P. S., McGovern, P. G., Finnegan, J. R., Forster, J. L., Wagenaar, A. C., & Wolfson, M. (1996). Project Northland: Outcomes of a communitywide alcohol use prevention program during early adolescence. *American Journal of Public Health, 86,* 956-965.

Pollitt, E. (1995). Does breakfast make a difference in school? *Journal of the American Dietetic Association, 95,* 1134-1139.

Porkka, K. V., Viikari, J. S. A., & Akerblom, H. K. (1991). Tracking of serum HDL-cholesterol and other lipids in children and adolescents: The cardiovascular risk in young Finns study. *Preventive Medicine, 20,* 713-724.

Satter, E. M. (1996). Internal regulation and the evolution of normal growth as a basis for prevention of obesity in children [Commentary]. *Journal of the American Dietetic Association, 96,* 860-864.

Serdula, M. K., Ivery, D., Coates, R. J., Freedman, D. S., Williamson, D. F., & Byers, T. (1993). Do obese children become obese adults? A review of the literature. *Preventive Medicine, 119,* 744-748.

Simeon, D. T., Grantham-McGregor, S. (1989). Effects of missing breakfast on the cognitive functions of school children of differing nutritional status. *American Journal of Clinical Nutrition, 49,* 641-653.

Story, M. (1992). Nutritional requirements during adolescence. In E. R. McAnarney, R. E. Kreipe, D. P. Orr, & G. D. Comerci (Eds.), *Textbook of adolescent medicine* (pp. 75-84). Philadelphia: W. B. Saunders

Story, M., & Neumark-Sztainer, D. (1996). School-based nutrition education programs and services for adolescents. In L. Juszczak & M. Martin (Eds.), Health care in schools [Special issue]. *Adolescent Medicine: State of the Art Reviews, 7,* 287-302.

Stunkard, A. J., & Burt, V. (1967). Obesity and body image: II. Age at onset of disturbances in body image. *American Journal of Psychiatry, 123,* 1443-1447.

Sullivan, S. A., & Birch, L. L. (1990). Pass the sugar; pass the salt: Experience dictates preference. *Developmental Psychology, 26,* 546-551.

Troiana, R. P., Flegal, K. M., Kuczmarski, R. J., Campbell, S. M., & Johnson, C. L. (1995). Overweight prevalence and trends for children and adolescents. *Archives of Pediatric and Adolescent Medicine, 149,* 1085-1091.

U.S. Department of Agriculture. (1992). *The food guide pyramid* (Home and Garden Bulletin No. 252). Hyattsville, MD: Human Nutrition Information Service.

U.S. Department of Agriculture. (1995). *Dietary guidelines for Americans.* Washington, DC: U.S. Department of Health and Human Services.

U.S. Department of Education. (1996). *Nutrition education in public school, K-12.* Washington, DC: Office of Educational Research and Improvement, National Center for Education Statistics.

U.S. Department of Health and Human Services. (1988). *The surgeon general's report on nutrition and health.* Washington, DC: Author.

U.S. Department of Health and Human Services, Public Health Service. (1991a). *Healthy people 2000: National health promotion and disease prevention objec-*

tives (DHHS Publication No. 91-50212). Washington, DC: U.S. Government Printing Office.

U.S. Department of Health and Human Services, Public Health Service, National Institutes of Health. (1991b). *Report of the expert panel on blood cholesterol levels in children and adolescents.* Bethesda, MD: Author.

U.S. Department of Health and Human Services, Public Health Service. (1995a). *Child health USA '94.* Washington, DC: U.S. Government Printing Office.

U.S. Department of Health and Human Services, Public Health Service. (1995b). *Healthy people 2000: Midcourse review and 1995 revisions.* Washington, DC: U.S. Government Printing Office.

Wagner, J. L., Winett, R. A., & Walbert-Rankin, J. (1992). Influences of a supermarket intervention on the food choices of parents and their children. *Journal of Nutrition Education, 24,* 306-311.

Webber, L., Nader, P., McKenzie, T., Luepker, R. V., Lytle, L. A., Nichaman, M., Edmundson, E., Osganian, V., Feldman, H., Cutler, J., & Wu, M. (1996). Cardiovascular risk factors in third to fifth grade students: Results from the Child and Adolescent Trial for Cardiovascular Health. *Preventive Medicine, 25,* 432-441.

Williams, C. L. (1995). Importance of dietary fiber in childhood. *Journal of the American Dietetic Association, 95,* 1140-1146.

• *CHAPTER 9* •

Prevention and Control of Injuries

BARBARA S. TUCHFARBER
JOSEPH E. ZINS
LEONARD A. JASON

Several years ago, when C. Everett Koop was U.S. surgeon general, he made the now widely quoted remark that "if a disease were killing our children in the proportions that accidents are, people would be outraged and demand that the killer be stopped." Childhood injury continues to be a major public health crisis in the United States, as injuries have replaced infectious diseases as the leading cause of childhood death (Baker & Waller, 1989). Although the pain and suffering associated with these injuries are distressing, it is fortunate that many of their causes are being identified and, consequently, that a number of effective and promising interventions have been developed to prevent and control their occurrence.

The terms *injury* and *accident* are often used interchangeably in both the lay and professional literature, but the term *injury* is preferred because *accident* implies that the trauma results from a twist of fate, is not within human control, and is therefore unavoidable. A large percentage of childhood injuries indeed *are* preventable and controllable, as illustrated throughout this chapter. Furthermore, the assumption is that children who are socially competent are less likely to engage in behaviors that lead to injury (Consortium on the School-Based Promotion of Social Competence [Consortium], 1994). Psychologists, social workers, counselors, physicians, teachers, nurses, and other human service providers are in positions to help parents, children, and communities decrease the number and the severity of injuries substantially, thereby cutting the enormous associated costs to individuals and society. Unless efforts to prevent the occurrence of injuries are undertaken, however, significant changes in injury morbidity and mortality rates are unlikely.

In this chapter, we first provide information related to understanding child and youth injury. Next, we outline developmental differences that influence the incidence of injury and its prevention. The following section describes injury control orientations and prevention strategies. We conclude with recommendations for practice and policy development. Our primary focus is on unintentional injury, although we include some discussion of intentional injury.

Understanding Child and Youth Injury: A Public Health Perspective

In this section, we review a number of issues that can help in understanding injury among young people. Application of this information to prevention strategies is included.

Injury among children and youth is a major public health issue because of the magnitude of the number of injuries, the potential years of life lost because of injury, and the associated costs to society. Injury is the leading cause of death during childhood, killing more children each year than all other diseases combined. Recent reports from the Centers for Disease Control and Prevention (CDC, 1995) indicate that 7,200 unintentional injury deaths occurred among children under the age of 15 years in 1991 and that an additional 1,600 deaths resulted from intentional injuries. To illustrate the extent of the problem, consider that in 1990, a national crusade was launched to eliminate measles in response to 40 deaths that year among unvaccinated children. In contrast, 24 children in the United States under the age of 15 years died *every day* that year from injury.

Approximately 13 million children are injured severely enough each year to require medical attention. About 1.4 million children are treated and released from emergency departments, but 360,000 children require hospitalization. Moreover, it is estimated that 50,000 children each year are permanently disabled by an injury

(CDC, 1995). Because of the large numbers of young victims, injuries claim more potential years of life each year than heart disease, cancer, and stroke combined (Rice et al., 1989). Almost 5.3 million potential years of life are lost annually to injuries, an average of 36 years per fatal injury (Robertson, 1992).

The financial, psychological, and social costs resulting from pediatric injury are great. The dollar costs associated with each injury death are higher than for any other disease, averaging about four times more than for cancer and more than six times that of cardiovascular disease. Annual medical costs and projected lost earnings associated with each death are estimated at $335,000 per injury death, $88,000 per cancer death, and $51,000 per cardiovascular disease death (Rice et al., 1989). Medical costs alone are estimated at $200 billion, an impressive figure in an era focused on health economics (Rice et al., 1989; Rosenberg, 1992). Yet the amount of federal spending for injury prevention and treatment is less than 17% of the total spent in cardiovascular research and 11% of the cancer research budget (Rice et al., 1989).

Psychological trauma also results from both unintentional and intentional injuries and can develop into short-term conditions such as acute stress disorders or more severe ones such as post-traumatic stress disorders. Social costs include the psychological and economic toll on the family, needless loss of promising and productive young people, and diversion of resources from beneficial educational and health programs to treatment efforts for pediatric injuries.

The public health model suggests that the epidemic of pediatric injury can be controlled through identification of risk factors, development of appropriate interventions, and evaluation of these efforts. The U.S. pediatric injury mortality rate has decreased steadily throughout this century with marked declines in the 1970s and 1980s. Among children under 20 years of age, injury death rates dropped about 27% between 1978 and 1991, from 40.22 per 100,000 to 29.58 per 100,000 (Rivara & Grossman, 1996).

Although the pediatric unintentional injury rate decreased by 38.9%, the death rate resulting from intentional injury increased by 47.1%. The homicide rate for persons of all ages increased from 1985 to 1991 and has declined since 1992 (CDC, Division of Violence Prevention, 1996). The January 28, 1994, *Morbidity and Mortality Weekly Report* ("Death Resulting From Firearms") projected that if current trends continue, the death rate from firearms will surpass that of motor vehicle crashes by the year 2003.

The importance of pediatric injury as a public health issue is emphasized further by the number of related goals included in *Healthy People 2000* (U.S. Department of Health and Human Services, Public Health Service [DHHS], 1991, 1995), which describes national health promotion and disease prevention objectives and opportunities. As shown in Table 9.1, the prevention of behaviors that can be related to intentional and unintentional injury is the focus of a substantial number of these objectives.

Risk Factors and Protective Mechanisms

Prevention and competence-enhancement approaches can help young people and their adult caregivers focus on (a) increasing skills that encourage the development of positive, health-enhancing behaviors such as defensive driving and anger control skills, (b) eliminating or reducing health-compromising actions such as driving after drinking and diving into shallow water, and (c) altering environments so they are more supportive of these activities. Particularly important to this discussion is that many behaviors associated with injuries are learned (often early in life) and, therefore, are amenable to change or modification. In other words, numerous factors that lead to injury are under the control of young people and their caregivers. In contrast to some of the topics in this volume, however, injury prevention efforts cannot solely be directed toward children and youth but also must involve adult caregivers because these individuals are important mediators of children's environments.

Risk factors place children in harm's way for injury and are associated with an increased likelihood of being injured. Benson (1993) surveyed 47,000 youth in grades 7 through 12 and identified a number of common risk indicators associated with negative health outcomes. Included were risks related to injury, such as having five or more drinks in a row during the last two weeks, attempting suicide, taking part in a fight, driving after drinking, and not using seat belts all or most of the time.

In contrast, protective mechanisms serve to buffer or protect an individual from injury. In Benson's (1993) study, he also found common protective factors associated with positive health out-

Table 9.1. Examples of *Healthy People 2000* Injury Risk Reduction Objectives for Children and Youth

Injury Related to Mental Health	
4.10	Increase the percentage of high school seniors who associate risk of physical or psychological harm with heavy use of alcohol to 70%.
6.1a & 7.2a	Reduce suicides among youth aged 15 to 19 to no more than 8.2 per 100,000 people.
6.2 & 7.2b	Reduce by 15% the incidence of injurious suicide attempts among adolescents aged 14 to 17.
Unintentional Injury	
9.12a	Increase the use of occupant protection systems such as safety belts, inflatable safety restraints, and child safety seats to at least 95% of children aged 4 and younger who are motor vehicle occupants.
9.3b	Reduce deaths among youth aged 15 to 24 caused by motor vehicle crashes to no more than 33 per 100,000 people.
9.5	Reduce drowning deaths to no more than 1.3 per 100,000 people.
Violent and Abusive Behavior	
7.1	Reduce homicides to no more than 7.2 per 100,000 people.
7.3	Reduce weapon-related violent deaths to no more than 12.6 per 100,000 people from major causes.
7.4	Reduce to less than 25.2 per 1,000 children the rising incidence of maltreatment of children younger than age 18.
7.7a	Reduce rape and attempted rape of women aged 12 to 34 to no more than 225 per 100,000.
7.9	Reduce by 20% the incidence of physical fighting among adolescents aged 14 to 17.
7.10	Reduce by 20% the incidence of weapon carrying by adolescents aged 14 to 17.

SOURCE: U.S. Department of Health and Human Services, Public Health Service (1995).

comes. Those related to injuries included parental monitoring of behavior, displaying assertiveness skills, and possession of friendship-making, decision making, and planning skills. Such skills may decrease children's and youth's susceptibility to injury. Environmental factors also play a role in risk reduction and protection.

Epidemiology of Injury

As noted earlier, injuries are not random events but result from predictable behaviors and disproportionately affect identifiable high-risk groups. The traditional model of host, agent, and environmental risk factors for disease is a useful construct in understanding the epidemiology of injury (Lilienfeld & Lilienfeld, 1980).

Host Factors. The host is the individual (e.g., child) who sustains the injury. Host factors are intrinsic characteristics that affect exposure, susceptibility, or response to an injury-producing agent or event. The developmental stage of the person is a key variable in determining exposure and response. Although young people are exposed to injury as motor vehicle passengers throughout all developmental stages, they are injured and killed at much higher rates when they start to ride with other teens or become drivers themselves. Mechanisms of injury vary by age, making assessment of developmental stage a key factor in developing interventions. Developmental influences affecting injury mechanisms and rates are discussed in more detail in a later section.

Injury patterns show distinct gender differences, with males at a much higher risk for most types of injury than females at all ages. Further, as age increases, so does the excess risk for males. During adolescence, males are four times more likely to die from an injury than are females (Rivara, 1992).

Lower socioeconomic status also has been associated with higher pediatric injury rates (Nersesian, Petit, Shaper, Lemieux, & Naor, 1985). Substandard housing with inadequate smoke detectors and poorly accessible evacuation routes, more playtime spent in or near streets, high traffic volume, and older cars with missing or inoperable safety belts increase exposure to many mechanisms of injury. In addition, living in low-income areas and having minority status place an individual at twice the risk of victimization (Singer, 1987).

Race is another risk factor for injury. Non-White children under 15 years of age die of intentional injuries almost twice as often as White children (CDC, 1995). Among African Americans, homicide is now the leading cause of death for males aged 15 to 34 (Rosenberg & Mercy, 1991), with male teenagers in this group five to six times more likely to die of homicide than their White peers, and female teens two to three times more likely than their White peers (Doren, Bullis, & Benz, 1996). Pediatric injury deaths are almost three times higher among Native American infants and preschool children than among the general population the same age (Rosenberg & Mercy, 1991). Race is related to exposure not only to injury-causing factors but also to physiologic response. The same amount of mechanical energy that results in only a soft tissue injury in an African American child may result in a fracture in a White child of similar age, height, and weight because of racial differences in bone mineral density (Li, Specker, Ho, & Tsang, 1989; Rupich, Specker, Lieuw-A-Ta, & Ho, 1996).

Agent Factors. Energy is the agent of injury. Exposure to mechanical, thermal, chemical, electrical, or radiation energy in doses that exceed the body's tolerance results in injury. For instance, being thrown against a car windshield when riding without a seat belt can lead to injury when the individual's tolerance for absorbing that force is exceeded. Injury can also result from events that deprive body tissues of oxygen, which interferes with the body's ability to produce energy, as in asphyxiation and drowning (Robertson, 1992). The amount of energy that is beyond body tissue tolerance levels determines the severity of the injury.

Environmental Factors. Pediatric injury incidence varies within the United States by geographic location. Warmer areas with higher numbers of swimming pools per capita have higher drowning rates among toddlers and preschoolers (American Academy of Pediatrics [AAP] Committee on Injury and Poison Prevention, 1993; Mann, Weller, & Rauchschwalbe, 1992; Wintemute, 1992), whereas colder regions have higher rates of skiing and snowmobile injuries. More serious falls occur in urban areas with high-rise residential buildings, more farm machinery-related injuries occur in rural areas, and interpersonal violence rates are higher in more densely populated, crowded areas.

Contingencies in the environment can also increase the probability of injuries. For example, traffic light patterns in busy, urban intersections can be timed either to increase the risk of a child pedestrian being injured by leading to more jaywalking (Jason & Liotta, 1982) or to reduce the risk of injury by influencing driver traffic rule compliance behavior (Jason, Neal, & Marinakis, 1985).

The interactions of host, agent, and environmental factors result in differential injury rates. Accordingly, at-risk groups can be identified and targeted for further study to determine why injury rates are higher and which interventions may be most likely to be effective. As discussed in the next section, developmental factors are important considerations, especially for pediatric injury deaths.

Developmental Factors Influencing Injury Incidence and Prevention

Examination of developmental factors associated with injury death can be a helpful element in designing effective preventive strategies. Our focus is on injury deaths, but in a comprehensive prevention program it also is important to address nonfatal injuries.

Infants (Younger Than 12 Months)

As shown in Table 9.2, homicide is the leading cause of both intentional and unintentional injury deaths in this age group. During 1991, unintentional injuries resulted in 961 deaths among infants under 1 year of age (CDC, 1995), with asphyxiation/suffocation being the most frequent mechanism of unintentional injury deaths and accounting for about 40% of all unintentional injury deaths in this age group. Most of these deaths result from choking on food or small items.

The next most frequent mechanisms of unintentional injury deaths during infancy are car crashes, fires and burns, and drowning. In 1993, 153 infants died in car crashes (AAP, 1994). Infants require adult intervention to restrain them properly in an appropriate child safety seat (CSS), and a properly used CSS reduces the risk of infant death in a crash by 69% (CDC, 1991). Although rate of use for CSS is approximately 76% among infants (Johnston, Rivara, & Soderberg, 1994), estimates of improper use of a CSS range as high as 82% (Bull, Stroup, & Gerhart, 1988). Studies of adult knowledge about proper use of a CSS have demonstrated a lack of accurate information, which can result in improper use of restraints (Ruffin & Kantor, 1992). The effectiveness of the CSS results from its ability to prevent ejection from the vehicle and to dissipate the mechanical energy generated in a crash through the seat components rather than to the infant's body. Improper installation of the seat in the vehicle or failure to appropriately harness the child into the seat impairs the ability of the CSS to adequately dissipate the energy forces.

Table 9.2 Leading Causes of Injury Death by Age

Less Than 1 Year	*1 to 4 Years*	*5 to 9 Years*	*10 to 14 Years*
Homicide	Fire/burns	Motor vehicle passenger	Motor vehicle passenger
Asphyxiation/ suffocation	Drowning	Pedestrian	Homicide
Motor vehicle passenger	Homicide	Fire/burns	Suicide
Fire/burns	Pedestrian	Drowning	Suicide
Drowning	Motor vehicle passenger	Homicide	Drowning

SOURCE: CDC (1995).

Drowning in infancy differs from drowning in school-age children. Infants are more likely to drown in a bathtub (it can occur with only a few inches of water) or to fall head first into a bucket (AAP, 1993; Fiser, 1993; Mann et al., 1992). Because of their proportionately larger heads and higher centers of gravity, they are unable to extract themselves from the containers.

Toddlers and Preschoolers (1 to 4 Years)

Fires and burns are the leading mechanism of injury death among children 1 to 4 years of age. Drowning, homicide, pedestrian injuries, and car crashes are the next most frequent mechanisms of fatal injuries (see Table 9.2).

The unchecked curiosity that is characteristic of toddlers often leads them to experimentation and exploration. Imitation of adult behaviors such as manipulation of cigarette lighters and matches results in tragic numbers of fatal fires each year, with 85% of the deaths resulting from burns and fires occurring in house fires (Rivara, 1994).

Many drownings in this age group also result from spontaneous, impulsive behavior. Most drownings involving toddlers and preschoolers occur in bathtubs or residential swimming pools, usually at the child's own home or that of a relative or friend (Fiser, 1993; Wintemute, 1990). In one California study, 89% of all drownings among 2- and 3-year olds occurred in neighborhood swimming pools (Wintemute, 1992). For most preschool drowning incidents, the history of the incident indicates that the supervising adult's attention was diverted from the child momentarily, such as by a telephone call or stove timer. Further, the majority (70%) of children in this age group who drown are wearing street clothes, indicating that the caretaker did not anticipate that the child would be playing in the pool (Present, 1987).

Pedestrian injuries are most likely to occur near a driveway or sidewalk. Toddlers playing or riding low tricycles in a driveway are at risk for having a car back over them, particularly if the family vehicle is a van or sports utility vehicle in which visibility for low objects may be difficult (Winn, Agran, & Castillo, 1991).

Although the majority of infants are restrained in a CSS, use rates for toddlers and preschoolers drop precipitously. Restraint use for preschoolers has been observed to range between 6.3% and 43% (Arneson & Triplett, 1990; Chang, Dillman, Leonard, & English, 1985; Morrow, 1989; Partyke, 1983; Roberts, 1986; Stuy, Green, & Doll, 1993). As a result, motor vehicle occupant injuries among children under 4 have been targeted as a national health priority by *Healthy People 2000* (DHHS, 1995), with a goal of 95% safety restraint use (see Table 9.1). Also important is that adult lap belts are estimated to be about 30% effective in preventing fatalities among 2- to 5-year-olds, primarily through preventing ejection from the vehicle or secondary collisions with the interior of the vehicle (Agran, Dunkle, & Winn, 1987; Hendey & Votey, 1994; Osberg & DiScala, 1992; Tso, Beaver, & Haller, 1993). There is general agreement that existing adult restraint systems are not adequate for toddlers and preschoolers. Therefore, the AAP (1995) recommends the use of a CSS for children up to 40 pounds and a booster seat for children from 40 to 60 pounds. Further, there is emerging concern about the safety of air bags when infants and toddlers ride in the front seat facing forward.

School-Age Children (5 to 9 Years)

Motor vehicle injuries are the leading cause of injury-related deaths in this age group. They are followed by pedestrian injuries, fires and burns, drowning, and homicides (see Table 9.2). Pedestrian injuries are more likely to result from midblock dart-outs (Agran, Winn, & Anderson, 1994; Malek, Guyer, & Lescohier, 1990; Winn et al., 1991). The impulsive behavioral characteristics of school-age children often lead to quick movements without an adequate search for oncoming traffic, and stopping in or returning to the roadway to retrieve a dropped or a missed item such as a ball.

Drowning deaths in this age group are four times higher among children with epilepsy or other seizure disorders (Diekma, Quan, & Holt, 1993). Such children are especially vulnerable for drowning in bathtubs and swimming pools.

Pre- and Early Teens (10 to 14 Years)

Motor vehicle occupant injuries continue to be the most common mechanism of injury deaths for 10- to 14-year-olds as they were for the previous group. Next are homicide, suicide, pedestrian injuries, and drowning. Intentional injuries are also a significant problem for these youth. If violence among youth continues to become more lethal (e.g., involving firearms), our concerns likewise will grow.

Drowning in this age group demonstrates a different pattern from that observed in younger children. Drowning is more likely to occur in natural bodies of water such as lakes and rivers (Orlowski, 1987), with alcohol increasingly identified as a contributing factor in a high percentage of these incidents (Wintemute, Teret, Kraus, & Wright, 1990).

Injury Control Orientations and Prevention Strategies

A variety of intervention methods have been applied to the prevention of injuries. In recent years, a multifaceted approach involving several different strategies has been the preferred approach when sufficient resources are available. A brief description of several perspectives and strategies is included here.

Conceptual Framework

Social Competence. As noted earlier and as might be anticipated on the basis of the contents of this volume, we assume that children and youth who are socially competent will be less likely to experience physical injury, particularly of a serious nature. Such individuals possess a number of characteristics that enable them to avoid engaging in behaviors that may lead to injury, as they gradually develop the cognitive, affective, and behavioral skills to engage in health-enhancing and health-protective behaviors (Consortium, 1994). Social competence for young children, however, who rely primarily on adult caregivers to ensure their safety, is much different from that for older children and adolescents who can take more responsibility for their own well-being.

Social competence also is related to factors beyond the individual. We believe that socially competent children tend to have more socially competent role models. These models help ensure that the children's environment is healthy and safe (e.g., provide adequate supervision and work toward adoption of laws conducive to health) and engage in behaviors themselves that reflect an awareness of safety issues (e.g., use seat belts and do not drink and drive), thereby further decreasing the number or severity of children's injuries.

There are several reasons why socially competent young people may be injured less often. They tend to possess skills that may serve as protective mechanisms against injury. For instance, they can generate effective solutions to problems, delay immediate gratification for longer-term rewards, identify the consequences of their actions, and resist negative peer pressures—skills that can be applied to help them avoid risk taking and injury. A junior high student may be able to apply his or her social problem-solving skills when confronted by a class bully, especially because many of these incidents involve increasing amounts of violence. Instead of responding with physical aggression or overly emotional responses that may provoke the bullying, the child may select a low-key approach. That is, he or she can avoid high-risk places when possible, use humor to defuse the situation, or respond assertively ("I don't like it when you take my backpack") and walk away. Or the child may recognize that the bully wants to be friends but does not have the social skills to initiate a relationship and thus respond accordingly. In contrast, those lower in personal/social skills have been found to be more likely to experience victimization (e.g., be beaten up) some time in their school career than those with higher skills in this area (Doren et al., 1996).

Social Learning Theory. Social learning theory (SLT; Bandura, 1977b) has been widely applied to understanding human behavior within a social context. It can be helpful in understanding childhood injury, and programs based on its principles have been shown to be successful (Pless & Arsenault, 1987). SLT is based on the notion that an individual's behavior can be understood only by examining interactions among the individual, other persons in the environment, and key aspects of the environment itself. Therefore, it is essential to consider the person from within an environmental context.

The model predicts that new behaviors are learned through a combination of (a) observations of competent models, (b) direct experiences in the performance of the desired behaviors (e.g., obtained through role playing and behavioral rehearsal) with corrective feedback, and (c) positive reinforcement for accurate performance. Modeling especially is seen as a powerful means of influencing learning or behavior change principally through its informative function; the modeled activities serve as guides for appropriate performance. Bandura (1977b) suggested that to learn from behavioral modeling, children must attend to what the model is doing, process and remember what the model did, practice what the model did and receive corrective feedback, and begin to use what they have learned at appropriate times.

Another key concept in SLT is reciprocal determinism, which suggests that individuals are influenced by their environment and, in turn, have an influence on it (Bandura, 1977a, 1982). SLT also recognizes the importance of intrapersonal variables such as thoughts, perceptions, and attributions. Further, individuals' behavioral histories affect their personal views of themselves, which reciprocally mediate how they behave. Thus, behavior results from interactive cycles of intrapersonal factors, behavioral actions, and reactions from others in their environment.

To further explain SLT, we present an example of its application to CSS use. SLT predicts that children and their parents learn to use safety seats through a combination of (a) observing their correct use by other children and adults, (b) direct experiences of the children in using the seats and of parents in placing their children in safety seats (e.g., which may be obtained through role playing and behavioral rehearsal) with corrective feedback, and (c) positive reinforcement for correct use and performance.

Reciprocal determinism also implies that health behaviors such as CSS use can be changed by altering any of the three elements, that is, intrapersonal factors, interactions with others, or the environmental context. Changing the environmental consequences for an action such as correctly using a CSS changes the children's behaviors and perceptions of themselves; similarly, changing the children's behaviors with respect to using safety seats changes the reactions of parents to the children. Correct modeling of CSS use by parents and other children likewise would be important.

Health Belief Model. The health belief model provides a framework for explaining why people do and do not practice health-related behaviors (Becker, 1974, 1979; Becker & Maiman, 1975). It suggests that people will take action when their behavior leads to an outcome that is valued and when they have an expectancy that the outcome can be achieved. The model has been extensively researched and applied to a number of preventive health behaviors, including compliance to medical regimes.

The health belief model is based on the assumption that health behaviors are more or less rationally determined by individuals' assessment of a potential health threat. From this perspective, people's readiness to engage in a health action is related primarily to perceptions of susceptibility, and perceptions of severity or seriousness of the injury. The likelihood of taking health actions is also determined by individuals' perceptions of the efficacy of their behavior. In other words, people proceed through a cost-benefit analysis associated with the preventive action. Finally, persons' sense of self-efficacy (Bandura, 1977a, 1982), that is, their belief that they can successfully accomplish the action required to achieve the goal, is an additional contributor to decisions concerning health behaviors (Rosenstock, Strecher, & Becker, 1988).

Several other mediating factors are related to health behaviors. Cues to action (e.g., being reminded or alerted about a potential problem) may increase preventive actions. Demographic variables (e.g., gender, age, race, and ethnicity), psychosocial factors (e.g., personality traits, social class, and social pressure), and structural variables (e.g., knowledge about or past experience with the health problem) also help determine the likelihood of taking preventive action.

In the example of car safety seats presented earlier, the health belief model predicts that the decision to use safety seats is determined by parents' perceptions of their children's vulnerability to injury and their perceptions of how severe these injuries might be. In addition, the decision may be influenced by cues to use safety seats, barriers such as the price of purchasing safety seats, the children's reaction to being placed in safety seats, and the ease with which the seats operate. Demographic, structural, and psychosocial factors may also be associated with seat use. In sum, parents who feel their children's health is threatened may use car safety seats, whereas those who do not have this belief would not use them.

Prevention Strategies

Environmental and Passive Methods. The most effective interventions tend to be those that require little behavioral change by the targeted group because they work automatically and require little effort on behalf of the target (Rivara, 1992). For instance, electric eyes that automatically stop garage doors when an object is in the way, fire retardant infant clothes, and reduced injury factor (soft) baseballs necessitate little effort after being installed or purchased, and therefore are in place in the event that a potential injury-producing event occurs. On the other hand, looking in all directions before crossing the street, wearing roller blade helmets and pads, and putting on a life jacket require an action each time a young person engages in the relevant activity, and as a result, they are not used with the same frequency as the other examples. Thus, intervention effectiveness is related to the amount or frequency of the behavioral change required (Cataldo et al., 1983), with the likelihood of use decreasing as more effort is needed.

Legislative Methods. A number of mandated or legislated methods have been adopted to prevent injury, and it is possible to use behavioral methods to influence legislation. For example, in recent years, every state has mandated some form of child passenger restraint system. As indicated earlier, thousands of children are injured or killed as a result of motor vehicle crashes each year. The majority of these injuries and fatalities could have been prevented if appropriate child restraints were used. Accordingly, legislation mandating use of such restraints represents a viable strategy for dealing with this pressing social problem. A variety of strategies were used by states to enact relevant legislation, and the following example (which also contains an educational component) is included because of its potential applicability to legislation for other interventions such as use of bicycle safety helmets.

Jason and Rose (1984) evaluated the effects of sending technical information regarding the number of children killed or injured in car crashes and the use of car safety restraints to Illinois legislators just prior to a vote on a child passenger restraint bill. They also provided legislators with data concerning the state's share of medical care costs following debilitating traffic injuries and with the results of a citizen survey that supported passage of the bill. Jason and Rose found that 79% of the senators receiving the information voted for passage of the bill, whereas only 53% of the senators not receiving the letter voted in favor of it.

Surveillance data indicated an increase in child restraint use, particularly for infants, just before enactment of the legislation; this was likely a result of the positive publicity that the media gave to the proposed legislation. Notably, with passage of the law, still higher rates in use were observed. Four observations taken before and after the law was passed indicated that infant use of appropriate restraints increased from 49% to 74%, whereas for children aged 1 to 4 years, use increased from 13% to 42%. Child deaths due to car crashes also decreased 53% during the 2 years before and 2 years after enactment of the law (Fawcett, Seekins, & Jason, 1987).

Educational Methods. These approaches motivate change by providing information about safety issues (e.g., risk of approaching cars with unknown drivers in them or of eating Halloween candy without having an adult inspect it), and often involve the use of prompts and reinforcement (e.g., school awards for best decorated bicycle helmets and free soft drinks from drive-through restaurants for patrons using seat belts). As noted earlier, one reason people engage in various health behaviors is related to their perceptions of vulnerability to injury and their views of how severe these injuries might be, along with the use of cues.

Although educational methods, particularly one-shot efforts, may produce some short-term benefits, change usually is not observed through long periods (Geddis & Pettengel, 1982). Consequently, to produce the best outcomes, educational efforts must be combined with other continuing approaches as discussed next, to increase the likelihood that sustained change will result (e.g., Pless & Arsenault, 1987; Rivara, 1996; Zins, Garcia, Tuchfarber, Clark, & Laurence, 1994).

Comprehensive Injury Prevention

Program Development. As the preceding discussion suggests, the use of a variety of intervention methods is clearly needed in a comprehensive injury prevention program. Environmental, educational, or mandated methods alone cannot solve all the problems but in combination can make a noticeable difference because most injury-producing events are too complex for simple, one-dimensional interventions (Zins et al., 1994). Furthermore, the better defined the target population and the mechanism of the injury, the more likely it is that the prevention program can be directed toward factors that will result in desirable behavioral changes and, ultimately, a reduction in injury rates. It usually is not cost-effective to target individual children because of resource constraints and the lack of success in identifying "high-risk" children, but at the same time, it may be inefficient to focus on the entire population when the incidence rate or the severity of a certain injury is low. Demographics such as geographic location may also influence the direction of efforts (e.g., swimming pool safety is more of a concern in Florida than in Montana). The challenge is in how to most efficiently and effectively direct the available resources, thereby having the greatest impact. Likewise, because so many potential injuries could be addressed, priorities need to be established related to the frequency and severity of a particular injury and also with regard to the known effectiveness of particular intervention strategies (Grossman & Rivara, 1992).

Another consideration has to do with intervention integrity. That is, to be maximally effective, injury prevention technology must be used as designed. It is not enough for a child to wear a bicycle safety helmet or to be placed in a child restraint system; the helmet must be worn properly (e.g., not too far back on the head or too loosely) and the restraint must be engaged appropriately (e.g., infants under 20 pounds should not face the front of the car; adult seat belts may be less effective with children under 8 years of age). There simply are too many instances in which available technology could have prevented an injury if it had been used or if it had been applied properly. Finally, injury prevention does not belong to one element of the community or to one profession. To be most effective, prevention efforts should involve a coalition of interested community members including parents, teachers, legislators, health care professionals, behavioral scientists, and so forth, as well as children, so that their various perspectives can be considered and their commitment energies focused.

Evaluation. A systematic, objective way of determining the effectiveness and limitations of any intervention is needed to determine whether it should be continued, modified, or discontinued. One aspect missing from many prevention programs, however, is an evaluation component that measures the extent to which a program is attaining its immediate objectives (so adjustments can be made if needed) and what overall goals are reached and that help direct future efforts (Consortium, 1994). Further, specific plans to examine these issues should be included when a program is first being developed.

With respect to injuries, measuring changes in injury mortality and morbidity rates is important, but these cannot be the only outcomes assessed. As noted earlier, the integrity with which the preventive intervention was provided must first be examined. If the technology is not used appropriately, then it is impossible to evaluate its efficacy. Furthermore, it is important to examine differences in risk and protective behaviors that may be associated with the injury prevention program. For instance, are children (and their caregivers) engaging in high-risk behaviors such as swimming without a lifeguard; keeping the temperature of the hot water heater above 120 degrees; or crossing the street without stopping and looking left, right, and left again? Can they be observed properly using injury prevention technology such as safety boundaries at bus stops; smoke, heat, and carbon monoxide detectors; flotation devices on a boat; and athletic safety glasses? Have relevant policies and regulations been enacted such as requiring that bicycle safety helmets be worn, window guards be installed in high-rise buildings, and gun cabinets be locked? Are children knowledgeable about safety-related behaviors and the steps they can take to ensure their own well-being? Multiple measures should be taken to evaluate the success of the program and to determine future directions.

Examples of Injury Prevention Programs

Successful injury prevention programs for children and youth have been conducted in a variety of settings. Examples of community-based programs include ones that targeted children's bicycle helmet use (Rivara et al., 1994), falls from high-rise windows and use of window guards (Barlow, Niemirska, Gandi, & Leblanc, 1983; Spiegel & Lindaman, 1977), and overall neighborhood safety (Davidson et al., 1994).

Schools are also excellent settings for establishing injury prevention programs in cooperation with community personnel and parents because they provide access to a large number of children and youth. A further advantage is that programs in schools have the potential to affect not only students but also out-of-school siblings, parents, and teachers.

In this section, two examples of our work with injury prevention in the classroom are provided. In the first, a single safety message is integrated throughout the curriculum, whereas the second strategy employs a short-term but highly engaging activity that addresses multiple safety issues. Both approaches can be implemented by a single institution, as detailed in the following section, and both illustrate use of social learning theory and the health belief model.

Integrated Car Safety Program

Preschool is developmentally an ideal time to teach safety skills such as use of the CSS to children. Programs designed specifically to increase use among preschoolers, however, have been generally ineffective. As might be anticipated, those with a relatively short-term educational intervention (2 to 4 weeks) have failed to demonstrate an increase in observed restraint use (Arneson & Triplett, 1990). Programs that reward parents, children, or both for buckling up produce only short-term gains; use rates quickly deteriorate to near baseline levels after the reward is removed (Geddis & Pettengel, 1982; Roberts, 1986; Roberts & Turner, 1986; Sowers-

Hoag, Thyer, & Bailey, 1987). On the other hand, there is increasing evidence that programs that employ extensive modeling, role playing, behavior rehearsal, performance feedback, clear consequences, positive reinforcement, and intermittent booster sessions can effectively produce behavioral change (Zins et al., 1994). These instructional techniques, incidentally, are commonly found in social competence promotion programs (Consortium, 1994).

The preschool car safety program developed by the Cincinnati Children's Hospital Medical Center (CHMC) is an example of a comprehensive program integrated throughout the activities of the school day (Garcia, Tuchfarber, Laurence, & Clark, 1995). Although Ohio state law mandates CSS use for children less than 4 years old or under 40 pounds, data from the hospital's trauma registry indicated that many preschoolers injured or killed in car crashes were unrestrained at the time of the crash. The preschool car safety program was developed to meet this community need by increasing the use of restraints. The safety curriculum was developed by educators and pediatric health care professionals. A curriculum manual detailing specific restraint activities and how to integrate the safety message into other areas of the general curriculum was prepared. Classroom teachers participated in developing the manual to ensure that the program was developmentally appropriate and able to be implemented in the real world of the classroom. Examples of specific activities are included in Table 9.3. The curriculum was implemented in October and continued formally through April.

Parental involvement is an important part of the success of any safety program, so relevant program information was included in newsletters sent home monthly to keep parents informed of classroom activities. Specific parent questions and concerns about proper restraint use were obtained by questionnaire and answered in the newsletters. Each school held a parent program that provided opportunities for interaction with experts regarding the selection and installation of a CSS.

Teachers received a curriculum manual and in-service training at the beginning of the school year. Additional support was provided through CHMC psychological services for teachers who identified children with fears of car crashes or injuries, and during the pilot program, car seats were available at no cost to families identified by teachers as in need.

Table 9.3. Examples of Curriculum Activities Rated Highly by Teachers During the Preschool Car Safety Pilot Program

Area	*Example of Specific Activity*
Whole language	*Journal activity:* One child per day is given a backpack containing a stuffed bear with a removable safety belt, a *Riding With Bucklebear* videotape, and a notebook. The child's "homework assignment" is to watch the video with his or her family and dictate a story about a car trip to an adult caretaker. The adult writes the child's story in the notebook. The teacher reads the child's story aloud during group time the next school day. For situations in which a child cannot perform the activity at home, a teacher or aide works with the child during the school day.
Dramatic play	*Safety Seats:* Infant, convertible, and booster seats are available in all classrooms. Children buckle their dolls into infant seats and themselves into the larger seats for pretend trips. Bags of special car toys are available for the children to use to amuse the dolls and keep them happy in their seats during long trips. The children teach the dolls and other child passengers songs to sing while in a CSS.
Gross motor	*Pedal Cars:* Safety belts are attached to plastic pedal cars which the children ride in the muscle room or outdoor play areas. Each child is issued a "driver's license" after demonstrating how to fasten the safety belt before "starting the car" and describing safe riding behaviors (staying in a CSS, keeping hands inside the car, not throwing things in the car, etc.).
Fine motor	*Flannel Board Stories:* Colorful felt pieces are used on flannel boards by the children to tell car safety-related stories. Felt car seat shapes can be put into the felt cars and child figures placed in the car seats. A variety of shapes, including animals and buildings, are used as scenery as the cars "drive" past.

SOURCE: Garcia et al. (1995).

Evaluation of the program was conducted through parent surveys, and comparisons were made by direct observations of restraint use in participating schools and in similar schools without the car safety program. During the program, restraint use increased significantly by 15.8%, from 71% (October) to 82% (April) at participating schools. Control schools demonstrated a statistically insignificant increase during the same period (66% to 72%).

Single Event Programming

The Safety Fair program, also developed by the CHMC, is another example of a school-based program. It provides several diverse injury prevention messages through a single event supplemented by additional classroom activities. The purpose is to reduce injury among elementary school children by teaching specific safety behaviors to students in kindergarten through fourth grade. The event provides hands-on activities at five separate safety stations: bicycle, pedestrian, motor vehicle occupant, home, and fire. The Safety Fair is supplemented by related classroom activities such as work sheets, videotapes, and discussions. In the evening, parents and siblings also participate and the *Safety Minutes* video is shown as an introduction to the fair.

Evaluation of the program demonstrated a significant increase in parental knowledge of safety issues 2 weeks following the Safety Fair. Students also demonstrated a significant increase in safety knowledge after the Safety Fair event but did not score significantly higher than students in control schools who had not yet attended the Safety Fair. In addition, consumer satisfaction data from students, parents, and teachers indicated that they rated the Safety Fairs as successful and useful in providing important safety information.

Conclusions, Policy and Practice Recommendations, and Challenges for the Future

At the beginning of the chapter, we stated that childhood injury largely is a preventable occurrence and noted that young people who are socially competent should engage in fewer behaviors that are likely to lead to injury, and should be more likely to engage in safe behaviors that prevent injury. We hope that the preceding discussion adequately demonstrated these points and provided some direction for the most effective ways to intervene to prevent injury.

It is commendable that the *Healthy People 2000* goal of reducing unintentional injuries was achieved in 1993 (DHHS, 1995). The challenge is to maintain that accomplishment. For instance, many states are increasing highway speed limits, so there is risk that crashes may become more serious. In addition, there is a need to use the knowledge we have gained to decrease injuries even further, such as by increasing the use of helmets by motor cyclists, decreasing the availability of firearms, teaching conflict resolution skills, and eliminating violence in the media.

Clearly, a number of policy implications can be derived from this discussion. Although educational and environmental strategies can affect the number of injuries sustained, these efforts will be improved substantially if supporting legislation is enacted and enforced. As suggested, the strategies used to pass CSS legislation appear applicable to other areas such as bicycle safety helmets (for which use is estimated to be 5% to 10%; DHHS, 1995) and installation of thermostatically controlled safety valves to regulate the temperature of the hot water flowing into bathtubs. Of course, such efforts should be part of a comprehensive injury prevention campaign. Needed also is more surveillance on injury morbidity and mortality to identify the causes and outcomes of injuries, as well as to evaluate the effectiveness of prevention programs. At this time, for instance, there are no national data on injury prevention instruction occurring in schools (DHHS, 1995), and little is known about its cost-effectiveness. Knowledge of protective mechanisms likewise is limited. Because of the scope of the problem and the need for coordinated efforts, the federal government should provide the leadership and funding to support such efforts.

In the absence of state or national legislation, it seems reasonable on the local level for schools or park boards to require those who ride their bikes or use roller blades to wear safety equipment. Other safety rules are adopted routinely by schools and other organizations serving youth. Local governments, community organizations, and schools could become partners in many of these injury prevention efforts. In addition, if the federal government continues to resist enacting legislation about handgun design to protect children, states must do so.

Promotion of social competence skills, similar to drug or AIDS education, also could be mandated by state departments of education. The incidence of interpersonal violence in schools is growing, and unless efforts to prevent its occurrence are undertaken, it is likely to escalate further. Social competence promotion programs also could include a focus on unintentional injury, similar to other areas of focus such as smoking, pregnancy, and child abuse prevention; there is overlap in the mechanisms that lead to these various problem behaviors. Parents and other community members must be involved in these efforts so that focused alliances of stakeholders can be formed. In addition, despite technological solutions to many of the problems, we must not lose sight of the role of personal and social values, behavior, and responsibility in the origin of the problems and in their solutions.

Coalitions of child care providers are also needed. Pediatricians increasingly are routinely including safety issues in their interactions with children and families (DHHS, 1995). Psychologists must continue to develop applications that are relevant to public health so that their ideas are incorporated into the public health infrastructure that provides much leadership for many injury prevention endeavors (Leviton, 1996). Those in other professions also have contributions to make. Ultimate success depends on using the contributions and perspectives of many disciplines and stakeholders.

The challenge to prevent injuries is clear. The question is not whether we, as a nation, must take up the challenge but rather who will do it and how it will be accomplished so that our communities—including children and families—are safe and healthy.

References

Agran, P. F., Dunkle, D. E., & Winn, D. G. (1987). Injuries to a sample of seatbelted children evaluated and treated in a hospital emergency room. *Journal of Trauma, 27,* 58-64.

Agran, P. F., Winn, D. G., & Anderson, C. L. (1994). Differences in child pedestrian injury events by location. *Pediatrics, 93,* 284-288.

American Academy of Pediatrics. (1994). *Safe ride news.* Elk Grove, IL: Author.

American Academy of Pediatrics. (1995, December/January). Safety update. *Healthy Kids,* 1-3.

American Academy of Pediatrics Committee on Injury and Poison Prevention. (1993). Preventing drowning in infants, children, and adolescents. *Pediatrics,* 92(2), 292-294.

Arneson, S. W., & Triplett, J. L. (1990). Riding with Bucklebear: An automotive safety program for preschoolers. *Journal of Pediatric Nursing, 5*(2), 115-122.

Baker, S. G., & Waller, A. (1989). *Childhood injury: State-by-state mortality facts.* Washington, DC: National Maternal and Child Health Clearinghouse.

Bandura, A. (1977a). Self-efficacy: Toward a unifying theory of behavioral change. *Psychological Review, 84,* 191-215.

Bandura, A. (1977b). *Social learning theory.* Englewood Cliffs, NJ: Prentice Hall.

Bandura, A. (1982). Self-efficacy mechanism in human agency. *American Psychologist, 37,* 122-147.

Barlow, B. B., Niemirska, M., Gandi, R. P., & Leblanc, W. (1983). Ten years of experience with falls from a height in children. *Journal of Pediatric Surgery, 18*(4), 509-511.

Becker, M. H. (Ed.). (1974). *The health belief model and personal health behavior.* Thorofare, NJ: Charles B. Slack.

Becker, M. H. (1979). Understanding patient compliance: The contributions of attitudes and other psychosocial factors. In S. J. Cohen (Ed.), *New directions in patient compliance* (pp. 102-122). Lexington, MA: D. C. Heath.

Becker, M. H., & Maiman, L. A. (1975). Sociobehavioral determinants of compliance with health and medical care recommendations. *Medical Care, 13,* 10-24.

Benson, P. (1993). *The troubled journey: A portrait of 6th-12th grade youth.* Minneapolis, MN: Search Institute.

Bull, M. J., Stroup, K. B., & Gerhart, S. (1988). Misuse of car safety seats. *Pediatrics, 81*(1), 98-101.

Cataldo, M. F., Derschewitz, R., Wilson, M., Christopherson, E., Finney, J., Fawcett, S., & Seekins, T. (1983). Childhood injury control. In N. A. Krasnegor, J. D. Araseth, & M. F. Cataldo (Eds.), *Child health behaviors: A behavioral pediatrics approach* (pp. 217-253). New York: John Wiley.

Centers for Disease Control and Prevention. (1991). Child passenger restraint use and motor vehicle related fatalities among children: United States, 1982-1990. *Morbidity and Mortality Weekly Review, 40,* 600-602.

Centers for Disease Control and Prevention, Division of Violence Prevention, National Center for Health Statistics. (1996). Trends in rates of homicide: United States, 1985-1994. *Morbidity and Mortality Weekly Review, 45*(22), 460-464.

Centers for Disease Control and Prevention, National Center for Injury Prevention and Control. (1995). *Childhood injury: Cost and prevention facts.* Washington, DC: U.S. Government Printing Office.

Chang, A., Dillman, A. S., Leonard, E., & English, P. (1985). Teaching car passenger safety to preschool children. *Pediatrics, 76*(3), 425-428.

Consortium on the School-Based Promotion of Social Competence (Elias, M. J., Weissberg, R. P., Hawkins, J. D., Perry, C. L., Zins, J. E., Dodge, K. A., Kendall, P. C., Gottfredson, D., Rotheram-Borus, M. J., Jason, L. A., & Wilson-Brewer, R. J.). (1994). The school-based promotion of social competence: Theory, research, practice, and policy. In R. J. Haggerty, L. Sherrod, N. Garmezy, & M. Rutter (Eds.), *Stress, risk, and resilience in children and adolescents: Processes, mechanisms, and interaction* (pp. 268-316). New York: Cambridge University Press.

Davidson, L. L., Durkin, M. S., Kuhn, L., O'Connor, P., Barlow, B., & Heagarty, M. C. (1994). The impact of the safe kids/healthy neighborhoods injury prevention program in Harlem, 1988 through 1991. *American Journal of Public Health, 84,* 580-586.

Deaths resulting from firearms and motor-related injuries: United States, 1968-1991. (1994, January 28). *Morbidity and Mortality Weekly Report, 43,* 37-42.

Diekma, D. S., Quan, L., & Holt, L. (1993). Epilepsy as a risk factor for submersion injury in children. *Pediatrics, 91*(3), 612-616.

Doren, B., Bullis, M., & Benz, M. (1996). Predictors of victimization experiences of adolescents with disabilities in transition. *Exceptional Children, 63,* 7-18.

Fawcett, S. B., Seekins, T., & Jason, L. A. (1987). Policy research and child passenger safety legislation: A case study and experimental evaluation. *Journal of Social Issues, 43,* 133-148.

Fiser, D. H. (1993). Near-drowning. *Pediatrics in Review, 14*(4), 148-151.

Garcia, V. F., Tuchfarber, B. S., Laurence, S. C., & Clark, K. M. (1995, April). *An effective school-based program for increasing restraint use among preschoolers.* Poster session presented at the meeting of the American Academy of Pediatrics Section on Injury and Poison Prevention, Philadelphia.

Geddis, D. C., & Pettengel, R. (1982). Parent education: Its effect on the way children are transported in cars. *New Zealand Medical Journal, 95,* 314-316.

Grossman, D. C., & Rivara, F. P. (1992). Injury control in children. *Pediatric Clinics of North America, 39*(3), 471-480.

Hendey, G. W., & Votey, S. R. (1994). Injuries in restrained motor vehicle accident victims. *Annals of Emergency Medicine, 24*(1), 77-84.

Jason, L. A., & Liotta, R. (1982). Pedestrian jaywalking under facilitating and nonfacilitating conditions. *Journal of Applied Behavior Analysis, 15,* 469-473.

Jason, L. A., Neal, A. M., & Marinakis, G. (1985). Altering contingencies to facilitate compliance with traffic light systems. *Journal of Applied Behavior Analysis, 18,* 95-100.

Jason, L. A., & Rose, T. (1984). Influencing the passage of child passenger restraint legislation. *American Journal of Community Psychology, 12,* 485-495.

Johnston, C., Rivara, F. P., & Soderberg, R. (1994). Children in car crashes: Analysis of data for injury and use of restraints. *Pediatrics, 93*(6), 960-965.

Leviton, L. C. (1996). Integrating psychology and public health: Challenges and opportunities. *American Psychologist, 51,* 42-51.

Li, J. Y., Specker, B. L., Ho, M., & Tsang, R. C. (1989). Bone mineral content in Black and White children 1 to 6 years of age: Early appearance of race and sex differences. *American Journal of Diseases of Children, 143,* 1346-1349.

Lilienfeld, A. M., & Lilienfeld, D. E. (1980). *Foundations of epidemiology* (2nd ed.). New York: Oxford University Press.

Malek, M., Guyer, B., & Lescohier, I. (1990). The epidemiology and prevention of child pedestrian injury. *Accident Analysis and Prevention, 22*(4), 301-313.

Mann, N. C., Weller, S. C., & Rauchschwalbe, R. (1992). Bucket-related drowning in the United States, 1984-1990. *Pediatrics, 89,* 1068-1071.

Morrow, R. (1989). A school-based program to increase seatbelt use. *Journal of Family Practice, 29*(5), 517-520.

Nersesian, W. S., Petit, M. R., Shaper, R., Lemieux, D., & Naor, E. (1985). Childhood death and poverty: A study of childhood deaths in Maine, 1975-1980. *Pediatrics, 75,* 41-50.

Orlowski, J. (1987). Adolescent drowning: Swimming, boating, diving and scuba accidents. *Pediatric Annals, 17,* 126-132.

Osberg, J. S., & DiScala, C. (1992). Morbidity among pediatric motor vehicle crash victims: The effectiveness of seat belts. *American Journal of Public Health, 82*(3), 422-425.

Partyke, S. C. (1983). *Infants and toddlers in passenger car crashes* (National Highway Traffic Safety Administration Tech. Rep.). Washington, DC: U.S. Department of Transportation, Mathematical Analysis Division.

Pless, I. B., & Arsenault, L. (1987). The role of health education in the prevention of injuries to children. *Journal of Social Issues, 43*(2), 87-103.

Present, P. (1987). *Child drowning study: A report on the epidemiology of drowning in residential pools to children under age 5.* Washington, DC: Consumer Product Safety Commission.

Rice, D. M., MacKenzie, E. J., Jones, A. S., Kaufman, S. R., deLissovoy, G. V., Max, W., McLoughlin, E., Miller, T. R., Robertson, L. S., Salkever, D. S., & Smith, G. S. (1989). *Cost of injury in the United States: A report to Congress.* San Francisco: University of California Institute for Health and Aging and Johns Hopkins University Injury Prevention Center.

Rivara, F. J. (1992). Prevention of injuries to children and adolescents. In H. M. Wallace, K. Patrick, G. S. Parcel, & J. B. Igoe (Eds.), *Principles and practices of student health: Vol. 1. Foundations* (pp. 89-102). Oakland, CA: Third Party.

Rivara, F. P. (1994). Unintentional injuries. In I. B. Pless (Ed.), *The epidemiology of childhood disorders* (pp. 369-396). New York: Oxford University Press.

Rivara, F. P. (1996, July). *Open forum on injury prevention.* Presentation at the Children's Hospital Medical Center, Cincinnati, OH.

Rivara, F. P., & Grossman, D. C. (1996). Prevention of traumatic deaths to children in the United States: How far have we come and where do we need to go? *Pediatrics, 97*(6), 791-797.

Rivara, F. P., Thompson, D. C., Thompson, R. S., Rogers, L. W., Alexander, B., Felix, D., & Bergman, A. B. (1994). The Seattle children's bike helmet campaign: Changes in helmet use and head injury admissions. *Pediatrics, 93*(4), 467-469.

Roberts, M. C. (1986). Rewarding elementary school children for their use of safety belts. *Health Psychology, 5*(3), 185-196.

Roberts, M. C., & Turner, D. S. (1986). Rewarding parents for their children's use of safety seats. *Journal of Pediatric Psychology, 11*(1), 25-36.

Robertson, L. S. (1992). *Injury epidemiology.* New York: Oxford University Press.

Rosenberg, M. L. (1992). Injury control: Meeting the challenge. *Archives of Physical Medicine and Rehabilitation, 73,* 1129-1132.

Rosenberg, M. L., & Mercy, J. A. (1991). Assaultive violence. In M. L. Rosenberg & N. A. Finley (Eds.), *Violence in America: A public health approach.* New York: Oxford University Press.

Rosenstock, I. M., Strecher, V. J., & Becker, M. H. (1988). Social learning theory and the health belief model. *Health Education Quarterly, 15,* 173-183.

Ruffin, M. T., & Kantor, R. (1992). Adults' knowledge about the use of child restraint devices. *Family Medicine, 24*(5), 382-385.

Rupich, R. C., Specker, B. L., Lieuw-A-Ta, M., & Ho, M. (1996). Gender and race differences in bone mass during infancy. *Calcified Tissue International, 58,* 395-397.

Singer, S. (1987). Victims in a birth cohort. In M. Wolfgang, T. Thornberggy, & R. Figlio (Eds.), *From boy to man, from delinquency to crime* (pp. 163-169). Chicago: University of Chicago Press.

Sowers-Hoag, K. M., Thyer, B. A., & Bailey, J. S. (1987). Promoting automobile safety belt use by young children. *Journal of Applied Behavior Analysis, 20*(2), 133-138.

Spiegel, C. M., & Lindaman, F. C. (1977). Children can't fly: A program to prevent childhood morbidity and mortality from window falls. *American Journal of Public Health, 67,* 1143-1147.

Stuy, M., Green, M., & Doll, J. (1993). Child care centers: A community resource for injury prevention. *Journal of Developmental and Behavioral Pediatrics, 14,* 224-229.

Tso, E. L., Beaver, B. L., & Haller, J. A. (1993). Abdominal injuries in restrained pediatric passengers. *Journal of Pediatric Surgery, 28*(7), 915-919.

U.S. Department of Health and Human Services, Public Health Service. (1991). *Healthy people 2000: National health promotion and disease prevention objectives* (DHHS Publication No. PHS 91-50212). Washington, DC: U.S. Government Printing Office.

U.S. Department of Health and Human Services, Public Health Service. (1995). *Healthy people 2000: Midcourse review and 1995 revisions.* Washington, DC: U.S. Government Printing Office.

Winn, D. G., Agran, P. F., & Castillo, D. N. (1991). Pedestrian injury to children younger than 5 years of age. *Pediatrics, 88*(4), 776-782.

Wintemute, G. J. (1990). Childhood drowning and near-drowning in the United States. *American Journal of Diseases in Children, 144,* 663-669.

Wintemute, G. J. (1992). Drowning in early childhood. *Pediatric Annals, 21*(7), 417-421.

Wintemute, G. J., Teret, S. P., Kraus, J. F., & Wright, M. (1990). Alcohol and drowning: An analysis of contributing factors and a discussion of criteria for case selection. *Accident Analysis and Prevention, 22,* 291-296.

Zins, J. E., Garcia, V. F., Tuchfarber, B. S., Clark, K. M., & Laurence, S. C. (1994). Preventing injury in children and adolescents. In R. J. Simeonsson (Ed.), *Risk, resilience, and prevention: Promoting the well-being of all children* (pp. 183-202). Baltimore: Paul H. Brookes.

• *CHAPTER 10* •

Academic Performance and School Success: Sources and Consequences

J. DAVID HAWKINS

The promotion of academic success in children is a national health goal (U. S. Department of Health and Human Services, Public Health Service [DHHS], 1991). Goal 8.2 of *Healthy People 2000* is to "increase the high school completion rate to at least 90 percent, thereby reducing risks for multiple problem behaviors and poor mental and physical health" (p. 253).

Promoting academic success has been designated as a national health goal because the available evidence suggests that academic success during childhood can be key to social and emotional wellness. Research indicates that academic success can reduce involvement in health risk behaviors that can compromise all forms of wellness (Dryfoos, 1990). *Healthy People 2000* (DHHS, 1991) states, "By addressing high school dropout rates as part of the nation's health promotion and disease prevention agenda, it may be possible to reduce unwarranted risk of problem behavior and improve the health of our young people" (p. 254). Moreover, certain methods of management and instruction in classrooms have been shown to accomplish the goals of both promoting academic success and promoting social and emotional competence. Teachers should learn and use these methods in classrooms to maximize the academic, social, and emotional skills of their students.

Finally, there is some evidence that the promotion of social and emotional competence in children can positively affect their academic performance. This evidence suggests that although often ignored in "back to the basics" movements in education, the promotion of social and emotional competence and the promotion of academic competencies are mutually reinforcing activities. Both should be included in the goals of schools.

This chapter briefly summarizes the evidence regarding the link between academic performance and health risk behaviors, including substance abuse, delinquency, teen sexual activity, and violence. This evidence suggests that the promotion of academic success in children vulnerable to health risk behaviors may reduce the likelihood of these behaviors. Next, the evidence regarding the mechanisms found in descriptive studies to characterize schools that are effective in promoting the academic performance of children is summarized. Then, a theory of behavior, the social development model, is outlined to organize this evidence on effective schools. The theory provides an example of a framework that can be used to select and implement school and classroom practices to promote the development of academic, social, and emotional competence in children. Finally, examples of practices that have been shown in intervention studies to be effective in promoting academic, social, and emotional competency are described in the context of the theory.

Predictors of Health Risk Behaviors

A number of factors have been shown to predict health risk behaviors during adolescence (see Dryfoos, 1990; Hawkins, Arthur, & Catalano, 1995; Institute of Medicine, 1994). Four of these are of interest here. Contextually, extreme economic disadvantage or poverty has been shown to increase risk for health risk behaviors such as crime (Dryfoos, 1990; Farrington, 1991; Institute of Medicine, 1994). Second, independent studies in different countries and cultures have shown that persistent physically aggressive behavior in the early elementary school grades (including fighting and bullying) predicts later crime, violence, and substance abuse (Farrington, 1991; Institute of Medicine, 1994; Kellam, Rebok, Ialongo, & Mayer, 1994; Robins, 1978). Finally, independent studies have found both academic failure and low commitment to schooling to increase risk for later substance abuse, delinquency, school dropout, teen pregnancy, and violence (see Dryfoos, 1990; Hawkins, Catalano, & Miller, 1992; Institute of Medicine, 1994; Maguin & Loeber, 1996). In their meta-analysis of the relationship of academic performance and delinquency, Maguin and Loeber found that academic performance makes an independent contribution to delinquency even after the effects of socioeconomic status or prior conduct problems are controlled.

Characteristics of Effective Schools

Simultaneous with the development of research on predictors of health risk behaviors has been a growing body of research on effective schools (for reviews, see Levine & Lezotte, 1990; Mortimore, 1995). Descriptive studies have shown specific mechanisms to be associated consistently with schools that are effective in producing better academic outcomes for students than would be expected from students' background characteristics.

Just as they are at greater risk for health risk behaviors, children raised in poverty are less likely to achieve academic success than are children of middle- and upper-class families (Mortimore, 1995). Schools must be effective in educating children of low-income families. Such children are more likely to be of ethnic minority status than the general population and more likely to be raised by a single female parent. Schools that can effectively ensure that these children succeed academically reduce their risks for health risk behaviors.

There is consistent evidence "that individual schools can promote positive or negative student outcomes; that those outcomes can include both cognitive and social behaviors; and that they are not dependent on the school receiving a favored student intake" (Mortimore, 1995, p. 341). What are the characteristics of schools that are effective in promoting learning and academic achievement? Mortimore has summarized eight that appear consistently across studies across continents. I have rearranged the order, but not the content, of Mortimore's list

1. Strong positive leadership of the school
2. Academic emphasis and a focus on learning
3. High expectations
4. The use of joint planning and consistent approaches toward students (consistent expectations)
5. Students' active involvement in schooling and school life
6. Parental involvement in the life of the school
7. Monitoring of student progress
8. Rewards and incentives (pp. 346-352)

Focused on a similar task, the Task Force on Defining a Disciplined Environment Conducive to Learning of the National Education Goals Panel (1995) identified the following key characteristics of effective school environments:

1. Clear discipline standards are provided that are firmly, fairly, and consistently enforced.
2. Staff express high performance expectations and demonstrate commitment to the academic success of all students.
3. The development of personal responsibility [and] social and emotional competence are promoted among students and staff.
4. Opportunities and incentives exist for all students and staff to become actively and continuously engaged in the learning process.
5. Reinforcement and recognition are given for students' and staff's efforts in the pursuit of learning.
6. Staff show concern and support for their students' intellectual and personal development.
7. Families and the larger community are successfully engaged in the work of the school and the education of their children.
8. The physical environment is safe, well-maintained and welcoming. (pp. 2-3)

Other reviews of the characteristics of effective schools have reached similar conclusions (Levine & Lezotte, 1990). The evidence suggests that if schools could successfully integrate all these characteristics into their operations, they would be more successful in educating their students.

Toward a Theory of Academic Performance and Social Development

Theory is needed to provide a framework for understanding how these characteristics interrelate in producing academic success and a commitment to learning. Theory can organize the existing evidence on the predictors of academic outcomes into plausible causal models. Theory is needed, ultimately, to guide the development, implementation, and testing of effective practices.

My colleagues and I have been working on a theory of human behavior, the social development model, for a number of years (Catalano & Hawkins, 1996; Hawkins & Weis, 1985). In this section, the social development model is used to link the current evidence on effective schools into a theoretical framework for both understanding and action to promote academic success.

The social development model seeks, ultimately, to explain why both healthy and health risk behaviors emerge during development. Here, the processes that relate to the promotion of academic success are described. I also seek to show how the promotion of academic success and of social, emotional, and physical health can be promoted through the use of the same theoretically specified processes or mechanisms. (For a complete exposition, see Catalano & Hawkins, 1996.)

Behavior is the product of the interaction between the individual and the environment (Hawkins & Weis, 1985; Moffitt, 1993). Generic processes of social development recur in different environments during the life course of the developing individual. From ages 6 to 18, schools are a major social environment experienced by children. Children who develop a commitment to succeed in school and who feel a sense of attachment to school and to their teachers are more successful academically than other children (Harachi, Abbott, Catalano, & Haggerty, 1996). Commitment and attachment are elements of a social bond to school.

The emphasis on the importance of social bonding is derived from Hirschi's (1969) theory of social control. Criminological research has shown that children who develop a bond of commitment and attachment to school are less likely to engage in serious crime and other health risk behaviors including violence and substance abuse (Hawkins, Catalano, & Miller, 1992; Hirschi, 1969; Maguin & Loeber, 1996). Similarly, Maguin and Loeber report that academic success has been shown across studies to protect against health risk behaviors during adolescence.

The social development model hypothesizes that bonding to school (i.e., commitment and attachment to schooling) is important both in promoting later academic achievement and in preventing health risk behaviors. The model hypothesizes that academic achievement contributes developmentally to later levels of bonding to school as well as to the prevention of health risk behaviors.

Bonding to school is, itself, the product of a process of interaction between the developing child and the school environment. The level of bonding between the individual child and the school depends on three elements. First is the degree to which the school itself provides opportunities to the developing child for active involvement in the educational process. Active student involvement in schooling is one of the characteristics of effective schools. Opportunities for active participation should be developmentally appropriate to the child's current level of skills to motivate the child to engage in the learning process (Csikszentmihalyi & Larson, 1980).

Skills or competencies are the second element in the interactive process by which bonding develops. Cognitive, as well as social and emotional, skills must be considered. Individual variation in intellectual skills is widely recognized (Herrnstein & Murray, 1994), but skills vary on a number of dimensions (Gardner, 1993; Goleman, 1995). To the extent that individuals possess and use behavioral, cognitive, emotional, and interpersonal skills required in confronting a particular opportunity in school, they are more likely to experience the opportunity as positive, both as a result of the internal satisfaction derived from the experience (Csikszentmihalyi & Larson, 1980) and as a result of the external reinforcement from the environment made more likely by a skillful performance.

In the social development model, reinforcement or recognition for skillful involvement is the third element in the process by which bonding to school develops. (See Mortimore, 1995, for a discussion of the role of rewards and incentives as mechanisms for eliciting positive behaviors.)

Since Plato set out to train youth in how to find pleasure in action that strengthens, rather than weakens, the bonds of human solidarity, the creation of social bonding has, itself, been a goal of education (Csikszentmihalyi & Larson, 1980). School personnel, and teachers in particular, have a great deal of influence over the degree to which children develop a bond to school, that is, over the degree to which they become committed to learning and like school and teachers. Teachers control the opportunity structure confronted by children through their selection of curriculum materials, their choice of methods for managing the classroom, and their choice of methods of instruction. Teachers also control many of the reinforcements experienced by students through the methods of classroom management and instruction they use. The job of teachers is to provide an opportunity and reinforcement system that promotes the development of desired skills in children. Success in that endeavor creates strong bonding to school. Commitment to educational pursuits and attachment to school motivate behaviors that are conducive to academic achievement. Strong bonding to school provides the motivation to work hard to live up to the norms or expectations held by school personnel.

To the extent that school personnel hold and communicate clear norms regarding high educational expectations for children in that school, these norms are likely to encourage children who are bonded to school to engage in behaviors consistent with learning, such as completing assignments. I will return to this topic of norms or standards for behavior later.

To this point, I have discussed the process by which bonding to school develops. Yet opportunities for active involvement, skills for participation, and reinforcement for skillful participation are elements in the process by which bonding develops to any social group, whether that group is a school class, a family, a group of peers, or a delinquent gang. This process can occur regardless of whether a group holds norms favorable or unfavorable to learning.

An alternative system of opportunity and reinforcement exists, in varying degrees, in the social environments of developing children and adolescents. Opportunities to engage in aggressive behavior and reinforcement for doing so are sometimes offered in the interactions of family members (Patterson, 1982, 1986) and peers (Pepler, Craig, & Roberts, 1995). Although some patterns of violent interaction may be learned (Patterson, 1982), aggressive and violent behaviors do not require the development of complex or difficult skills.

Individual constitutional differences affect both academic performance and the propensity to engage in health risk behaviors. It is hypothesized that these differences manifest themselves in differential perceptions of opportunities, differential levels of skills, and different perceptions regarding reinforcement among individuals (see Catalano & Hawkins, 1996). In general, the extent to which individuals engage in behaviors consistent with academic achievement or in health risk behaviors is influenced, in part, by the relative balance of opportunities, skills, and reinforcements they experience during development.

To the extent that individuals develop bonds of commitment and attachment to individuals and social groups that hold high expectations for learning and achievement, they are more likely to pursue academically focused activities. To the extent that they do not develop such bonds, they are less constrained from substance use, crime, early sexual activity, and other health risk behaviors. As a result of opportunities and reinforcements experienced in social groups that model, condone, or approve of these behaviors, individuals may be encouraged to engage in such behaviors (Bourgois, 1995).

Norms that assert that "school is a White thing" or that academically successful adolescents are "nerds" denigrate achievement and contribute to academic failure. Schools must counteract these norms to be successful in promoting achievement of students. This suggests one reason that involving parents in school life is important. A goal of parental involvement is to build consensus about the importance of academic achievement and school success for children between parents and schools. The society cannot afford inconsistency between schools and families regarding norms about the importance of a good education.

This view of the etiology of school achievement and health risk behaviors suggests that the development of a social bond of commitment and attachment to schooling by students is, in part, a responsibility of schools. This is accomplished through the provision of appropriate opportunities for active participation and skill development and the use of appropriate reinforcement for skillful performance both inside and outside the classroom. The development of bonding to school is essential both to ensure successful academic achievement and to create the motivation to live according to norms or standards for healthy behavior promoted by school personnel (i.e., non-drug use, nonviolence, abstinence from early sexual activity and unprotected sex, etc.).

From this perspective, the promotion of social, emotional, and physical wellness in the schools is more fundamental than a new curriculum laid on top of the three Rs. The promotion of social, emotional, and physical wellness is a function of the way teachers manage and teach in their classrooms and on playgrounds. Schools that fail to create the conditions that bond students to school fail to promote a strong protective factor against health risk behaviors.

In this context, the importance of strong positive leadership of the school becomes apparent. School leaders must clearly establish expectations for behavior. Leaders must express explicit commitment to strong academic performance, setting high expectations for all staff and all students. At the same time, school leaders must assert and maintain standards for healthy behavior for schools to become "free of drugs, violence, and the unauthorized presence of firearms and alcohol" (National Education Goals Panel, 1995, p. 13). Establishing, exemplifying, and enforcing high academic expectations and behavior standards are primary functions of school leaders.

Yet it is also clear that the task of establishing and maintaining high standards is best accomplished by using social development processes to ensure that those affected by the standards will be committed to upholding them. If expectations are developed through a process that extends opportunities for active involvement to include faculty, staff, students, and parents; if the endeavor helps develop skills for participation in the process; and if those who participate are recognized for their participation, commitment to the school and its standards and their maintenance should be broadened (Mortimore, 1995). This is consistent with the emphasis on joint planning and faculty cohesion identified as a characteristic of effective schools (Levine & Lezotte, 1990). In sum, school leaders can act to establish clear, high standards for academic performance and student behavior and to promote commitment and attachment to school among staff, students, and their families.

Effective Interventions to Promote Academic Success and Healthy Behavior

What do researchers know about practices that promote the previously discussed academic and behavioral outcomes? Clearly, cognitive, emotional, and social development begins before birth and is affected by factors and experiences from conception onward (Institute of Medicine, 1994). Effective interventions for promoting children's academic success and healthy behaviors are not confined to K-12 schools. Interventions with economically disadvantaged mothers during pregnancy and their children's infancy, interventions for low birth weight and preterm babies, and early childhood education and family support interventions before children enter the elementary grades have shown positive effects on the cognitive development of children (Hawkins, Catalano, & Brewer, 1995; Institute of Medicine, 1994; Kagan & Neuman, 1997). This chapter, however, is limited to discussion of school-based interventions that promote academic performance during the elementary and secondary grades. The focus is on practices and policies of schools and classrooms that have been shown to be effective in promoting academic achievement and healthy behavior.

Classroom Interventions

Teaching is fundamental to the academic development of children. The research on teaching is extensive. Significant literatures are focused on the teaching of specific subject matters, on teaching to different learners, on teaching for different developmental stages, and on teaching methods themselves (see Berliner & Calfee, 1996; Wittrock, 1986). I do not attempt to summarize that literature here but rather illustrate practices shown to be effective for promoting achievement and healthy behavior.

Good teaching begins with good classroom management. There is strong experimental evidence of the effectiveness of behavioral techniques for classroom management, such as the establishment of clear rules and directions, the use of contingent approval and reinforcement, and the involvement of students in specifying contingencies and reinforcing themselves (O'Leary & O'Leary, 1977). Proactive classroom management strategies are aimed at establishing an environment that is conducive to learning and that promotes appropriate student behavior and minimizes disruption to classroom activities (Cummings, 1983). Proactive classroom management requires that teachers act in advance to anticipate and avoid classroom discipline problems in managing entire groups or classes of students. Classroom routines are established at the beginning of the year to create consistent expectations for both academic and social behavior for all students in the classroom. Teachers and students develop clear and explicit expectations for behavior, for teacher monitoring of behavior, and for consequences of acceptable and unacceptable behavior. Teachers recognize students' attempts to meet these expectations with frequent, appropriate specific encouragement or praise that identifies the student behavior being rewarded. Teachers also use strategies such as "the law of least intervention" for keeping minor classroom disruptions from interrupting instruction and decreasing opportunities for learning.

Intervention studies have shown that teachers can learn to use proactive classroom management methods and that their use produces less student misbehavior in class and more on-task academically focused behavior (Evertson, 1985; Evertson, Emmer, Sanford, & Clements, 1983; Kellam & Rebok, 1992). By promoting clear expectations for both academic and social behavior that are firmly, fairly, and consistently enforced; by involving students in developing behavioral standards for the classroom and emphasizing personal responsibility for adhering to them; and by consistently using incentive and rewards, proactive classroom management illustrates a number of the characteristics of effective schools (National Education Goals Panel, 1995). It also illustrates the use of social development processes to increase commitment to learning and adherence to classroom expectations for behavior.

With regard to classroom instruction itself, continuous progress instruction and cooperative learning methods have been found to be consistently effective across a number of studies in increasing academic success for elementary grade students at risk of failure (Slavin, Karweit, & Madden, 1989; Slavin, Karweit, & Wasik, 1994). Continuous progress instruction is a form of mastery-based learning in which students proceed through a defined hierarchy of skills and are tested at each level to assess their readiness to advance. Corrective instruction and tutoring are provided for those who need it to achieve mastery of a skill. Teachers deliver most instruction to groups of students at the same instructional level who may be grouped or regrouped for instruction depending on their skills in different subjects.

In cooperative learning, after teachers have provided instruction to groups of students or the class as a whole, students work in learning teams composed of four or five members of mixed skill levels, to help each other learn and to assess one another's progress in preparing for tests and teacher assessments. Students are tested individually but contribute to team recognition if their scores show increasing mastery, thereby increasing motivation to help teammates learn. Cooperative learning provides opportunities and reinforcement for active involvement of all children in academically focused learning groups in the classroom. Positive effects of cooperative learning on achievement have been shown in both short- and long-term experimental tests in elementary schools and in short-term tests in secondary schools (Slavin & Madden, 1989).

In social development terms, both continuous progress instruction and cooperative learning methods increase opportunities and reinforcement for active involvement in schooling, which should, in turn, increase academic achievement and commitment to learning. Both methods seek to increase time allotted to instruction and learning and to provide opportunities for practice to achieve mastery (that is, opportunities for active involvement in learning), to provide a structured hierarchy of learning tasks adjusted to students' current levels of skills, and to use frequent monitoring of student progress both to allow for adjustment of instruction and to provide specific information for recognition and reinforcement of student progress.

A related approach to improving achievement has been to change the demographics of instruction, that is, to alter the number and/or characteristics of students being instructed by a teacher. Reductions in class size have been advocated, for example, to provide greater opportunity for student-teacher interaction for each student. Tutoring is an extreme example of this in which the student-teacher ratio is reduced to one-to-one. Academic achievement has been affected consistently and positively by one-on-one tutoring of elementary students. Tutoring by older students, adult community volunteers, trained paraprofessionals, and certified teachers has produced substantial long-term improvements in students' achievement in reading and math (Wasik & Slavin, 1994). Positive results of tutoring have been found regardless of whether the tutoring was preventive or remedial, or structured or unstructured, in design. Tutoring provided by other students has positive effects on both tutors' and tutees' academic achievement and attitudes toward the subject covered across all achievement levels (Cohen, Kulik, & Kulik, 1982). Tutoring of elementary grade students has been shown to positively affect achievement for 2 years following tutoring (Coie & Krehbiel, 1984; Greenwood, Terry, Utley, Montagna, & Walker, 1993).

In social development terms, one-on-one tutoring provides extensive opportunities for active involvement and interaction focused on learning and provides a source of immediate and continuous reinforcement for effort and improvement in performance. When delivered by other students, tutoring provides these conditions for both tutors and those being tutored, and both have benefited academically from tutoring.

With respect to reductions in class size more generally, Slavin's (1990a) meta-analysis showed that substantial reductions in class size (greater than 20%) had small positive effects on reading achievement in kindergarten and first grade. Reductions in class size at later grades, however, have produced no reliable effect on achievement.

Another example of the approach of changing the demographics of instruction is grouping students for instruction on the basis of ability. Ability grouping across classes and grades for reading in the elementary grades has shown consistent moderate positive effects on reading achievement. Ability grouping for mathematics instruction in the middle and late elementary grades has also shown moderate positive effects (Slavin, 1987). Ability grouping in secondary schools, however, has not shown consistent positive effects on achievement (Slavin, 1990b).

A final example of this approach is the use of diagnostic-prescriptive pullout strategies for students in need of remedial instruction. Again, where specific learning needs are clearly identified and instruction appropriate to these needs is given by a teacher to individuals or small groups of about three to eight students, positive effects on achievement have been consistently observed (Madden & Slavin, 1989).

Methods of classroom management, instruction, and regrouping for instruction have been combined in classroom-based interventions focused on promoting academic achievement and reducing behavior problems of children. Two examples are described here: Success for All (Madden, Slavin, Karweit, Dolan, & Wasik, 1993; Slavin et al., 1995) and the Seattle Social Development Project (Hawkins, Catalano, Morrison, et al., 1992).

The Success for All program developed by Slavin et al. (1995) combines continuous progress instruction, one-on-one tutoring, and cooperative learning methods with other intervention methods to improve the academic success of children in the elementary grades. The comprehensive intervention seeks to enable all students to achieve academic success by providing a half-day preschool and/or a full-day kindergarten focused on language development and academic and social readiness, followed in the primary grades by small-group reading instruction using an empirically based reading curriculum and cooperative learning methods. Students are assessed by teachers every 8 weeks to reconstitute ability-based reading groups and determine which students should receive individual tutoring in 20-minute daily sessions provided by certified tutors focused on helping students master the reading curriculum. In addition, a family support team involves parents in actively helping their children to succeed academically by supporting learning at home. A representative school advisory committee oversees the program.

Evaluations of the Success for All intervention have shown positive effects on achievement, as measured by reading tests, by reductions in special education placements, and by reductions in rates of retention in grade, with greatest effects shown for those children initially in the lowest quartile of achievement (Madden et al., 1993; Slavin et al., 1995).

Explicitly guided by the social development model, the Seattle Social Development Project was a multicomponent intervention designed to prevent delinquency and other problem behaviors. The project employed a package of classroom management and instruction methods in the elementary grades including cooperative learning, proactive classroom management, and interactive teaching (Hawkins, Catalano, & Morrison, et al., 1992; O'Donnell, Hawkins, Catalano, Abbott, & Day, 1995).

Proactive classroom management consisted of establishing expectations for classroom behavior; using methods of maintaining classroom order that minimized interruptions to instruction and learning; and giving frequent, specific, and contingent praise and encouragement for student effort and progress. Interactive teaching involved clear specification of learning objectives, continuous monitoring of students, and remediation, requiring students to master specific learning objectives before proceeding to more advanced work. Structured cooperative learning groups were used in experimental classrooms from grades 2 through 6. In the experimental intervention, teachers of the elementary grades were trained to use these three methods of instruction. These methods were tested in combination with a social competence curriculum and parent training during the 6 years of elementary school.

The intervention was tested with a multiethnic urban sample. By the end of grade 2, boys in intervention classrooms were rated as significantly less aggressive than boys in control classrooms (Hawkins, Von Cleve, & Catalano, 1991). By the beginning of grade 5, experimental students were significantly less likely to have initiated delinquent behavior and alcohol use than were controls (Hawkins, Catalano, Morrison, et al., 1992). By the end of grade 6, intervention boys from low-income families had significantly greater academic achievement, better teacher-rated behavior, and lower rates of delinquency initiation than did control boys from low-income families (O'Donnell et al., 1995). A 6-year follow-up at age 18 found significantly higher achievement and lower rates of lifetime violent delinquent behavior among children exposed to the full intervention compared with controls (Hawkins et al., 1996). The studies summarized here provide consistent evidence that interventions to improve classroom management and teaching practices in elementary schools can promote the academic performance of students, including those at greater risk of academic failure and health compromising behaviors.

To this point, I have reviewed innovations that seek explicitly to enhance the academic success of children. There is some evidence that the teaching of social and emotional skills in schools also can have long-term effects on academic achievement (Elias, Gara, Schuyler, Brandon-Muller, & Sayette, 1991). The Improving Social Awareness-Social Problem Solving project sought to promote social and emotional competence in elementary school children through an instruction and application phase. In the instruction phase, teachers used scripted lessons involving the following steps: group sharing of interpersonal problems, successes, and feelings to create a mental set for the lesson; teacher-led presentation of the cognitive, affective, and behavioral skills to be taught; written and video presentations modeling use of the skills in applicable situations; class discussions of the situations and ways to use the new skills;

role playing of the skills by students; and summary and review. In the application phase, teachers encouraged students to problem solve difficult interpersonal encounters and to use the skills in daily situations confronted in the classroom and other environments. In a quasi-experimental study, this problem-solving skills program in grades 4 through 6 was followed by positive effects on academic achievement at grade 10 (Elias et al., 1991).

The social development model suggests that the successful development of skills for participation in the classroom contributes to the development of commitment to schooling and to academic success. The intervention studies reviewed above used similar methods of instruction to promote the development of cognitive/academic skills and the development of social and emotional skills. Regardless of the skills to be learned, skills are acquired when students are motivated to learn them, when skills are broken into manageable components, when successful performance of the skills is demonstrated or modeled, when students have an opportunity to actively practice the skills, and when they receive specific feedback and reinforcement for their performance of the skills (Stallings & Stipek, 1986; W. T. Grant Consortium on the School-Based Promotion of Social Competence, 1992).

These findings suggest that an important task for schools and teachers is to integrate the teaching of academic and social and emotional skills in the classroom. Two initiatives currently under way seek to accomplish this goal. The Child Development Project conducted by Battistich, Schaps, Watson, and Solomon (1996) seeks to help schools to become

> "caring communities of learners"—social contexts in which all students feel supported and valued, can actively participate in and contribute to school life, and where there is a common commitment not only to learning, but to fairness, respect, responsibility, and concern for others. (p. 8)

The project uses cooperative learning; proactive classroom management methods that seek to foster responsibility, establish prosocial norms, and strengthen conflict resolution skills; classroom and schoolwide community building activities; activities for students and parents to do at home together; and a literature-based language arts program that emphasizes students' critical thinking about relevant social and ethical issues.

A longitudinal, multisite quasi-experimental test of the Child Development Project involving 12 intervention and 12 comparison elementary schools across the United States found significant increases in student attachment and commitment to school and academic achievement, increases in conflict resolution skills and prosocial behaviors, and significant reductions in alcohol use among fifth and sixth grade students (Battistich et al., 1996; Battistich, Solomon, Watson, & Schaps, in press).

In Raising Healthy Children, a third-generation intervention study growing from the Seattle Social Development Project, Catalano, Haggerty, and their colleagues are testing methods for integrating five classroom strategies for promoting academic, social, and emotional growth through the use of integrated curricula. The Raising Healthy Children project is an experimental test of these strategies involving all first- and second-grade children in five experimental and five control schools. The strategies include (a) proactive classroom management; (b) use of effective instructional techniques including motivational and active student involvement in learning activities; (c) interpersonal and social problem-solving skills training; (d) cooperative learning methods; and (e) reading strategies that balance guided reading, shared reading, reading aloud, and reading alone. Because children often come to the classroom unprepared for the social environment in which learning occurs, and because cooperative learning techniques require interpersonal and problem-solving skills for successful implementation, a major focus of the teacher training intervention is on helping teachers integrate social and emotional skills into the classroom environment and curricula. During teaching workshops, teachers identify how to integrate interpersonal and problem-solving skills training into the daily schedule.

Participating elementary school teachers identified these interpersonal skills as prerequisites to academic success: listening, how to give compliments, problem solving, anger management, recognizing and sharing feelings, tattling versus reporting, and manners. Literature units have been created to assist in skill development through direct instruction, practice, reinforcement, and generalization. The units are designed to be used in conjunction with the Get-Along series (Cummings, 1993), a set of interpersonal and problem-solving skill storybooks for children in the primary grades that are integrated with reading units. Each unit takes approximately 1 month to teach, including an introductory lesson and 5- to 10-minute lessons for the following days. Teachers plan and practice integrating social and emotional skills training into the reading curriculum. Teachers use a variety of short activities, designed to eliminate dead time during transitions to keep the focus on the social and emotional learning environment of the classroom. For example, while focusing on listening and waiting for the recess bell to ring the teacher asks, "Let's brainstorm all the times you will need to listen in one day." As students develop, social skills are highlighted in conjunction with reading assignments. For example, third graders reading *Charlotte's Web* learn to map Wilbur's social network and then to ask, "Who are good friends and who aren't such good friends?" Fifth-grade students focus on journal writing their feelings as if they were Philip, the main character in their reading novel, *The Cay*. Teachers also use class meetings to facilitate problem solving and discuss relevant issues regarding the classroom learning environment.

One day of instruction is provided to teachers for each of the five Raising Healthy Children strategies, 1 to 2 years before children in the study panel enter their classrooms. Teachers practice using the skills in the classroom and are provided coaching and advanced workshops in each topic.

After 1.5 years of exposure of the study panel to these integrated teaching practices, academic and behavior outcomes have been examined, using hierarchical linear modeling of growth and level differences between experimental and control groups. In the academic area, students in the experimental condition have shown significantly higher commitment to school and academic achievement. In the behavioral area, both social competency and appropriate social interaction have shown growth and level changes favoring intervention students. Measures of antisocial behavior also have shown significant level and growth differences favoring the intervention group. Experimental students had lower levels of antisocial behavior and decreasing rates compared with increasing growth rates of antisocial behavior for control students (Catalano, Harachi, Haggerty, & Abbott, 1996).

The early results of both the Child Development Project and Raising Healthy Children study indicate that the teaching of academic and socioemotional skills can be integrated in the classroom with positive effects on academic achievement, social and emotional skills, and student behavior. Schools are likely to maximize results if they seek to develop both academic and emotional competencies of their students. Development of the cognitive skills required for academic success is accomplished using methods similar to those used for the development of social and emotional skills. High and consistent expectations for behavior must be established. Teaching and learning are done in a way that requires active involvement of the learners, that is, participation with others in tasks and activities requiring both cognitive and interpersonal skills for successful completion. Continual monitoring and reinforcement are essential for learning both types of skills. The best practice is likely to integrate the teaching of both types of skills in planned developmental sequences that complement each other.

Schoolwide Approaches

Although classrooms are environments of social development for students, classrooms are nested in schools that by virtue of their leadership and organizational arrangements affect expectations and standards, opportunities and rewards, and the degree of consistency in these across the school. Several investigators have intervened to change the organization of schools to make them more effective.

Comer (1988) developed a comprehensive elementary school intervention involving four components: (a) a social calendar that integrated arts and athletic programs into school activities; (b) a parent program in support of school academic and extracurricular activities that fostered interaction among parents, teachers, and other school staff; (c) a multidisciplinary mental health team that provided consultation for school staff in managing student behavior problems; and (d) a representative governance and management team composed of school administrators, teachers, support staff, and parents that oversaw the implementation of the other three components. A number of elements of the intervention, including the active involvement of parents, illustrate the elements of effective schools listed earlier. Originally implemented in two New Haven inner-city elementary schools serving predominantly African American children from families in poverty, the intervention is now widely used. From a social development perspective, by providing greater opportunities for teachers, other school staff, and parents to interact and to become involved in clarifying and setting expectations through governance and management activities, the intervention should create greater commitment to schooling among all involved and establish shared high expectations for student achievement and behavior.

Follow-up studies of students from the original intervention elementary schools and matched comparison students have shown significantly better middle school grades, achievement test scores, and self-rated social competence in intervention students when compared with matched comparison students (Cauce, Comer, & Schwartz, 1987; Comer, 1988).

Gottfredson (1986) evaluated a comprehensive school organization intervention for secondary schools in low-income, predominantly African American areas in Charleston County, South Carolina. The six main components were (a) teams composed of teachers, other school staff, students, parents, and community members that designed, planned, and implemented school improvement programs, with the assistance of two full-time project staff; (b) curriculum and discipline policy review and revision, including student participation in the development of school and classroom rules and continuing in-service training for teachers in instructional and classroom management practices; (c) schoolwide academic innovations, including study skills programs and cooperative learning methods; (d) schoolwide climate innovations, including expanded extracurricular activities, peer counseling, and a school pride campaign intended to improve the overall image of the school; (e) career-oriented innovations, including a job-seeking skills program and a career exploration program; and (f) special academic and counseling services for students who were low achieving and disruptive.

The intervention was implemented and evaluated for 2 years in three middle schools and for 1 year in three high schools. A middle school and a high school served as comparisons in the quasi-experimental design. Although the general population of students in intervention schools significantly improved in grades, alienation, attendance, and self-concept, these changes were matched by similar improvements on these outcomes among students in comparison schools. Because Gottfredson does not directly compare the experimental and comparison schools, it is difficult to ascertain the effects of the schoolwide intervention. The low-achieving and disruptive students in intervention schools who received special academic and counseling services, however, scored significantly higher on standardized tests of basic academic skills and were significantly less likely to report drug involvement or repeat a grade than were control group students in the experimental school. Seniors who received these services were significantly more likely to graduate (76%) than were seniors in the corresponding control group (42%). There were no significant differences, however, between students who received special services and control students on delinquency, court contacts, or other educational or behavioral measures. Probably the clearest implication from the Gottfredson (1986) study is that in the context of a whole-school improvement effort, selective and indicated preventive interventions with students at greatest risk of school failure and health-compromising behaviors can have beneficial effects on academic success and on a major health and education goal, that is, high school completion, even when implemented late in development.

Gottfredson has continued to develop and test schoolwide interventions that seek to reduce health-compromising behaviors by increasing commitment to education. In 1987, she reported results of a schoolwide intervention implemented in the context of the Program Development Evaluation organizational development activity. The school improvement activities consisted of training for teachers in classroom management techniques and cooperative learning as well as a parent volunteer program, a community support and advocacy program, and other components from the Charleston project. Although no direct comparisons were made between the experimental and comparison groups, the evaluation indicated that when the intervention was well implemented, students reported significantly more rewards from academic involvement and less delinquent and rebellious behavior than did comparison school students (Gottfredson, 1987).

Felner and his colleagues (1993) have implemented broader interventions seeking to ease the transition to high school to create greater bonding to school among students from disadvantaged low-income backgrounds. Students entering ninth grade were assigned to units of 65 to 100 students in a "school within a school." Homeroom and academic classes were composed only of students in the same unit, and classrooms for the same unit were located in proximity to each other. Academic subject teachers also served as homeroom teachers and as the main administrative and counseling link between the students, their parents, and the rest of the school. Homeroom teachers contacted parents before the school year and also held brief check-in sessions with homeroom students once a month.

The intervention increased bonding to school. Experimental students had significantly more positive perceptions of school, teachers, and other school personnel than did comparison students at the end of the yearlong intervention. Moreover, intervention students showed significantly smaller decreases in academic performance and attendance during the transition between junior and senior high school. With respect to the *Healthy People 2000* goal of high school completion, intervention students had a significantly lower dropout rate (24%) than did comparison students (43%).

The Comer, Gottfredson, and Felner intervention studies provide evidence that elementary and secondary schools can be reorganized to achieve key characteristics of effective schools. Each of these interventions explicitly involved faculty in more joint planning and the use of consistent approaches toward students, emphasized learning, and explicitly involved parents more actively in school life and the education of their children.

This summary of research evidence on effective interventions to promote achievement, emotional competence, and prosocial behavior shows that there are tested methods for installing the characteristics of effective schools in other schools. When key policies and practices in schools and classrooms are changed, student achievement, social and emotional competence, and behavior improve. There is evidence that this can be accomplished in schools serving disadvantaged and minority populations.

Conclusion

At the present, the United States is not achieving the health and education goals of academic achievement that we have set for ourselves as a society. In 1990 and again in 1994, 86% of 19- to 24-year olds had obtained high school credentials, indicating little movement toward the goal of 90% (DHHS, 1995). Other measures of the academic competence of students in the United States show greater reason for concern. Goal 3 of the National Education Goals Panel (1995) asserts,

> By the year 2000, all students will leave grades 4, 8, and 12 having demonstrated competency over challenging subject matter including English, mathematics, science, foreign languages, civics and government, economics, arts, history, and geography; and every school in America will ensure that all students learn to use their minds well, so they may be prepared for responsible citizenship, further learning, and productive employment in our Nation's modern economy. (p. 11)

The 1995 National Education Goals Panel scorecard showed less than a third of students reading at the performance standard for grades 4 and 8 and no increase in this rate since 1992. No more than a quarter at grades 4, 8, or 12 were achieving at standard in mathematics at the most recent assessment. Other subject areas showed similar results.

High-quality public education that guarantees success for all children, regardless of race or socioeconomic status, is feasible. This society has developed the technology to organize schools and classrooms to promote academic achievement, emotional competence, and healthy behavior of students. But to make it happen, everyone has to want to do it.

That includes parents expecting more from public education but also doing more to be actively involved in the schools, classrooms, and learning experiences of their children. It includes teachers working together to master management and instructional methods that promote more active involvement of students as learners and that promote the development of reasoning and problem-solving skills for both academic and social problems.

It includes school administrators who view their role as leadership in the creation of a community of commitment to learning and positive social development through the communication of high expectations for achievement and behavior; the modeling of instructional and personal leadership; and the development of opportunities and recognition for involvement of parents, students, teachers, helping professionals, and community residents in the life of the school. It includes central administrative systems that ensure access for school leaders and staff to the best practices for school and classroom management, instruction and organization, and reinforcement for change in pursuit of excellence.

Most of all, it includes a public that is serious about education. Taxpayers should be entitled to expect schools to use the best methods available to organize and manage themselves so that students achieve academic and social competence and avoid health-compromising behaviors.

Schools should be provided the resources to do that and the flexibility to organize and manage their activities to achieve the academic outcomes, emotional competencies, and behavioral standards they and the taxpayers seek as outcomes. Schools should, in turn, be accountable for implementing improvements that can be expected to achieve the specified outcomes and for monitoring student progress related to these goals.

Taxpayers should be prepared to provide resources to support the changes in schools that can make a difference. All the effective interventions reviewed here involved costs, some more than others. Teaching, itself, must again be valued in the society, both financially and as a calling.

Today, nations across the world disintegrate into ethnic and religious struggles while others overtake the United States with cost-efficient production and manufacturing. It is hard to imagine that this society can ensure its future cohesiveness in the face of increasing diversity and promote its competitiveness in the world economy without a healthy and effective system of universal public education. We should stop arguing about this and secure its creation using the tools at hand and committing the resources necessary. We can and should ensure that all American public schools are effective in promoting the academic competence, emotional competence, and healthy behaviors of all students.

References

Battistich, V., Schaps, E., Watson, M., & Solomon, D. (1996). Prevention effects of the Child Development Project: Early findings from an ongoing multisite demonstration trial. *Journal of Adolescent Research, 11,* 12-35.

Battistich, V., Solomon, D., Watson, M., & Schaps, E. (in press). Caring school communities. *Educational Psychologist.*

Berliner, D. C., & Calfee, R. C. (1996). *Handbook of educational psychology.* New York: Simon & Schuster Macmillan.

Bourgois, P. (1995). *In search of respect: Selling crack in el barrio.* New York: Cambridge University Press.

Catalano, R. F., Harachi, T. W., Haggerty, K. P., & Abbott, R. D. (1996, August). Proximal effects of a comprehensive risk and protective factor prevention strategy. In *School-based risk and protective factor-focused drug abuse prevention.* Symposium conducted at the 104th annual convention of the American Psychological Association, Toronto, Ontario, Canada.

Catalano, R. F., & Hawkins, J. D. (1996). The social development model: A theory of antisocial behavior. In J. D. Hawkins (Ed.), *Delinquency and crime: Current theories* (pp. 149-197). New York: Cambridge University Press.

Cauce, A. M., Comer, J. P., & Schwartz, D. (1987). Long-term effects of a systems-oriented school prevention program. *American Journal of Orthopsychiatry, 57,* 127-131.

Cohen, P. A., Kulik, J. A., & Kulik, C. C. (1982). Educational outcomes of teaching. *American Education Research Journal, 19,* 237-248.

Coie, J. D., & Krehbiel, G. (1984). Effects of academic tutoring on the social status of low-achieving, socially rejected children. *Child Development, 55,* 1465-1478.

Comer, J. P. (1988). Educating poor minority children. *Scientific American, 259,* 42-48.

Csikszentmihalyi, M., & Larson, R. (1980). Intrinsic rewards in school crime. In K. Baker & R. J. Rubel (Eds.), *Violence and crime in the schools.* Lexington, MA: D. C. Heath.

Cummings, C. (1983). *Managing to teach.* Edmonds, WA: Teaching, Inc.

Cummings, C. (1993). *The get-alongs: A guide for teaching social skills.* Edmonds, WA: Teaching, Inc.

Dryfoos, J. G. (1990). *Adolescents at risk: Prevalence and prevention.* New York: Oxford University Press.

Elias, M. J., Gara, M., Schuyler, T., Brandon-Muller, L. R., & Sayette, M. A. (1991). The promotion of social competence: Longitudinal study of a preventive school-based program. *American Journal of Orthopsychiatry, 61,* 409-417.

Evertson, C. M. (1985). Training teachers in classroom management: An experimental study in secondary school classroom. *Journal of Educational Research, 79*(1), 51-58.

Evertson, C. M., Emmer, E. T., Sanford, J. P., & Clements, B. S. (1983). Improving classroom management: An experiment in elementary school classrooms. *Elementary School Journal, 84*(2), 173-188.

Farrington, D. P. (1991). Childhood aggression and adult violence: Early precursors and later-life outcomes. In D. J. Pepler & K. H. Rubin (Eds.), *The development and treatment of childhood aggression* (pp. 5-29). Hillsdale, NJ: Lawrence Erlbaum.

Felner, R. D., Brand, S., Adan, A. M., Mulhall, P. F., Flowers, N., Sartain, B., & DuBois, D. L. (1993). Restructuring the ecology of the school as an approach to prevention during school transitions: Longitudinal follow-ups and extensions of the School Transition Environment Project (STEP). *Prevention in Human Services, 10,* 103-136.

Gardner, H. (1993). *Multiple intelligences: The theory in practice.* New York: Basic Books.

Goleman, D. (1995). *Emotional intelligence.* New York: Bantam.

Gottfredson, D. C. (1986). An empirical test of school-based environmental and individual interventions to reduce the risk of delinquent behavior. *Criminology, 24,* 705-731.

Gottfredson, D. C. (1987). An evaluation of an organization development approach to reducing school disorder. *Evaluation Reviews, 11,* 739-763.

Greenwood, C. R., Terry, B., Utley, C. A., Montagna, D., & Walker. (1993). Achievement, placement, and services: Middle school benefits of classwide peer tutoring used at the elementary school. *School Psychology Review,* 22(3), 497-516.

Harachi, T. W., Abbott, R. A., Catalano, R. F., & Haggerty, K. P. (1996, October). *The effects of risk and protective factors on antisocial behavior and academic success in the early primary grades.* Paper presented at the meeting of the Life History Research Society, London.

Hawkins, J. D., Arthur, M. W., & Catalano, R. F. (1995). Preventing substance abuse. In M. Tonry & D. Farrington (Eds.), *Building a safer society: Strategic approaches to crime prevention* (Crime and Justice: A Review of Research, Vol. 19). Chicago: University of Chicago Press.

Hawkins, J. D., Catalano, R. F., & Brewer, D. D. (1995). Preventing serious, violent, and chronic juvenile offending: Effective strategies from conception to age six. In J. Howell, B. Krisberg, J. Hawkins, & J. Wilson (Eds.), *A sourcebook: Serious, violent, and chronic juvenile offenders* (pp. 47-60). Thousand Oaks, CA: Sage.

Hawkins, J. D., Catalano, R. F., Kosterman, R., Abbott, R. D., Hill, K. G., & Janosz, M. (1996, October). *Promoting academic success and preventing adolescent health risk behaviors: Six year follow-up of the Seattle Social Development Project.* Paper presented at the meeting of the Life History Research Society, London.

Hawkins, J. D., Catalano, R. F., & Miller, J. Y. (1992). Risk and protective factors for alcohol and other drug problems in adolescence and early adulthood: Implications for substance abuse prevention. *Psychological Bulletin, 112,* 64-105.

Hawkins, J. D., Catalano, R. F., Morrison, D. M., O'Donnell, J., Abbott, R. D., & Day, L. E. (1992). The Seattle Social Development Project: Effects of the first four years on protective factors and problem behaviors. In J. McCord & R. Tremblay (Eds.), *The prevention of antisocial behavior in children* (pp.9-161). New York: Guilford.

Hawkins, J. D., Von Cleve, E., & Catalano, R. F. (1991). Reducing early childhood aggression: Results of a primary prevention program. *Journal of the American Academy of Child and Adolescent Psychiatry, 30,* 208-217.

Hawkins, J. D., & Weis, J. G. (1985). The social development model: An integrated approach to delinquency prevention. *Journal of Primary Prevention, 6,* 73-97.

Herrnstein, R. J., & Murray, C. M. (1994). *The bell curve: Intelligence and class structure in American life.* New York: Free Press.

Hirschi, T. (1969). *Causes of delinquency.* Berkeley: University of California Press.

Institute of Medicine. (1994). *Reducing risks for mental disorders: Frontiers for preventive intervention research.* Washington, DC: National Academy Press.

Kagan, S. L., & Neuman, M. J. (1997). Defining and implementing school readiness: Challenges for families, early care and education, and schools. In R. P. Weissberg, T. P. Gullotta, R. L. Hampton, B. A. Ryan, & G. R. Adams (Eds.), *Healthy children*

2010: Establishing preventive strategies (Issues in Children's and Families' Lives, Vol. 9). Thousand Oaks, CA: Sage.

Kellam, S. G., & Rebok, G. W. (1992). Building developmental and etiological theory through epidemiologically based preventive intervention trials. In J. McCord & R. Tremblay (Eds.), *Preventing antisocial behavior: Interventions from birth through adolescence* (pp. 162-195). New York: Guilford.

Kellam, S. G., Rebok, G. W., Ialongo, N., & Mayer, L. S. (1994). The course and malleability of aggressive behavior from early first grade into middle school: Results of a developmental epidemiology-based preventive trial. *Journal of Child Psychology and Psychiatry and Allied Disciplines, 35*(2), 259-281.

Levine, D., & Lezotte, L. (1990). *Unusually effective schools: A review of research and practice.* Madison, WI: National Center for Effective Schools Research and Development.

Madden, N. A., & Slavin, R. E. (1989). Effective pull-out programs for students at risk. In R. E. Slavin, N. L. Karweit, & N. A. Madden (Eds.), *Effective programs for students at risk.* Boston: Allyn & Bacon.

Madden, N. A., Slavin, R. F., Karweit, N. K., Dolan, L. J., & Wasik, B. A. (1993). Success for all: Longitudinal effects of a restructuring program for inner-city elementary schools. *American Educational Research Journal, 30,* 123-148.

Maguin, E., & Loeber, R. (1996). Academic performance and delinquency. *Crime and justice: A review of research, 20,* 145-264.

Moffitt, T. E. (1993). Adolescence-limited and life-course-persistent antisocial behavior: A developmental taxonomy. *Psychological Review, 100*(4), 674-701.

Mortimore, P. (1995). The positive effects of schooling. In M. Rutter (Ed.), *Psychosocial disturbances in young people: Challenges for prevention* (pp. 333-363). Cambridge, UK: Cambridge University Press.

National Education Goals Panel. (1995). *National education goals report: Building a nation of learners.* Washington, DC: U.S. Government Printing Office.

O'Donnell, J., Hawkins, J. D., Catalano, R. C., Abbott, R., & Day, L. E. (1995). Preventing school failure, drug use, and delinquency among low income children: Effects of a long-term prevention project in elementary schools. *American Journal of Orthopsychiatry, 65,* 87-100.

O'Leary, K. D., & O'Leary, S. G. (1977). *Classroom management: The successful use of behavior modification* (2nd ed.). New York: Pergamon.

Patterson, G. R. (1982). *Coercive family process.* Eugene, OR: Castalia.

Patterson, G. R. (1986). Performance models for antisocial boys. *American Psychologist, 41,* 432-444.

Pepler, D. J., Craig, W. M., & Roberts, W. L. (1995). Social skills training and aggression in the peer group. In J. McCord (Ed.), *Coercion and punishment in long-term perspectives* (pp. 213-228). Cambridge, UK: Cambridge University Press

Robins, L. N. (1978). Sturdy childhood predictors of adult anti-social behavior: Replications from longitudinal studies. *Psychological Medicine, 8,* 611-622.

Slavin, R. E. (1987). Ability grouping and student achievement in elementary schools: A best-evidence synthesis. *Review of Educational Research, 57,* 293-336.

Slavin, R. E. (1990a). Class size and student achievement: Is smaller better? *Contemporary Education, 42,* 6-12.

Slavin, R. E. (1990b). *Cooperative learning: Theory, research, and practice.* Englewood Cliffs, NJ: Prentice Hall.
Slavin, R. E., Karweit, N. L., & Madden, N. A. (Eds.). (1989). *Effective programs for students at risk.* Boston: Allyn & Bacon.
Slavin, R. E., Karweit, N. L., & Wasik, B. A. (1994). *Preventing early school failure.* Needham Heights, MA: Allyn & Bacon.
Slavin, R. E., & Madden, N. A. (1989). Effective classroom programs for students at risk. In R. E. Slavin, N. L. Karweit, & N. A. Madden (Eds.), *Effective programs for students at risk* (pp. 23-51). Boston: Allyn & Bacon.
Slavin, R. E., Madden, N. A., Dolan, L. J., Wasik, B. A., Ross, S., Smith, L., & Dianda, M. (1995, April). *Success for all: A summary of research.* Paper presented at the meeting of the American Educational Research Association, San Francisco.
Stallings, J. A., & Stipek, D. (1986). Research on early childhood and elementary school teaching programs. In M. C. Wittrock (Ed.), *Handbook of research on teaching* (3rd ed., pp. 727-753). New York: Macmillan.
U. S. Department of Health and Human Services, Public Health Service. (1991). *Healthy people 2000: National health promotion and disease prevention objectives* (DHHS Publication No. PHS 91-50212). Washington, DC: U.S. Government Printing Office.
U. S. Department of Health and Human Services, Public Health Service. (1995). *Healthy people 2000: Midcourse review and 1995 revisions.* Washington, DC: U.S. Government Printing Office.
Wasik, B. A., & Slavin, R. E. (1994). Preventing early reading failure with one-to-one tutoring: A review of five programs. In R. E. Slavin, N. L. Karweit, & B. A. Wasik (Eds.), *Preventing early school failure: Research, policy, and practice* (pp. 143-174). Boston: Allyn & Bacon.
Wittrock, M. C. (Ed.). (1986). *Handbook of research on teaching* (3rd ed.). New York: Macmillan.
W. T. Grant Consortium on the School-Based Promotion of Social Competence. (1992). Drug and alcohol prevention curricula. In J. D. Hawkins, R. F. Catalano, & Associates (Eds.), *Communities that care* (pp. 129-148). San Francisco: Jossey-Bass.

Index

About the Editors

Gerald R. Adams is Professor in the Department of Family Studies at the University of Guelph, Ontario, Canada. He is an associate editor for the series **Advances in Adolescent Development** and **Issues in Children's and Families' Lives.** He is a Fellow of the American Psychological Association, the American Psychological Society, and the American Association of Applied and Preventive Psychology. His research focuses on family psychology, adolescent development, family-school connections in predicting adjustment and academic success, and aspects of primary prevention and social interventions. He is the coauthor of five textbooks, more than a dozen books, and many research reports, chapters, and public journalist articles. He is on the editorial boards of journals in sociology, psychology, human development, family science, and education.

Thomas P. Gullotta is CEO of the Child and Family Agency in Connecticut. He currently is the Editor of the *Journal of Primary Prevention.* He is a book editor for the **Advances in Adolescent Development** series and is the senior book series editor for **Issues in Children's and Families' Lives.** In addition, he serves on the editorial boards of the *Journal of Early Adolescence* and *Adolescence* and is an adjunct faculty member in the psychology and education departments of Eastern Connecticut State University. His published works focus on primary prevention and youth.

Robert L. Hampton, Ph.D., is Associate Provost for Academic Affairs, Dean for Undergraduate Studies, and Professor of Family Studies and Sociology at the University of Maryland, College Park. He has published extensively in the field of family violence and is editor of *Violence in the Black Family: Correlates and Consequences* (1987), *Black Family Violence: Current Research and Theory* (1991), *Family Violence: Prevention and Treatment* (1993), and *Preventing Violence in America* (1996). His research interests include interspousal violence, family abuse, male violence, community violence, resilience, and institutional responses to violence.

Bruce A. Ryan is Associate Professor in the Department of Family Studies at the University of Guelph, Ontario, Canada. He earned a doctorate in educational psychology from the University of Alberta and has served in numerous positions of responsibility at the University of Guelph and in child and family service associations and agencies in Ontario. His current research interests and most recent publications are focused on the relationship between family processes and school outcomes for children.

Roger P. Weissberg is Professor of Psychology at the University of Illinois at Chicago (UIC), where he is Director of Graduate Studies in Psychology and Executive Director of the Collaborative for the Advancement of Social and Emotional Learning (CASEL). He also directs the NIMH-funded Predoctoral and Postdoctoral Prevention Research Training Program in Urban Children's Mental Health and AIDS Prevention. He also holds an appointment with the Mid-Atlantic Laboratory for Student Success, funded by the Office of Educational Research and Improvement of the U.S. Department of Education. His research interests include school and community preventive interventions, urban children's mental health, and parent involvement in children's education. He has been President of the American Psychological Association's Society for Community Research and Action. He is a recipient of the William T. Grant Foundation's 5-year Faculty Scholars Award in Children's Mental Health, the Connecticut Psychological Association's 1992 Award for Distinguished Psychological Contribution in the Public Interest, and the National Mental Health Association's 1992 Lela Rowland Prevention Award.

About the Contributors

Bruce E. Compas is Professor of Psychology and Director of Clinical Training at the University of Vermont. He received his Ph.D. in clinical psychology from the University of California, Los Angeles. He is a Fellow of the American Psychological Society and the American Psychological Association and serves as Consulting Editor for several journals, including the *Journal of Consulting and Clinical Psychology, Health Psychology, Developmental Psychology,* and the *Journal of Personality and Social Psychology.* His research, supported by the William T. Grant Foundation and the National Institute of Mental Health, focuses on stress and coping during childhood and adolescence, depression during adolescence, the psychological effects of cancer on patients and their families, and psychological interventions for women with breast cancer.

Jennifer Connor is a doctoral student in clinical psychology at the University of Vermont. She received her undergraduate degree in psychology from Duke University. Her research and clinical interests are focused on developmental psychopathology. Her current research is concerned with the measurement, nature, and course of depression during adolescence and coping with stress during childhood and adolescence.

Joy G. Dryfoos is an unaffiliated researcher, writer, and lecturer from Hastings-on-Hudson, New York. She has received support from the Carnegie Corporation since 1984 for a long-term "youth-at-risk" project with a focus on the integration of the knowledge base in four prevention fields: substance abuse, delinquency, school failure, and teen pregnancy. Her volume *Adolescents at Risk: Prevalence and Prevention* (1990) presents strategies for developing more comprehensive programs at the community, state, and federal levels. *Full-Service Schools: A Revolution in Health and Social Services for Children, Youth, and Families* (1994) documents the proliferation of school-based youth and family resource centers. *Safe Passage: Making It Through Adolescence in a Risky Society* (1997) focuses on effective approaches to helping adolescents grow into responsible adults. She is a consultant to foundations including Carnegie, Grant, Dewitt Wallace-Reader's Digest, and Wellness and is a Trustee of the Milton Eisenhower Foundation. She has served on the Committee on Comprehensive School Health of the Institute of Medicine, the Panels on High-Risk Youth and Adolescent Pregnancy of the National Academy of Sciences, and the Carnegie Task Force on Youth Development and Community Programs and is a member of the editorial boards of the *Journal of Adolescent Health* and the *Journal of At-Risk Youth.*

Linda Dusenbury is a Clinical Associate Professor of Psychology in the Department of Public Health at Cornell University Medical College. She received her B.A., M.A., and Ph.D. from the University of Vermont, where her adviser was George W. Albee, one of the leaders in the field of primary prevention. Her research has included longitudinal field trials of school-based drug abuse prevention curricula, as well as evaluations of drug abuse prevention programs for homeless youth and AIDS education. She has managed projects involving more than 150 schools and 10,000 students in New York City and has trained more than 700 teachers and administrators in drug education. Her research in the past decade has focused primarily on drug education among multiethnic youth, as well as dissemination of drug education teaching techniques. She has served on numerous state and federal review panels and is frequently invited to speak throughout the country about drug abuse prevention. She recently completed an in-depth review of nationally available drug education curricula for Drug Strategies, a nonprofit research institute in Washington, D.C.

Mathea Falco, J.D., is President of Drug Strategies, a nonprofit research institute in Washington, D.C., that identifies effective approaches to substance abuse. The author of *The Making of a Drug-Free America: Programs That Work* (1994), she comments frequently on drug policy in the media and in public speeches across the country. Until her move to Washington, D.C., in 1993, she was Director of Health Policy, Department of Public Health, Cornell University Medical College in New York City. From 1977 to 1981, she was Assistant Secretary of State for International Narcotics Matters. In earlier positions, she served as Chief Counsel and Staff Director of the U.S. Senate Judiciary Committee Juvenile Delinquency Subcommittee and Special Assistant to the President of the Drug Abuse Council. She has been a member of the Board of Overseers of Harvard University, a Trustee of Radcliffe College, and the Chair of the Visiting Committee on Harvard University Health Services. She has also served on the national boards of Girl Scouts, USA; Big Brothers of America; the International Women's Health Coalition; the Ploughshares Fund; and the National Council on Crime and Delinquency. She is a graduate of Radcliffe College and Yale Law School.

Nancy G. Guerra, Ed.D., is Associate Professor of Psychology at the University of Illinois at Chicago. Her interests include programs directed at the prevention of aggressive and antisocial behavior, particularly in urban settings. Her research activities include a large-scale prevention research trial with more than 9,000 children in 15 urban elementary and middle schools. This trial is designed to evaluate the effectiveness of teacher training, classroom curricula, small-group peer training, and family counseling on behavioral outcomes, including aggression and delinquency.

J. David Hawkins is Professor of Social Work and Director of the Social Development Research Group, University of Washington, Seattle. He received his B.A. from Stanford University and his Ph.D. in sociology from Northwestern University. His research focuses on understanding and preventing child and adolescent health and behavior problems. He seeks to identify risk and protective factors for health and behavior problems across multiple domains; to understand how these factors interact in the development or prevention of problem behaviors; and to test comprehensive prevention strategies to promote social development and reduce risk through the enhancement of protective factors in families, schools, peer groups, and communities. Since 1981, he has been conducting the Seattle Social Development Project, a longitudinal prevention study based on his theoretical work. He is codeveloper of the Social Development Model, a theory that provides a foundation for positive development and delinquency and drug abuse prevention, and is coauthor of Preparing for the Drug (Free) Years, a prevention program that empowers parents to strengthen family bonding and reduce the risks for drug abuse in their families. He is also coauthor of *Communities That Care: Action for Drug Abuse Prevention,* coeditor of *A Sourcebook on Serious, Violent, and Chronic Juvenile Offenders,* and editor of *Delinquency and Crime: Current Theories.* He has served as a member of the National Institute on Drug Abuse's Epidemiology, Prevention and Services Research Review Committee and the Office for Substance Abuse Prevention's National Advisory Committee. He currently serves on the National Education Goals Panel Resource Group on Safe and Drug Free Schools and was a member of the Committee on Prevention of Mental Disorders of the Institute of Medicine at the National Academy of Sciences. He was awarded the NPN Seventh Annual Award of Excellence for Outstanding Contribution to the Field of Prevention and was also named the University of Washington Lecturer for the 1996-1997 academic year. He is committed to translating research into effective practice and policy to improve adolescent health and development.

Leonard A. Jason is Professor of Psychology at DePaul University. He received his Ph.D. in clinical and community psychology from the University of Rochester. He is a former President of the Division of Community Psychology of the American Psychological Association and a past Editor of *The Community Psychologist.* He has published more than 250 articles on preventive school-based interventions; the prevention of alcohol, tobacco, and other drug abuse; media interventions; and program evaluation. He has been on the editorial boards of seven psychological journals, and he has edited or written nine other books. He has served on review committees of the National Institute on Drug Abuse and the National Institute of Mental Health and has received more than $6 million in federal grants to support his research. He has received three media awards from the American Psychological Association and is frequently asked to comment on policy issues for numerous media outlets.

John Kalafat is currently on the faculty of Rutgers Graduate School of Applied and Professional Psychology. He is a Fellow of the American Psychological Association, a member of the Board of

Directors of the American Association of Suicidology (AAS), and Director of the Prevention Division of AAS. He is a Consulting Editor of *Suicide and Life-Threatening Behavior* and the coauthor of *Lifelines: A School-Based Adolescent Suicide Response Program,* as well as author of articles and chapters on youth suicide prevention, crisis intervention, and school-based family support programs. He has been involved in the development of and consultation to crisis centers for more than 25 years and has been developing and evaluating school-based suicide prevention programs since 1980. He is also currently involved in the evaluation of school-based family resource/youth service centers.

Carol Bartels Kuster is Associate Director for the Collaborative for the Advancement of Social and Emotional Learning (CASEL) at the University of Illinois at Chicago. She received her Ph.D. in clinical/community psychology from the University of Maryland at College Park. Her research interests include social and emotional learning, family violence, parent training and education programs, and prevention of child abuse and neglect.

Leslie A. Lytle, Ph.D., R.D., is Associate Professor in the Division of Epidemiology at the University of Minnesota School of Public Health. She is a registered dietitian and has a master's degree from Purdue University in education and a doctoral degree from the University of Michigan in health behavior and health education. She also did postdoctoral work at the University of Minnesota in cardiovascular health behavior. Her work experience includes a private practice as a dietitian counseling individuals and families on eating behavior change. Her research interests include school-based health promotion and the design of eating behavior change interventions and evaluation strategies for children and adolescents. She serves as Co-Principal Investigator and Project Officer of the Minnesota site of the Child and Adolescent Trial for Cardiovascular Health (CATCH). She wrote the content and was the primary presenter for the 1996 Centers for Disease Control television conference on effective school nutrition programs.

Mary E. Murray is a graduate student in community and prevention research at the University of Illinois at Chicago. Her interests focus on addressing the needs of children living in poverty and include the development and evaluation of school- and community-based preventive intervention and social policy planning for children, youth, and families.

Roberta L. Paikoff is Associate Professor of Psychology in the Department of Psychiatry at the Institute for Juvenile Research, University of Illinois, Chicago. She completed her B.S. in human development and family studies at Cornell University and received her Ph.D. in child psychology from the Institute of Child Development at the University of Minnesota. Her postdoctoral training was completed in psychology at the Hebrew University of Jerusalem and in education policy research at the Educational Testing Service. Her current research interests focus on understanding the preadolescent and young adolescent years by emphasizing the interplay among biological, cognitive, and social relational factors in contributing to individual outcomes. In particular, she is interested in understanding the relationship of early sexuality to other normative developmental processes and in using information derived from research to create more effective programs and services to reduce high-risk sexual behavior among youth. Her work is supported by the National Institute of Mental Health Office on AIDS and the William T. Grant Faculty Scholar Award.

Cheryl L. Perry is Professor in the Division of Epidemiology, School of Public Health, at the University of Minnesota. She began her career as a junior high and high school teacher and junior high school vice-principal in Davis, California. She then received her Ph.D. from Stanford University and worked with the Stanford Heart Disease Prevention Program prior to joining the faculty at the University of Minnesota in 1980. At the University of Minnesota, she served as Director of Youth Health Promotion Research and was responsible for the youth and parent component of the Minnesota Heart Health Program from 1980 to 1993. She has published more than 100 articles in the peer-reviewed literature on health promotion programs with children and adolescents, including articles on health promotion theory, design, implementation, and outcomes. She was the Senior Scientific Editor of the 1994 *Surgeon General's Report on Preventing Tobacco Use Among Young People.* Currently, she serves as Principal Investigator of the University of Minnesota site of the Child and Adolescent Trial for Cardiovascular Health (CATCH), the 5-a-Day Power Plus Study in Saint

Paul, Minnesota, and Project Northland, a 28-community trial to reduce alcohol use among adolescents.

Lynda M. Sagrestano is a postdoctoral fellow in the Prevention Research Training Program in Urban Children's Mental Health and AIDS Prevention at the University of Illinois at Chicago. She completed her B.S. in psychology at Duke University and received her Ph.D. in social psychology from the University of California at Berkeley. She received postdoctoral training in health psychology at UCLA before training in prevention. Her current research reflects two main theoretical interests. The first focuses on power and conflict in interpersonal relationships, including the use of social influence in peer and marital relationships and parent-child conflict during adolescence. The second focuses on psychosocial factors in reproductive health, including the role of social support, relationship factors, and mental health factors during pregnancy and contextual and psychosocial factors affecting high-risk sexual behavior among urban youth.

Mary Story, Ph.D., R.D., is Associate Professor in the Public Health Nutrition Program, Division of Epidemiology, School of Public Health, University of Minnesota. She received her Ph.D. in human nutrition from Florida State University. In 1980, she joined the Adolescent Health Program in the Department of Pediatrics at the University of Minnesota. As Nutrition Director in this program, she worked extensively with adolescents and their families in a variety of multidisciplinary clinical and community-based settings, including school-based clinics. Her experience included working with adolescents with eating disorders and obesity and with pregnant teenagers. She has published more than 50 peer-reviewed articles on child and adolescent nutrition. Currently, she is the Principal Investigator of an NHLBI-funded multisite school-based study, Pathways, which focuses on obesity prevention among American Indian children through culturally appropriate behavioral curricula, parental involvement, and school food service and physical education changes.

Barbara S. Tuchfarber, R.N., is a Ph.D. candidate in epidemiology/biostatistics at the University of Cincinnati. She currently is an epidemiologist with the Cincinnati Children's Hospital Medical

Center (CHMC), Division of Health Policy and Clinical Effectiveness. Her previous work includes pediatric injury prevention research with the CHMC Trauma Service and clinical pediatric nursing.

Martha Wadsworth is a doctoral student in clinical psychology at the University of Vermont. She received her undergraduate degree in psychology from the University of Vermont. Her research and clinical interests are focused on developmental psychopathology. Her current research interests include coping with stress during childhood and adolescence, the impact of poverty on child development and psychopathology, and families coping with the stress of cancer.

Kirk R. Williams, Ph.D., is Associate Director of the Center for the Study and Prevention of Violence at the University of Colorado. His research interests have focused on documenting patterns and trends in youth violence and applying these data to help communities develop effective violence prevention strategies.

Joseph E. Zins, Ed.D., is Professor in the College of Education at the University of Cincinnati and a psychological consultant with the Beechwood Independent Schools. He is a licensed psychologist in Ohio and Kentucky and a nationally certified school psychologist. He has published more than 100 articles, chapters, and books on consultation, prevention, and related topics. He coedited the *Handbook of Consultation Services for Children: Applications in Educational and Clinical Settings* and coauthored *Helping Students Succeed in the Regular Classroom: A Guide for Developing Intervention Assistance Programs.* His work has been funded by the U.S. Office of Education and the Ohio Board of Regents. He is editor of the multidisciplinary *Journal of Educational and Psychological Consultation* and consulting editor for the **Guidebooks for School Practitioners Psychoeducational Interventions** book series. He has been a member of seven editorial boards. In addition, he is a Fellow of the American Psychological Association (Divisions 13, 16, 27, and 37) and past Secretary of the National Association of School Psychologists.